Modern medicine is engaged in a struggle to find its heart, soul, and spirit. This task must begin with physicians themselves. Dr. David Kopacz's *Re-Humanizing Medicine* is an excellent guide in how this urgent undertaking can unfold.

Larry Dossey, MD, author of *Reinventing Medicine* and *Healing Words*; executive editor of *Explore: The Journal of Science and Healing*

Brilliant, well-written, practical and inspiring, *Re-humanizing Medicine* provides clarity and understanding of the most pressing issues facing doctors (and patients) today. All doctors, including future doctors, should read this book and empower themselves to be the change that is so needed in our current systems of health care. As we physicians transform ourselves, we will transform the practice of medicine and be better able to serve those who seek our help.

Rama Thiruvengadam, MD, founder of Physician Heal Thyself Retreats™

Dr. David Kopacz bears exquisite witness to medical dehuman-ization and puts his heart and soul into a thoughtful, reflective, yet practical guide for countering its contemporary ills. This book can change lives, careers, and systems.

Stevan M. Weine, MD, author of *When History is a Nightmare* and *Testimony after Catastrophe*; director, International Center on Responses to Catastrophes, University of Illinois at Chicago.

Re-humanizing Medicine is a marvelous book about one person's journey to find meaning and quality of life in the practice of medicine. Dr. David Kopacz presents a very human account of his frustrations within the conventional health care system and inspires us with his search for solutions. His analysis of the underlying philosophies of the kind of care we provide was illuminating for me and helped me understand why conditions only worsen despite our collective (as physicians and patients) complaints. His proposals for how to move forward into a sustainable health care future are solid, well supported by science, and promise to integrate the poetic, mystical, compassionate side of medicine with its science. In a world of no time, this book is well worth the time to read it.

Lewis Mehl-Madrona, MD, PhD, author of *Healing the Mind through the Power of Story: The Promise of Narrative Psychiatry*; Core Faculty, Union Institute & University, Clinical Psychology; Executive Director, Coyote Institute for Studies of Change and Transformation, Brattleboro, Vermont

In *Re-humanizing Medicine*, David Kopacz offers an informed and committed corrective to the loss of soul that has occurred in the practice of Western medicine over the past century. Central to his understanding is the notion that the broader transformation of medicine turns on the personal awakening and transformation of the physician. Until such time as the biomedical curriculum gives as much attention to the cultivation of sensitivity, empathy and holistic consciousness as it does to the transmission of the reductionist principles on which it is based, *Re-humanizing Medicine* will remain a welcome source of nourishment for all within the profession of medicine who are searching for ways to deepen their connection to the historic mission of medicine, which is to heal not only the ills of the body, but also those of the entire nexus of relationships within which we find ourselves.

Vincent Di Stefano, DO, ND, MHSc, author of *Holism and Complementary Medicine: Origins and Principles*

If this informative, readable and practical book encourages doctors to put into practice even half of what is being put forward here, the world will be a better place.

Dr. Patte Randal, Licentiate of the Royal College of Physicians (LRCP), Membership of the Royal College of Surgeons (MRCS), DPhil, co-editor and co-author of *Experiencing Psychosis: Personal and Professional Perspectives*

Simple yet complex, idealistic and realistic, this book turns a spotlight onto human connection, a fundamental factor that is too readily neglected in today's technology-driven medical practice. Thoughtfully bringing his personal experience and a rich collection of literature, Dr. David Kopacz offers an excellent 'portable' holistic framework that can be applied ecologically to cultivate an authentic wholeness in both practitioners and patients. Notably, the book differentiates itself from the crowd through the 'organic' incorporation of autobiographical narrative which demonstrates abundant universal qualities through the most individualized perspective. I heartily endorse this book as a must-read, particularly for people like myself who are considering creating a private practice in holistic medicine.

Qi Liu, Postgraduate Diploma in Chinese Integrative Medicine, Nanjing University of Traditional Chinese Medicine, China; New Zealand Registered Occupational Therapist (NZROT); Postgraduate Certificate in Mental Health (PgCertMH)

Our world currently faces great challenges that require each individual to commit to a process of growth and renewal. Kopacz's book provides a thoughtful and practical account of how to inspire greater well-being by transforming managerial medicine into a place of personal and social healing.

Guiding the reader through a wealth of insight into the history of scientific and alternative approaches, he convincingly argues for holistically-oriented medicine that encompasses objective knowledge, compassion, and intuitive guidance.

His call for reintroducing attention to the human condition in an increasingly corporatized world has far reaching impulses, not only for medicine, but also for education, the business world and society.

Leading by example, Kopacz enriches any reader's understanding of their own responsibility to change themselves and the world.

Anke Pinkert, Ph.D., author of *Film and Memory in East Germany*; Illinois Program for Research in the Humanities Fellow 2012-2013: "Transforming the Humanities Through Higher Education in Prison;" director of Undergraduate Studies; Associate Professor of German, Media and Cinema Studies, University of Illinois Urbana-Champaign

I am grateful this book has been written, and a voice has been given to this vital message, reminding us of the 'care' aspect of health care, for practitioner and patient alike. Confronting, honest and transparent ... written with a wisdom rarely seen.

Chrissy Diamond, BHS NMT, Dip CST, DIP CTM, Neuromuscular Therapist, Holistic Alignment, New Zealand College of Massage

This book is essential for establishing a refreshed approach inside medicine and brings new insights about the practice of psychiatry. Dr. Kopacz addresses different modes of involvement in patient care, all of which facilitate a therapeutic alliance and optimal treatment outcome through empathy, intuition, and spiritual awareness.

Dr. Georgiana Antoce, Fellow of the Royal Australian and New Zealand College of Psychiatrists; Senior Lecturer with University of Queensland; Private Practice, Brisbane, Australia

Re-humanizing Medicine has reinforced my own commitment to the importance of holistic leadership. I am confident that practitioners trained in biomedical and holistic health practices will feel this same kinship. This book brings both topics dynamically to the table for discussion.

I was deeply moved by Kopacz's inspiring words and reflections on his own personal experiences. There is a major cultural shift on the horizon in the fields of medicine and business to cultivate connection with the whole person and a holistic way of being. Kopacz's research on Gandhi, Youngson, Palmer and other enlightened leaders further supports the concept of a compassion revolution. I hope that *Re-humanizing Medicine* will be required reading for all future generations of physicians and health care providers. Dr. Kopacz's open mind and open heart will inspire many to 're-humanize and re-connect.'

Sara Holmes, BS RA LMT NCTMB; Complementary Therapies, Massage and Aromatherapy Instructor Parkland College, Champaign, Illinois; www.botanicalhealingarts.com

As a physician in private practice, I know first-hand the effect of long-term stress and never-ending demands on the practicing doctor—a guarantee for poor health and burnout. In *Re-humanizing Medicine*, Dr. Kopacz makes a well-argued case that doctors need to begin healing patients by healing themselves first. Preventive care is the recommended prescription for doctors who want to remain as energized and caring as they were when they entered medical school. This book illuminates a path to enjoying a long and fulfilling career as a physician who practices what he should be preaching.

Rich Berning, MD; creator of PrivatePractice.MD Website; Pediatric Cardiologist, Sandy Hook, Connecticut

It gives me great pleasure to review this informative text that will hopefully become essential reading to all medical practitioners and related clinicians working in the healing arts. David sets out a coherent and well-articulated background to the current issues that face medical practice in a global environment which has witnessed a significant loss of essential human interactions in the healing process. David's review of the outcomes of physician burnout are a startling reminder to us all of the risk that this leads to – not only for ourselves as doctors but also for our patients.

Modern medical practice has developed a profound arrogance over the recent past choosing to ignore the time old lessons from our traditional healer colleagues who have been trained in the art of healing from a different perspective that engages overall health and well-being through a fundamental understanding of human systems, culture and social environments. David's book challenges us to re-examine these issues, sets out coherent and articulate arguments for the benefits of changing and places patients at the centre of engaging in an integrated and holistic new paradigm of healing based on a compassionate under-standing of the frailty of the human predicament. I would whole-heartedly recommend this book to both existing practitioners and those embarking on a medical career.

Dr Gary Orr, Consultant Psychiatrist in New Zealand and Research Director of Health Empowerment Through Nutrition (www.hetn.org), a foundation that supports bio-available nutri-tional interventions to overcome the issues of hidden hunger. Gary was originally born in South Africa, and qualified as a medical doctor and completed his postgraduate studies in Psychiatry in the United Kingdom.

Re-humanizing Medicine

A Holistic Framework for Transforming Your Self, Your Practice, and the Culture of Medicine

Re-humanizing Medicine

A Holistic Framework for Transforming
Your Self, Your Practice, and
the Culture of Medicine

David R. Kopacz, MD

**AYNI
BOOKS**

Winchester, UK
Washington, USA

First published by Ayni Books, 2014
Ayni Books is an imprint of John Hunt Publishing Ltd., Laurel House, Station Approach,
Alresford, Hants, SO24 9JH, UK
office1@jhpbooks.net
www.johnhuntpublishing.com
www.ayni-books.com

For distributor details and how to order please visit the 'Ordering' section on our website.

ISBN: 978 1 78279 075 4

A CIP catalogue record for this book is available from the British Library.

Design: Lee Nash

Printed and bound by CPI Group (UK) Ltd, Croydon, CR0 4YY

We operate a distinctive and ethical publishing philosophy in all
areas of our business, from our global network of authors to
production and worldwide distribution.

CONTENTS

Permissions

Quote from Vaclav Havel's *Disturbing the Peace*, translated by Paul Wilson, used by permission of Random House.

'Healing,' by D.H. Lawrence used by permission of Penguin Group (USA) Inc.

Foreword

(Internal dialogue of a busy academician)

'Why on earth should I read this book? I've got five articles to write, an accreditation visit to plan for, and a large new curricular element to roll out. Who has time for this? The darn thing is so long!'

'But you thought Dave Kopacz was one of the singularly most talented psychiatry residents you have ever had the pleasure of supervising! And you promised! And who knows what interesting things he has gotten himself into in the intervening years – after all, he made a gigantic trek to New Zealand just for starters!'

'Fine ... fine. I'll skim it. The touchy-feely title is a little off-putting, but hey, you promised! Let's just do it and get it over with.'

Several hours later, so totally engrossed in the book that I asked my assistant to lock in reading time to my appointment schedule, I had totally changed my opinion about David Kopacz's book, entitled *Re-humanizing Medicine: A Holistic Framework for Transforming Your Self, Your Practice, and the Culture of Medicine*. It should be required reading for every medical student, resident, and practicing physician.

Medical education, and medicine itself, easily becomes a dehumanizing process. There are so many facts to be learned, so many procedures to be memorized, so many treatments to be continuously updated, just *so many*. It is easy to lose oneself in the process and fall prey to the stereotype of the physician who is always available, has all the answers, and has no personal life (or for that matter existence) outside the hospital. Physicians bemoan the limitations of the 80-hour work week as the loss of the days when 'patients came first.' Dave's book offers a compelling argument why losing oneself, however, is simply *not* in the best interest of the patient, the practice, or the physician him- or herself.

The book divides itself neatly into five parts. The first points out the dehumanization of contemporary medicine through multiple examples, and the analysis of a variety of paradigms of medical models. The second part of the book describes the paradigm of holistic medicine more fully, while the third is a clearly written, step-by-step self-help section that helps the reader develop his or her deeper sense of humanity. The fourth part of the book builds on the third, describing how to take the new holistic viewpoint and put it to use in one's own practice. The fifth, closing the book, describes how the holistic paradigm, if used broadly, might re-humanize the culture of medicine itself.

Throughout the book, Dave uses very personal examples that put a real face on the dehumanization that trainees experience. Never bitter or accusatory, he is skilled at pointing out the system's many flaws without ever 'throwing out the baby with the bathwater' and calling for a mass revolution in an angry tone (to which the authors of many previous books have resorted when facing the massive issues in health care today, by the way). On top of the excellent personal examples, David draws on his impressive depth and breadth of knowledge in such diverse topics as psychotherapy, medical economics, health care reform, poetry, culture, holistic medicine, pharmaceutics, religion, and science to make very persuasive arguments. While the book at times may use terms unfamiliar to the physician, it becomes a 'cliff note' version of a huge body of literature that is deftly summarized and clearly written, something absolutely invaluable to the reader (and thus the large blocks of time currently in my schedule to read the book again more slowly, regardless of other obligations).

Particularly useful, and practical, for those already committed to the idea of a more holistic existence and practice, are Parts III and IV, full of exercises to transform elements of the self through a series of clearly described exercises, and thoughtful writing on using this new holistic framework as a tool for transforming one's medical practice. As the Associate Dean of an innovative medical school in the United States, I am strongly considering these sections (at least) to be required reading for our medical students.

It is clear that David Kopacz is a thoughtful, intelligent, well-read author with a great deal of important messages to convey. What also comes through clearly is the *person* behind the words, as generous, kind, and human as he was even in the midst of a demanding psychiatry residency several decades ago. It was this positive impression that made me promise to (and ultimately to) read this book, and I (and perhaps several forthcoming generations of medical students) will be the richer for it.

Debra Klamen, MD, MHPE
Associate Dean for Education and Curriculum
Southern Illinois University School of Medicine

Acknowledgments

I would like to acknowledge all those who have contributed to my life and education and directly or indirectly influenced this book. This includes everyone who has helped me maintain, and at times regain, my humanity. First of all, I thank my parents, Tom and Linda Kopacz, for creating an environment that supported questioning, the love of nature, and encouragement to follow one's own dream, no matter how eccentric. I thank my sister, Karen Kopacz, as a co-conspirator and inspiration in writing, from my un-publishable *In the Shadow of the Slaughterhouse: Silence Is the Only Crime against Humanity*, to her *Minneago Belladonna Journal* and more reputable *Mental Contagion*. Also, thanks to Karen for the professional help (developing my website and blog through her business, Design for the Arts). I thank my wife, Mary Pat Traxler, who is always up for adventure and misadventure. You are a kindred spirit on the path of personal growth. Mary Pat also did an initial edit of the book and greatly helped me to better organize my ideas. Thanks to our cat, Sofia, for all her support and words of encouragement. I also thank my 'other' sister, Melanie Traxler, for her friendship over the years. Thank you also to the whole Traxler family: Anthony, Pat, Julie, Nick Heynen, Anthony Jr., Theresa, Ben and Layne. Mollie Barker provided a professional edit of the book that really focused my writing and made the book more readable, thanks for that!

I thank all of my teachers through the years: 'Chuck' Potts for giving me a firm foundation in science, Gail Mitchell for encouraging me to ask the big questions in life, and Peter Gregory for an introduction to Buddhism and Taoism. The following people I consider as much life mentors as teachers. I am grateful to Bob Molokie for his dedication to teaching, his ability to seamlessly teach medicine and literature, and for expanding my capacity to carry on multiple conversations at the same time. I would like to thank Deb Klamen for being such a positive influence early in my career and for being a role model of independent thought as well as for academic success. Thank you to Steve Weine for being an incredibly dedicated teacher and mentor who helped me to see how it is possible to undertake a serious study of punk rock, as well as to combine interests in biography, literature, trauma and creativity with academic and scholarly work. Thanks to Robert Coleman for an education in poetry and pinot noir.

I often seem to find myself questioning the mainstream, yet still trying to be accepted by it. I would like to thank all the friends I have found through the years who I can relate to as 'insider/outsiders': Jack Scott, Bob Wagner, Todd Walper, Dan Guyer, John Snow, Dan Griggs, Pete Eggleson, Andy Switzky, Paul Ripp, Mike Barry, Rick Valentin, Rose Marshack, Rich Giulliani, Gene Dillon, Steve Aug, Sam Smucker, Lynn Canfield, Karen Kopacz, Judge Tom Chapman, Mike Tulis, Milan Seth, Gary Henderson, Suzie Gude, Kirsten Pond, Matt Brown, Jill Anderson, Ed Byars, Phil Pan, Garrick Martin, Gary Orr, Jen Harris, Carl Reisman, Sara Holmes, Kevin Elliot, Rama Thiruvengadam and Bernie Howarth. Darin Dougherty belongs in this group as well, but deserves special mention as a fellow practitioner of the counter-curriculum of re-humanization in medical school. Thanks to 'Iron Man' Roberto Jimenez who encouraged me to believe anything is possible and that you can always reinvent yourself.

I would like to acknowledge those who have supported me in my move to New Zealand and in my acculturation: Dawn Bannister, Debbie Antcliff, Ian Soosay, Adele Wakeham, Christine Rigby, Dianne Bartlett, Gary Orr, Berni and David Solomon, Fiona Wilson, Kirsten Holiday-White, Chris White, Nick Hoeh, Dorothy Lami, Rex Hoeh, Phil Venables, Kirsten McDonald and Louise de Candole. Thanks to Ian and Gary for many conversations filled with creative ideas. Thanks to Gary for keeping the dream alive and always being positive and hopeful. Special thanks to Tricia Lewicki and Don Lonam for their help and support during our move from New Zealand back to the States.

Thanks to the Auckland Holistic Writing Group: Qi Liu, Sneh Prasad, Mary Pat Traxler, Gary Orr, Patte Randal, Helen Florence, Chrissy Diamond, Kath Courtenay, Susan MacGregor and Josephine Stanton.

Thanks to Shamshad Karatela, the other member of the Auckland Café Writers Group. Also thanks to Freddino's café for excellent food and coffee, an inspiring atmosphere and a great space to write. Thanks to the staff at Mission Bay Café, Sea Cow, Fiesta and Mud Pie Deli for their great coffee that supported for my writing. I would like to thank the band Doves for their album *Kingdom of Rust*, which I regularly used as a soundtrack when I sat down to write.

Namaste to Sneh Prasad, Arishma Narayan, and Bernie Howarth for their work in stirring up peace and trouble in the Exploring Mental Health through Yoga group. I would also like to thank the people, the building, and the land of Buchanan Rehabilitation Centre in Auckland.

Thank you to Jessica Watson for her advice on writing and book publishing.

Thank you to all the extraordinary healers I have worked with over the years: Chrissy Diamond, Susan Matz, Martia Nelson and Antonia Herbstreit. Also, thanks to Steve Suddens from Les Mills for all your help with the physical dimension. Thanks to Trevor Harbrow for keeping things in alignment.

I would also like to thank Sam Smucker, Melanie Traxler, Anke Pinkert and Mary Pat Traxler, as well as all our respective pets for an incredible journey and great camaraderie during our years in Champaign-Urbana, Illinois.

A big thank-you to everyone who helped make my private practice a success. Even though it was primarily a micropractice model, I had a lot of behind-the-scenes help: Kathy Melchior, Kathy O'Brien, Mary Pat Traxler, Susan Matz, Martia Nelson, Chris Cottet, Priscilla Sullivan, Kevin Elliott, Sara Holmes and Lynn Canfield.

Thank you to all my students over the years for helping me to remember what I know and to realize what I do not know.

A really big thank you to all my patients and clients over the years who have shared their pain, trusted me with their sorrows and shown me that healing is always possible.

Dave Kopacz
Mission Bay Café
Auckland, New Zealand
November 20, 2012

Introduction

Only connect! ... Live in fragments no longer.
E.M. Forster[1]

The great error of our day in the treatment of the human body
is that physicians first separate the soul from the body.
Plato[2]

Dehumanization in Contemporary Medicine

This book takes on the task of re-humanizing medicine. We start
by recognizing that there is a problem with how medicine is
currently practiced: it dehumanizes staff and clients, creating
dissatisfaction, suffering, poor performance and medical errors.
Dehumanization is an iatrogenic effect of the dominant
paradigms in contemporary medicine – the economic/business
model and the reductionist and materialistic approach of
biomedicine. In the day-to-day practice of medicine, doctors are
expected to see more patients in less time and to efficiently
reduce people to symptoms, diagnostic codes, prescriptions,
procedures and billing codes. This leaves little time or space for
people – physician or patient.

Future doctors are attracted to medicine for idealistic and
humanitarian reasons, but through training they often lose this
idealism.[3,4] *How can we preserve idealism and humanitarianism in
medicine?* Practicing physicians have high rates of burnout and
job dissatisfaction. *How can we reinvigorate the practice of medicine
and make it sustainable?*

A Counter-Curriculum of Re-Humanization

In medical school, I realized that I had to engage in a parallel
education process in addition to the standard scientific
curriculum. We could even call this a 'counter-curriculum',

focusing on re-humanization. At times I found teachers, mentors, and fellow students who practiced this counter-curriculum, but often I had to seek it out on my own in order to balance my education. *This book is about that counter-curriculum of re-humanization.* Science and evidence-based interventions are one paradigm of medicine, but as human beings working with human beings, we must have a human framework as well as a scientific one.

As a medical student, the first research project I worked on was with Deb Klamen and Linda Grossman at the University of Illinois at Chicago. Our study examined symptoms of Posttraumatic Stress Disorder (PTSD) in relation to medical training and found that 13% of trainees in the study reported sufficient symptoms (relating to their internship year) to potentially qualify for a PTSD diagnosis.[5] The findings provide evidence supporting the need to change postgraduate medical education to reduce stress and to enhance the well-being of trainees. I went on to work with Linda and Deb on three other papers that examined medical students' beliefs and their attitudes toward the controversial issues of homosexuality, abortion, and AIDS.[6,7,8] These papers examined how medical student beliefs can shape attitudes that adversely impact medical care. The studies also allude to the fact that people are not purely rational beings, and beliefs, fears and stigma can undermine scientific reasoning or professional ethics. Even my student research experience was concerned with the counter-curriculum of exposing dehumanization and seeking re-humanization.

To re-humanize medicine, the people who work in medicine must be well-rounded, well-developed human beings, as well as safe and effective technicians. A great deal of time, energy, and money is spent in making sure that physicians are good technicians, but are they good human beings? Being a good technician (objective, detached, unaffected by emotion, protocol-driven) can actually interfere with being a good human being. Clinicians should not stop being technicians or scientists, but they have a responsibility to attend to their own humanity, as well as that of the client. The counter-curriculum provides a holistic framework for being a human being, for working with human beings, and for creating systems that deliver care by human beings to human beings.

A Holistic Framework for Medicine

A holistic framework is founded on multiple interacting and mutually influencing sub-systems. Scientific medicine and the objective, observable body make up just one dimension of human health. Sometimes the physical dimension is primary, for instance in physical trauma and surgery. Sometimes other human dimensions are more important. Emotion, mind, love, self-expression, intuition, spirituality, context and time all play a role in health and illness.

A holistic framework is a paradigm for understanding and interacting with human beings. It is a human systems approach and a way of being in the world. Holistic medicine is a philosophy, or a paradigm for understanding what it is to be human, to suffer, to be ill, to be healthy; what it is to change, grow and live. It helps us understand how disconnection can lead to suffering and how connection can lead to healing. Holistic medicine is not defined by using an herb instead of a medication, or by any specific technique or intervention. Being a good technician (whether biomedical or 'natural') is part of being a good physician, but being a good physician is more than just being a good technician.

It is hard work to maintain a complex identity that includes being a technician and a human being, but that is what being a medical professional involves: balancing different roles for the purpose of alleviating suffering and treating disease. Re-humanization reconnects the art and science of medicine, the heart and the mind. A holistic framework encourages integration.

When you start to connect in a different way, you change the health care delivery system in which you work. What starts as personal dissatisfaction can become personal transformation, which changes systems. Institutions will always drift toward promoting their own interests over human interests. It is the responsibility of health professionals to ensure that they stay human, help their clients stay human, and ensure that health care delivery systems promote humanization rather than dehumanization.

Intended Audience and Purpose of the Book

I wrote this book for people who are looking for different ways of thinking about and practicing medicine. Dehumanization in medicine occurs throughout the world, particularly as business models replace humanitarian models of care. Many of the examples in the book are specific to the United States or New Zealand, drawing on my experience of practicing medicine in various settings in both countries; but whether dehumanization results from the profit motive of an insurance company (as in the US) or the bureaucratic processes of a national health system (as in New Zealand), the effect is the same. Re-humanizing medicine is a universal need.

This book is written specifically for clinicians, doctors, and physicians,[9] who face daily humanitarian[10] challenges in their roles, but is of interest to any health care professional or administrator. There are many fields where the application of a trained technique interferes with human connection, so teachers, trainers, educators and business people will find it relevant too. Of course, so will anyone interested in being a whole human being!

Since holistic medicine is a philosophy and a mode of being, I do not list diagnoses and alternative treatments. There are already a number of excellent books that review various complementary, alternative, and integrative medical techniques. The foundation of a holistic medical practice is you, not the services and techniques that you offer. Therefore, this is a book for people who are willing to change at a personal level in order to be better doctors and clinicians.

Contemporary medicine and holistic medicine are not inherently in conflict. My hope is that by defining holistic medicine as a paradigm, rather than as a specific technique, its benefits can be integrated with those of contemporary medicine. My primary argument is that the human elements of medicine need to be valued so that technical interventions occur within a human context.

Holistic Medicine, Re-humanization and the Quality Revolution in Health Care – A Convergence?

There is a worldwide trend in health care that, interestingly, overlaps with the philosophy of holistic medicine. This trend is a focus on quality, efficacy and safety, stimulated by the continual increase in the cost of health care. Experts are calling for a 'revolution in health care delivery,'[11] and 'system-wide change.'[12]

Many of the suggestions involve cost-cutting and standardization of treatment. The 'Quality Revolution' also raises issues related to re-humanization, such as putting the patient at the center of treatment, making decisions collaboratively, and establishing a 'continuous healing relationship.'[13] These are the strengths of a holistic framework – not only is it patient-centered, but it includes the concept of *healing* in addition to *treatment*, and it often encourages low-cost, low-risk lifestyle changes and preventative medicine. It may be that it is time for a Compassion Revolution and a Quality Revolution to join forces in order to make medicine more affordable, safe and effective, as well as more compassionate, caring and human.

Structure of the Book

The book is divided into five major parts. The first discusses the underlying paradigms of the biomedical and economic models of contemporary medicine and how these models have side effects of dehumanization. This critique does not mean that there is no benefit in the contemporary paradigm; rather it is an examination of the strengths and weaknesses of the underlying paradigms of the current system. The second part describes the paradigm of holistic medicine as a way of understanding the whole person. The third part is a 'self-help' section that outlines how you, as a clinician, can develop a more holistic and deeper sense of your own humanity. The fourth part is a 'how-to' component that describes how to create a holistic practice in any setting and how to re-humanize your practice. The last part describes the benefits of a holistic paradigm for re-humanizing the culture of medicine.

Part I

PERSPECTIVES ON CONTEMPORARY MEDICINE

Overview

How has contemporary[1] medicine come to be dehumanizing for staff and clients? We will review the history of medicine and see how it has been influenced by different conceptual and theoretical models, often with contradictory values.

In his book, *Humanizing Healthcare Reforms*, anthropologist Gerald Arbuckle describes different models of health care that inform different core value systems that lead to different priorities in reform discussions. The *traditional model* includes indigenous and pre-scientific understandings of health and illness in an environmental and spiritual context. The *foundational model* is based on the values of Western medicine: compassion, social justice and care for the sick and impoverished. The *biomedical model* is the predominant model in medicine today and is based on principles of biological reductionism, objective observation and the scientific method. The *economic rationalist model* views medicine as a commodity that must be managed through business principles in order to make a profit or control costs.[2]

A discussion of these different, and at times contradictory, models helps us to understand why contemporary medicine is practiced the way it is. The biomedical and economic rationalist models are those with the most current influence in contemporary medicine.

While the biomedical model has led to many scientific advances in treatment, it has a side effect of fragmenting our view of the whole person and leading to a technician mentality for doctors. The economic rationalist model has brought about standardization of care and focused on safety and regulation, but it has also led to de-professionalization and has de-emphasized personal human relationships in favor of provider-consumer business exchange relationships. Many doctors and health professionals feel increasingly marginalized by administrative bureaucracies and miss the values of ethics, care and compassion of the foundational model, as these values are not prominent in the biomedical and economic rationalist models of care.

Chapter one provides an examination of how the biomedical and economic rationalist models (when not sufficiently counter-balanced by other more holistically-oriented models) lead to dehumanization in contemporary medicine.

Chapter two provides a critique of the biomedical and economic rationalist models by exploring philosophical perspectives within science; perspectives from religion, poetry and mysticism; and socio-cultural perspectives. The purpose of this critique it not to negate or eliminate the values of these models, but to simply provide a counter-balance by pointing out crucial aspects of health and illness which are not accounted for by these models.

Chapter 1

Dehumanization in Contemporary Medicine

> The relentless urgency that characterizes most corporate cultures undermines creativity, quality, engagement, thoughtful deliberation, and, ultimately, performance.
> Tony Schwartz, Jean Gomes and Catherine McCarthy[1]

The first research project I worked on as a student examined symptoms of Posttraumatic Stress Disorder (PTSD) related to the internship year of medical training. I was drawn to this topic, although I did not know why at the time. In retrospect, the concerns characterizing this project have been defining my work ever since.

The PTSD symptoms experienced by medical interns could partly be explained by the occupational hazards of being a physician, such as exposure to death and illness and the sense of helplessness at not being able to prevent such suffering. However, I believe that some of physicians' distress is iatrogenic – it is caused by the system in which treatment is delivered. We cannot change the occupational hazard of exposure to intense existential situations in medicine. Existential engagement *is* the job of medicine. We can, however, change components in the system which are iatrogenic causes of dehumanization for doctors and patients alike.

Physician Dissatisfaction and Burnout

Stephen Bergman, aka Samuel Shem, dramatizes the trauma of medical training in his book, *The House of God*. He writes, 'I struggle to rest, and cannot, and I struggle to love, and I cannot for I am all bleached out, like a man's shirt washed too many times.'[2] He goes so far as to call medical education the 'doctor's disease.'[3] He details a list of ten rules for the House of God, such as 'the only good admission is a dead admission,' and 'the patient is the one with the disease.'[4] The cost of these cynical rules for self-preservation is that, in an attempt to save themselves, the trainees end up losing their own humanity. While *The House of God* is semi-fictional autobiography, it captures the dilemmas of dehumanization that face trainees and doctors.

Up to 60% of physicians in the US report symptoms of burnout, defined as emotional exhaustion, depersonalization (treating patients as objects) and a low sense of accomplishment.[5,6,7] High rates of burnout and stress have also been found in physicians in New Zealand,[8,9,10] Australia,[11,12] in the National Health Service in the UK[13,14] and in Canada.[15,16]

A number of recent books by physicians describe burnout and suggest ways to address it. Robin Youngson's *Time to Care: How to Love Your Patients and Your Job* focuses on how we can regain compassion and humanity.[17] Youngson is originally from the UK, but has worked in New Zealand for the past 20 years. American physician Lee Lipsenthal, in *Finding a Balance in a Medical Life*, examines the effects of stress on physicians' health, and how to counteract them.[6] Allan Peterkin, a Canadian physician, lists four major domains of burnout in his book, *Staying Human During Residency Training*: physiological, psychological and emotional, behavioral and organizational.[7] It is important to recognize that the effects of physician burnout are multidimensional, affecting both doctors and patients, and also the treatment that is given. It has been found to be related to poorer quality of care, patient dissatisfaction, increased medical errors and increased malpractice claims.[6,7,18,19]

Burnout is becoming a major concern even for health care organizations that employ physicians, as illustrated by Britt Berrett and Paul Spiegelman in their recently published book, *Patients Come Second*.[20] As they point out, in any business, 'you cannot take care of customers if you do not take care of employees. Healthcare is no different. We must find ways to engage ... (our employees) ... so that they WANT to provide great service to their patients.'[21]

The opening quote to this chapter, by Schwartz and colleagues, lists the effects of chronic time pressure in corporate environments, claiming that it *undermines creativity, quality, engagement, thoughtful deliberation, and, ultimately, performance*. We will look at what happens to the human beings working in a system when their work is affected in these ways.

Organizational effects create high levels of dissatisfaction in physicians. A 2001 Kaiser Foundation study of 2,608 US physicians showed that 58% reported decreased enthusiasm for the practice of medicine, 87% said that morale had decreased in the last five years, and 46% were dissatisfied due to lack of autonomy.[22]

Miller, Goodman and Norbeck's book, *In Their Own Words*, is based on a 2008 survey of 12,000 physicians in the US by the Physicians Foundation, and it includes both the statistical findings and many direct quotes by the doctors themselves. The purpose of the study was to 'determine whether or not how physicians think about medicine is affecting access to care and, by extension, quality of care for all patients.'[23]A few of the disturbing findings: 94% of physicians report that paperwork demands have increased in the past three years and 63% said this led to spending less time with patients; 76% said they were at 'full capacity' or were 'over-extended and overwhelmed'; 78% characterized the practice of medicine as 'less satisfying' and 'less rewarding.'[24] Similar surveys in other English-speaking countries also show concerning levels of job dissatisfaction and burnout in physicians.

Richard Fernandez, in his book, *Physicians in Transition: Doctors Who Successfully Reinvented Themselves*, interviewed 25 physicians who left clinical practice. The doctors describe levels of dissatisfaction that led to career change. For instance, in the foreword, Michelle Mudge-Riley asks how someone would feel who was unhappy in medicine after all the sacrifice and years of training. She asks, 'Would you feel trapped? Like you'd lost yourself somewhere along the way? Maybe that you were a failure? ... That's what I felt like.'[25]

Models of Medicine

The term 'model' designates a set of underlying ideas, concepts and values that shape a particular attitude and approach. For instance, in the US, we could say that there are two primary models of politics, the Republican and the Democratic. The Republican model is founded on principles such as: the role of government is to stay out of the way of the individual, and government should not limit individual rights. In this model, 'good' government is 'small' government. The Democratic model is founded on different principles, such as: individual rights are important, but sometimes the common good of society should come before the good of the individual.

There are many other values that make up a political party, but those serve as a good introduction to how there can be two different models for the same thing which are sometimes in contradiction with each other. The fundamental assumptions of the Republican and Democratic models share some overlap, but they have significant differences. They both represent legitimate American values; however, each model focuses on different values and as a result prioritizes spending differently. An American citizen may be a proponent of one model over the other, however, the core values of each model of individual freedom and social responsibility are equally consistent with "American" values.

Contemporary medicine is also made up of different models with different beliefs and values about what 'good' medicine is and what the doctor's role should be. While medical students and doctors are taught that medicine is a unitary construct (evidence-based biomedicine), there are different legitimate models of medicine, with different values and priorities. These values shape how health care delivery systems function, how doctors conceptualize their role and responsibilities, and even shape debates about how health care should be reformed.

Anthropologist and international medical organizational consultant Gerald Arbuckle has described a number of health care models, four of which will be used as a framework for understanding the influences in contemporary medicine. These are the *traditional*, the *foundational*, the *biomedical* and the *economic rationalist* models. Each will be briefly discussed in the following paragraphs.

The Traditional Model

In the *traditional model*, 'mental, physical and social health are profoundly interrelated.'[26] Stretching back into ancient times, medicine was embedded in religious, spiritual, cultural and mythopoetic domains. There was a degree of what we would consider scientific medicine that had evolved through cause-and-effect observations of the use of certain plants and herbs that we know today do have bioactive and therapeutic properties. However, the traditional model did not understand the efficacy of these treatments in terms of alterations of biochemicals; rather it focused on the therapeutic element as re-balancing vital energy; harmonizing what had been disconnected (heaven, spirit, body, earth); and bringing the internal into a new relationship with the external. This was a holistic, but non-scientific era of medicine in which health was understood as balance and harmony, and illness was understood as imbalance and disconnection. Ancient Greek and Egyptian medicine grew out of this 'traditional' matrix of the interconnectedness of individuals, environment, society and religion/spirituality. Indigenous cultures around the world today are very much

influenced by this 'traditional model' of understanding health
and illness in relationship to unseen forces, gods and Nature.

The Foundational Model

Arbuckle describes the *foundational model* of health care as rooted
in the story of the Good Samaritan and grounded in values of
'holistic health, equity, social justice, respect, compassion, hospi-
tality, courage and dialogue.'[27] He traces the history of this model
from the early Christian era to the founding of health care
systems in the US, UK, Canada, New Zealand and Australia.
Whether through the development of religiously based health
care systems or national public health systems, the foundational
values of compassion, the universal right to health care and the
goal of alleviating suffering influenced health care institutions in
the 19th and early 20th centuries. Core values of this model are
that health care is a basic human right, and that individuals, institutions and societies have the responsibility to give the gift of
compassion and healing to those who are suffering. This era
greatly influenced our ideals of humanitarianism in medicine.

The Biomedical Model

The *biomedical model* is the primary model that doctors and health
care workers are trained in today. It is founded on science and
technology; however, its emphasis on objectivity and detachment
is at odds with the interpersonal, social and compassionate
aspects of the *foundational model*. What is gained with the
biomedical model is the ability to intervene with technology to save
lives, particularly in acute situations such as infections, accidents,
birth defects and tissue and organ injury. What is lost is the
holistic aspect of the traditional model: viewing the whole person
in relationship to their inner and outer contexts. The *biomedical
model* has limitations in treating chronic conditions (which form
the bulk of primary care visits) that do not have a quick and easy
technological cure. The explosion of technology has come with a

financial cost and this can be seen as a primary contributor to the development of the new, economic rationalist model in the late 20th century.

The Economic Rationalist Model

Arbuckle calls the next model the *'economic rationalist model'* of health care, and describes how it has led to the 'corporatization' and 'privatization' of medicine.[28] It is concerned with the business of medicine, such as profit and loss. He rightly points out that the 'American economic rationalist model is diametrically opposed to the foundational model.'[29] This model can be implemented to maximize profits, as in the for-profit sector in the US; or to minimize costs, which is more common in the national health services of most other industrialized nations. The motto of the economic rationalist model is that 'medicine is a business and it should be run like any other business.'

Models of Health Care in Action

Contemporary medicine in the US is increasingly influenced by the economic rationalist and biomedical models, while many doctors and patients complain about the loss of values of the foundational model and the holistic approach of the traditional model. There are other models of medicine, but these four will help us understand why contemporary medicine is the way it is and why dehumanization, burnout and dissatisfaction are so common today. Any given organization or country will have different percentages of influence from the different models. For instance, in the for-profit sector in the US, the order of influence might be economic rationalist, biomedical and foundational. In an academic medicine setting the biomedical model might be greater or equal to the economic rationalist influence. The traditional model has little influence in the US, although if the patient population was Native American, or heavily influenced by recent immigrants, an understanding of this model would become more important. In the US, aspects of the traditional model do appear through an interest in 'natural' medicine and traditional medicine systems, such as Traditional Chinese Medicine. Perhaps the spirit of traditional medicine is reappearing in the growing interest of both doctors and patients in alternative, complementary, integrative and holistic medicine.

When I started a holistic private practice, I did so because I felt I could not practice 'good' medicine within existing work settings because of the overwhelming influence of the economic rationalist and biomedical models. I created a new health care delivery system that was much more balanced regarding holistic (with elements of the traditional), foundational, biomedical and economic rationalist models of medicine.

Another example, contemporary medicine in New Zealand, contains all four of Arbuckle's models. The traditional model is emphasized in regard to Maori health and has some influence even in mainstream services. Many doctors still subscribe to the values of the foundational model. The biomedical model has a strong place in practice. The economic rationalist model comes into effect with government-led planning through the Ministry of Health and through the national pharmaceutical formulary (Pharmac). Different services within New Zealand have a different balance of the models, particularly if they are cultural services for Maori or Pacific Islanders.

Countries that have national health systems, like Canada, the UK, Australia and others, may have a similar balance to for-profit health care organizations in the US; however, rather than maximizing profits, the economic rationalist model's influence may be more focused on containing costs. The creation of national health services was largely an influence of the foundational model; however in recent years, with the global increases in health care costs, economic rationalist models have begun to have increasing influence in regard to allocation of resources and cost containment.

We will now examine in more depth the dehumanizing side effects of the biomedical and economic rationalist models in contemporary medicine.

Contemporary Medicine

The great gain ... (of the adoption of laboratory science as the primary approach in medicine) ... had been a widespread dissemination and utilisation of scientific knowledge of disease and rational methods of treatment. The great loss was a severe eclipsing of the art of physicianship that had been slowly won over many thousands of years.
Vincent Di Stefano[30]

Contemporary medicine has elements of all four of Arbuckle's models of medicine. But in the US, and increasingly in developed countries around the world, it is largely influenced by biomedical and economic rationalist values, while the values and approaches of the traditional and foundational models have receded into the background. These diminished values include compassion, viewing patients holistically and having the time to really listen to and understand patients.

The biomedical model of medicine has led to the rapid increase in expensive, technological studies and interventions. These in turn have driven up the costs of health care worldwide, to the point where health care systems in the 21st century are in economic crisis and increasingly enticed into an economic rationalist 'solution' in an effort to contain costs.

Both the biomedical and economic rationalist models grow out of the philosophical position of 'logical positivism.'[31] The reductionist position of positivism could be stated as 'the only thing that matters is matter.' This means that both models value 'things' that can be observed, counted and measured. Concepts or values that are not reducible to the status of 'things' are considered irrelevant or non-existent from a positivist perspective. While the *economic* part of the economic rationalist model refers to profit and loss as primary motivators, the *rationalist* perspective is characterized by the notion 'if you cannot measure it, you cannot manage it.'[32] It is this emphasis on 'things' that objectifies and dehumanizes doctors and patients when it is not tempered by models that value aspects of people that are not reducible to things.

As we shall see, the scientific method and its counterpart, evidence-based medicine (EBM), have led to many advances in medicine at a cost of many things that make medical care warm, caring and human. The belief that good health care can be achieved through counting and measuring things with an eye always on profit translates into the enormous influence wielded by insurance companies and government bureaucracies, as well as pharmaceutical companies. In this regard, the control of medical care has gradually shifted away from the doctor.

The Scientific Method

The biomedical model of contemporary medicine is based on science, a method of studying and explaining how things happen in the world. Science takes the whole of something and then breaks it down into its component parts. Thus, the field of biology (the study of life) can be broken down into gross anatomy (parts of the body that can be seen with the eye), histology (microscopic anatomy) and physiology (the study of organs and biochemical interactions). The body can be broken down into many different levels, but each level is mutually interdependent with the others. No level can exist apart from the others. In reality, there is no such thing as a living kidney or heart existing outside the larger context of a human being with emotions, dreams and spiritual experiences.

One side effect of science is that it creates more fields of study as technology provides new ways of dividing up reality. The study of life was once limited to what the naked eye could see. Around the 1600s, the microscope was invented, opening many new dimensions that previously had not been known to exist. With the discovery of bacteria and microorganisms and their role in some diseases, the fields of microbiology and infectious disease emerged. There were many early theories of how life processes occurred, but eventually the study of organic chemistry came about through the analysis of chemical structures and reactions. Molecules were eventually 'discovered,' then atoms, then subatomic particles, then all sorts of bizarre subparticles and forces. The search for the most fundamental building block of nature and life has been elusive and could possibly be an infinite regress. Each new level of discovery opens many new doors.

As medicine has become more scientific, specialties and subspecialties have proliferated. In the first half of the 20th century, most physicians in the United States were primary care doctors. However, by the end of the 20th century, there was a shortage of primary care doctors as most medical students chose specialty training.[33] The trend toward sub-specialization can be viewed as a natural progression of greater scientific understanding of subsystems in the human body. (The financial incentive to make more money as a sub-specialist also drives this choice.) This has led to the development of a vast number of different medical specialists for different parts of the body. Whereas a family doctor used to treat most concerns from birth to death, we now have obstetricians for pregnancy and delivery, pediatricians for childhood and geriatricians for old age. Additionally, there are doctors for every organ in the body: psychiatry studies the brain and behavior; hematology studies the blood; cardiology studies the heart; oncology studies cancer; surgical oncology specializes in cutting out cancer from the body; and radiation oncology specializes in killing cancer cells with focused beams of radiation. Now, we have the growing field of genetics which studies DNA and illness. With increasing technological advances in MRI, fMRI, SPECT and PET scans, new sub-specialties of radiology are developing that can not only study static tissue, but also measure various functional states of internal aspects of the human body. The level of detail in which we can analyze the human body is constantly increasing.

The tendency to break things down into small parts which are managed by sub-specialists fragments medical care. This is one of the primary complaints of patients in today's medical system: no one is in charge and no one is coordinating care. In other words, no one sees them as a whole person. Patients feel 'bounced around' from doctor to doctor. As the depth of focus in sub-specialties increases, there has been a corresponding loss of breadth. An analogy is the zoom feature on your camera. The more you zoom in on an image, the more fine detail you can see. But this occurs at the cost of losing sight of the bigger picture and the context. I, myself, remember periodically being disturbed while doing my surgical rotations in medical school when I would suddenly remember that the 'thing' I was leaning on for leverage to hold a surgical retractor was in fact a person, not an armrest.

Another side effect of medical science is that it studies the individual in relation to large groups, rather than the individual as themselves. Statistics are used to calculate whether a given treatment has a better chance of helping a group of patients than a placebo treatment tested on a different group of comparable patients. It may be that a treatment only helps 50% of people, but it still could be considered an effective treatment and be approved by the US Food and Drug Administration if this 50% is statistically significantly higher than the percentage of people helped by placebo, 30% for instance. A treatment does not have to help everyone, or even most people. It only has to prove itself to be statistically superior to no treatment at all (placebo). Also, a treatment effect may only be a 10% improvement in symptoms, but if a large enough number of people have this improvement, it can be statistically significant. Scientific medicine focuses on the people it can treat, but there are substantial numbers of people who do not respond to standard treatments. While there are many protocols for 'treatment-resistant' patients, the lack of efficacy of standard treatments should be an indication to review the diagnosis as well as an invitation to include other dimensions of intervention beyond the pharmaceutical.

Under the influence of the biomedical model, contemporary medicine attempts to standardize treatments by dictating what the 'best' medications are, what the best dose of medication is and how long a patient should take it. These determinations are based on statistics and averages and published as evidence-based guidelines. Many people still do not respond to the 'best' medication, and an individual may do very well on a medicine that is not considered the 'best.' Also, the average dose of a medication may be too high or too low for a particular person. In this way, medical science is an abstraction from the individual. The guidelines of medical science will always have to be tailored to fit the individual. Science is so respected, deified even, that sometimes doctors end up treating numbers and abstractions and lose sight of the actual person. The chronic time-pressure can lead doctors to take shortcuts by automatically following a guideline, rather than using their own clinical decision-making abilities.

Science's emphasis on objectivity, numbers and measurement has contributed to a devaluation of individualization of treatment approaches, subjectivity and the human and interpersonal aspects of the doctor–patient relationship.

Evidence-Based Medicine (EBM)

Clinical algorithms ... discourage physicians from thinking independently and creatively. Instead of expanding a doctor's thinking, they can constrain it.
Jerome Groopman[34]

Currently, there is a lot of attention given to 'evidence-based medicine.' We can see this as a logical outgrowth of the conceptual systems of the biomedical model and the economic rationalist model in which good medicine is that which is measurable, objective, repeatable, standardized and unvarying from individual to individual. To practice in an evidence-based way is to prioritize treatments that have been scientifically proven to help patients, but the danger is that this can replace critical thinking and decision-making. As the Groopman quote suggests, excessive reliance on algorithms can dumb us down. If everything is a protocol and the practice of medicine is simply following a guideline, one should be able to make a simple computer program that would diagnose and recommend treatment. Indeed Groopman draws this conclusion regarding contemporary medical education: 'the next generation of doctors was being conditioned to function like a well-programmed computer that operates within a strict binary framework.'[35] There may also be a loss of individualized treatment.[36] The risk is that EBM may become less human and more cold and machine-like.

I will use the example of depression to look at the benefits and shortcomings of evidence-based medicine. There are many treatments that are scientifically proven to help alleviate symptoms of depression, including various forms of psychotherapy, exercise, socialization, dietary changes or supplements, medication and the treatment recommended by my favorite study: swimming with dolphins.[37] However, physicians tend to jump to medication as the first option. Scientific studies favor pharmaceutical interventions because it is easy to have a placebo control group, whereas this is more difficult for exercise, acupuncture, or meditation. Also, pharmaceutical companies are the major funding source for studies of treatment efficacy, leading to more research on medication than on non-medication modalities. (To my knowledge, dolphins have not funded any research on their natural anti-depressant effect on people.)

To be diagnosed with major depression a person must meet five out of nine clinical criteria for two weeks or more. One issue with scientific medicine, and particularly in psychiatry, is that people can have similar symptoms and yet have different conditions. For instance, the same symptoms of fatigue, weight change, insomnia, sad mood and social withdrawal could be caused by hypothyroidism, prednisone or beta interferon treatment, grief, the break-up of a relationship, substance abuse, the depressed phase of bipolar disorder, personality disorder, dysthymia (low-level depression), major depression and a lot of other conditions as well. Because of these complexities, physicians are taught to use the biopsychosocial model which takes into account multiple dimensions of cause and effect. However, the appeal (for both doctor and patient) of a quick and powerful intervention like a pharmaceutical often takes precedence over interventions that are equally effective but sometimes longer-lasting and less expensive. While I cite depression as an example of a medical condition that has many other determinants in addition to the biological, similar arguments can be used for any chronic condition such as obesity, high blood pressure, diabetes, high cholesterol and pain conditions.

When doctors blindly follow protocols and guidelines, they stop being clinicians and become technicians. Technicians relate to people through the application of techniques, which are standardized methods of intervening to promote a particular outcome. In his book, *The Illusion of Technique*, the philosopher William Barrett defines a technique as a 'standard method that can be taught. It is a recipe that can be fully conveyed from one person to another. A recipe always lays down a certain number of steps which, if followed to the letter, ought to lead invariably to the end desired.'[38] While Evidence-Based Medicine and the Quality Revolution strive for standardized treatment interventions, science-fiction writer Philip K. Dick cautions that standardization can lead to a loss of humanity, what he calls 'androidization.' He writes that, 'Androidization requires obedience. And, most of all, predictability. It is precisely when a given person's response to any given situation can be predicted with scientific accuracy that the gates are open for the wholesale production of the android life form.' [39] According to Philip K. Dick, we must be careful not to lose the 'human' as we strive for predictable and replicable behavior. His distinction between the android and the human sounds a lot like Groopman's critique that younger generations of doctors are being taught to be more machine than human.

Barrett cautions against over-reliance on technique. He states that it

has become a general faith, widespread even when it is unvoiced, that technique and technical organization are the necessary and sufficient conditions for arriving at truth; that they can encompass all truth; and that they will be sufficient, if not at the moment, then shortly, to answer the questions that life thrusts upon us.[40]

Barrett's cautions address recent cultural belief systems, of which contemporary medicine is one example, in which the over-emphasis on technique obscures other sources of truth and other dimensions of humanity.

Economics and Time Pressure

The economic aspects of medicine are not taught in medical school, yet economics play a major role in shaping how physicians practice today. Look at a simple breakdown of how much money a physician can bill for seeing patients for different session times. In many practices, how much you bill determines your salary. This may seem completely irrelevant to those who have only worked in public systems on a fixed salary. However, your employer (whether public, private, or NGO/non-profit) will want you to see enough patients to make sure that the clinic is not losing money, so the economics of medicine affect all practice settings. Let us use the following numbers for a comparison, which were, incidentally, the fees in US dollars I used when I first opened my private practice (I include the psychiatric billing code):

60-minute visit (90807): $150
30-minute visit (90805): $100
15-minute visit (90862): $75

This leads to an hourly income/productivity (assuming collections are equal to billing) of:

One patient per hour: $150
Two patients per hour: $200
Four patients per hour: $300

There is the old saying that 'time is money,' and in medicine we can quickly see that there is a relationship between time spent with patients and money earned. A physician who sees four times as many patients a day will bill twice as much as a physician who sees one patient per hour. This means that if a physician sees four times as many clients, writes four times the number of notes and does four times the administrative work, they will make twice the income. This simple fact is an issue that all physicians must appreciate, because how they prioritize their values has a major impact on how they practice medicine. If physicians make income their top priority over other values (the economic rationalist model) they will have less time to spend with each patient. There is a point where a physician cannot provide the same quality of care to more clients in shorter visits. A physician cannot provide the same quality of care in a 10–15-

minute appointment as they can in a 30-minute appointment. The less time a physician spends with clients, the more he (or she) will rely on a reductionist biomedical model and the less he will be aware of holistic factors in health and healing. If a physician has other values they hold higher than money or science (or if they strive for a balance of values), they may see fewer patients and make less money, but have a better quality of life and be better able to provide high-quality health *care*. One problem in contemporary medicine is that individual physicians feel they have a diminished ability to make decisions about how they spend their time. Reimbursement by Medicare has been decreasing in the US; employers want physicians to see more patients to generate more billing; and physicians want to pay off all those student loans. All of this can contribute to a powerful feeling that external agencies are 'forcing' physicians to practice in a certain way. This is also the acculturation pressure exerted by the economic rationalist model.

Insurance Companies and Government Bureaucracies
Insurance companies in the United States are commonly criticized by doctors and patients alike for the bureaucracy they introduce into health care. Private insurance pays for about one-third of all health care (36%) in the US. The federal government pays for roughly another third (34%), out-of-pocket payment is 15%, states pay for 11% and private funds 4%.[41]

Insurance companies play lesser roles in the delivery of health care in other countries. In New Zealand, only 5% of all health care is paid for by private insurance companies, while 66% is through the Ministry of Health (national government), 16% is out of pocket and about 10% is through ACC (Accident Compensation Corporation).[42] ACC is a government-run accident insurance agency in New Zealand. In the UK, private health insurance accounts for 11.5% of health care.[43] Although insurance companies play smaller roles outside of the US, nationalized health care often introduces complex administrative bureaucracies that can interfere with the doctor–patient relationship. For instance, burdensome paperwork, medication formularies and the shifting emphasis of programs and initiatives with each election can still come between doctor and patient. Many administrative systems can take on a life of their own and there is the risk that the doctor will become more focused on trying to navigate the system than on connecting with patients. Dehumanization will be the side effect.

Countries around the world are struggling to create affordable and effective health care delivery systems. The amount of money spent on health care does not directly translate into how 'good' a country's health care system is, at least in terms of life expectancy. For instance, in 2007 the US spent US$7,290 per person on medical care, yet the average life expectancy was 78 years, less than most other developed nations. The UK spent less than half than the US (about US$3,000 per person) but had a slightly higher life expectancy of 79 years. New Zealand spent even less, about one-third of the US (US$2,500 per person) and had an even higher life expectancy of over 80 years. Japan, perhaps the best value for money, spent about US$2,500 per person and yet had a life expectancy of almost 83 years. Another thing to consider is that people in Japan had an average of 12 visits to a doctor per year, residents of the UK and New Zealand had an average of four visits, while in the US, the average was less than four visits per year.[44]

Why is the US spending more than twice that of other countries on health care? Are we really getting our value from that expenditure? It appears that higher cost and fewer doctor visits are side effects of the US health care system when compared worldwide. There are many reasons for the rising costs of insurance, which are beyond the scope of this book, but rapid increases in expensive medical technology, 'defensive' medicine to avoid lawsuits, multiple layers of health care businesses each with their own profit motive and layers of administrative bureaucracy surely contribute. This dramatic difference in the cost of the US health care system was recently made clear to me when I was pricing international travel health insurance and found that there are two rates: the most expensive rate includes the US and the entire world; the less expensive rate is for the entire world, excluding the US.

As insurance companies in the US have come to play a larger role in the day-to-day practice of medicine, they have introduced a style of doctor–patient interaction that is at odds with the humanitarian aspects of medicine. Insurance companies grow out of the economic rationalist model, with its values of efficiency, cost-savings and productivity. As we have seen, this model has values that are diametrically opposed to those of the foundational model of medicine, which are compassion, connection, universal right to health care and a focus on the whole person. Insurance companies view payment for health care as 'loss' rather than as a positive health benefit. When the language of 'loss' is taken to the extreme, and applied in the short term of quarterly profits, spending money is to be avoided at any cost (pun intended: the 'cost' of the economic rationalist model is human cost, as economic values are placed above human values). Insurance companies have, increasingly, taken on the role of deciding which tests and treatments are indicated. This frustrates doctors as it takes decision-making out of their hands. Similar feelings are expressed by doctors in New Zealand working with ACC, the government-funded accident insurance program. Some models of insurance, such as managed care and capitated care, have 'incentivized' doctors to become 'gatekeepers' who stand between the person who is ill and the provision of services, and are rewarded for providing less care. When doctors and health care delivery systems interact daily with insurance companies, they start to think like insurance companies, viewing the provision of health care as a 'loss' rather than a benefit.

Historically, the HMO model of health insurance grew out of a previous American health care crisis in the early 1970s. Paul Ellwood, director of the American Rehabilitation Foundation, proposed the concept of a 'Health Maintenance Organization.' His goal was to shift the focus of health care from tertiary care to preventative care, which a plethora of research shows is more cost effective. In practice, however, the HMO concept became more of a cost-containment policy than a preventative health policy. While US Senator Ted Kennedy was calling for a national health plan, the Nixon administration opted for the HMO model with a call to 'change the incentives in health care.'[45] The health care system today in the US reflects these changed incentives, and physicians have experienced a diminished sense of control in the daily practice of medicine. Furthermore, the language of business has been hybridized with that of medicine. The insurance industry became an intervening agent between the doctor and the patient.

Managed care has not successfully contained costs in the US and it created layers of bureaucracy that interfere with the doctor–patient relationship. Physicians and patients alike have experienced interference as care is limited or denied. Managed care has effectively taken away doctors' role of being the primary decision-makers about medical treatment and evaluation, while doctors still carry all the liability for treatment outcomes. HMOs and insurance companies have also increased the amount of paperwork for physicians, such as filling out treatment request forms. When ordering a test, the physician must consider whether it is covered under the HMO and maybe even place a call through the interminable automated phone tree to reach an agent of the HMO to try to request 'prior authorization' for a procedure. HMOs often dictate which medications a physician can prescribe, and this 'formulary' is constantly changing. The aversive experience of interacting with insurance companies can condition the physician into prescribing certain medications for people under certain insurance plans because it is easier than constantly pushing back on the encroaching system.

Even after a patient leaves the office, the physician may still have more administrative work to do, sometimes stretching out over weeks of phone calls and faxes. The pharmacy may call, stating that a medication is no longer covered or that it requires prior authorization. Sometimes the reason for denial is readily apparent, but other times it is obscure, such as getting prior authorization for an inexpensive generic medicine or for a 'quantity limit' override in which a doctor has prescribed more pills a day of a medication than the insurance company will routinely pay for, such as an arbitrary limit of 100 pills per month. If a patient is prescribed four pills a day of a medicine (120 pills/month), they have to pay a second copayment to get the 20 pills beyond the 100/month that the insurance company will cover. So the physician has to fill out more forms or make more calls, which takes more time out of their day and competes with the patient for attention. Most clinics in the US do not schedule time for physician paperwork, so this time ends up being taken out of face-to-face time spent with patients and/or personal time (as completing necessary paperwork is not a billable procedure).

While many doctors feel they can effectively multi-task, any patient knows that human beings really are not very good at multi-tasking, as they sit patiently while the doctor calls pharmacies, insurance companies, prepares faxes, takes phone calls about other issues, is interrupted by office staff and in-between all this speaks to the patient. Chabris and Simons, in their book, *The Invisible Gorilla*, present a great deal of research on how people cannot multi-task effectively. Perhaps the best known and most dramatic example is their study in which subjects count the number of passes a basketball team makes. About 50% of people concentrating on this task miss seeing a person in a gorilla suit walk on to the middle of the court.[46] Research such as this has profound implications for health care delivery systems in which doctors are bombarded by information and interruptions while trying to perform numerous clinical and administrative tasks and speaking with their client. It also makes one wonder what kind of gorillas in our midst we are missing as we count lab results and procedure codes.

Even once doctors have completed all of their work providing services, there is still the issue of collecting payment. In the US, doctors and clinics can set whatever price they want for a given procedure or service. However, they rarely get paid this amount. Every insurance company, as well as government-funded Medicare and Medicaid, can independently decide how much they will actually pay. So doctors may do the same work, but get paid vastly different amounts depending on the insurance coverage of a particular client. Take for example a 30-minute psychotherapy session with medication management (90805). For instance, take a service that has a fee of US$100. One private insurance company might pay the full amount, while another company pays $85.17, Medicare might pay $48.09, while Medicaid might pay $25.34. This creates an accounting nightmare to try and keep track of billing and collections. The frustration that these differential billing systems invoke is another source of distress and dissatisfaction for physicians and can, again, distract the physician from connecting with the patient.

Personal Example

What can be done in the face of this dehumanizing pressure of an unchecked economic rationalist model? This book will explore different responses in later chapters, but I'll give one personal example. In my private practice, I worked with an insurance company that distorted the meaning of an extended-release, 'once daily' medication to mean that they would only authorize one pill a day per prescription. Even though the FDA-approved maximum dose was higher than the strength of one pill, the company would only authorize one pill per day. To get the maximum dose of the medication, which the patient was taking, I had to prescribe four different prescriptions with four different pill strengths and the patient had to pay four separate co-payments. This was after numerous phone calls back and forth between the pharmacy, the patient, myself and the insurance company.

What I did in response to this company's practice: first, I appealed the declined prescription (which was denied using circular reasoning); second, I did my best to ensure that the patient could get the medication dose they had been on for years for the lowest expense possible; third, a number of different patients with this insurance plan had similar problems, so I filed a series of complaints with the state insurance regulatory agency (which did not see a problem with the practice); fourth, for this, and several other reasons, I dropped out of this particular insurance network, as I considered it unethical. Not every doctor can decide whether or not to participate in an insurance network, but you always have a voice, even if you cannot make the final decision. A question to ask yourself is, 'Have I done everything I can to challenge this injustice?'

Pharmaceutical Companies

Conflicts of interest between physicians' commitment to patient care and the desire of pharmaceutical companies and their representatives to sell their product pose challenges to the principles of medical professionalism.
Troyen Brennan and colleagues[47]

Pharmaceutical companies straddle two paradigms, the biomedical and the economic rationalist. They use a biomedical model to create many useful medications that alleviate pain and suffering and sometimes cure disease. However, the primary interest of pharmaceutical companies is to sell more medication and to make more money – not necessarily the best interests of the patient. They want physicians to prescribe the 'newest' and 'best' medicine, which really means the medicine that their company makes. Pharmaceutical representatives try to appear as emissaries of science, but they are really well-paid sales people who are highly trained to influence doctors' prescribing practices. Of particular significance is the way that pharmaceutical companies become another layer of competing interests between the doctor and the patient.

Do We Even Need a Pill at All?

Some authors express concern about 'the medicalization of everyday life' in which pharmaceutical interventions are used to address issues that are normal or might be addressed more effectively and less expensively in other ways. For instance, Moynihan and Cassels, in their book *Selling Sickness*, describe the expansion of approved uses for pharmaceuticals for more and more conditions, often with only shaky scientific evidence. They make a good argument that the pharmaceutical companies are actively working to expand their markets (recent lawsuits penalizing companies for false marketing also attest to this), while at the same time, people are more and more willing to accept a medical explanation for what was previously viewed as a problem of life. In their book, they describe how medications for aging, menopause, obesity, hyperactivity and other 'syndromes' have been approved through the US Food and Drug Administration (they also point out the conflicts of interests in the FDA in that pharmaceutical companies are now partly bankrolling the salaries of those who are supposed to be objectively evaluating scientific evidence). Moynihan and Cassels see this problem as going beyond that of greedy industry profit-motives, arguing that 'the $500 billion dollar pharmaceutical industry is literally changing what it means to be human.'[48] A recent *Reuters Business Insight* report designed for drug company executives argued that the ability to 'create new disease markets' is bringing untold billions in soaring drug sales. One of the chief selling strategies, said the report, is to change the way people think about their common ailments, to make 'natural processes' into medical conditions ... The coming years will bear greater witness to the corporate sponsored creation of disease.[49]

Many syndromes have well-documented evidence for non-medication interventions, such as irritable bowel syndrome (IBS), hypertension, high cholesterol, obesity, type II diabetes, metabolic syndrome, fibromyalgia and chronic fatigue syndrome. In some cases, lifestyle changes (diet, exercise, stress management) may actually 'cure' these conditions, meaning that the person no longer has the syndrome. A good argument can be made that using preventative, mind–body and lifestyle approaches is more humane, has fewer costs long term, has fewer medication side effects and has positive side effects of empowering people in regards to their health and their lives.

The Cost of Pharmaceuticals
The amount spent on prescriptions in the US doubled from 1999 to 2008, up to $234 billion per year. Almost 50% of Americans were reported to have used a prescription medication in the previous month.[50] According to Wazana, in the year 2000, the pharmaceutical industry was spending US$5,000,000,000 per year on sales representatives, and an estimated US$8000–13,000 per year per physician.[51] Brennan and colleagues reported that in 2000 the pharmaceutical industry sponsored 314,000 events specifically for physicians.[52] Dana and Lowenstein report that between 1989 and 2000, the US FDA

judged 76 percent of all approved drugs to be no more than moderate innovations over existing treatments, with many being a modification of an older product with the same ingre-dient. All of this money is spent with the goal of convincing doctors to prescribe a given pharmaceutical company's product, which may not even be any better than generic alternatives.[53]

What Will All That Money Buy? How the Pharmaceutical Industry Influences Doctors
Studies show that physician prescribing patterns are influenced by pharmaceutical representatives, regardless of whether or not physicians consciously believe that they are influenced. Dana and Lowenstein review social science research on this topic and discuss the concept of *self-serving bias*, which states that individuals will unconsciously make decisions that maximize their own personal benefit. The article concludes that, first,

> individuals are unable to remain objective, even when they are motivated to be impartial, demonstrating that self-serving bias is unintentional. Second, individuals deny and succumb to bias even when explicitly instructed about it, which suggests that self-serving bias is unconscious. Third, the studies show that self-interest affects choices indirectly, changing the way individuals seek out and weigh the infor-mation on which they later base their choices when they have a stake in the outcomes.[54]

Wazana's review of 29 studies on gift giving and pharmaceutical company interactions with physicians concludes that,

> although some positive outcomes were identified (improved availability to identify the treatment for complicated illnesses), most studies found negative outcomes associated with the interaction. These included an impact on knowledge (inability to identify wrong claims about medication), attitude (positive attitude toward pharmaceutical representatives;

awareness, preference, and rapid prescription of a new drug), and behavior (making formulary requests for medications that rarely held important advantages over existing ones; nonrational prescribing behavior; increasing prescription rate; prescribing fewer generic but more expensive, newer medications at no demonstrated advantage).[55]

Embracing 'evidence-based medicine' has created a tremendous business opportunity for pharmaceutical companies as well as a booming industry for the physicians who draft these guidelines. If a pharmaceutical company can prove that their medication is the best (or, even better, the only) treatment for a certain condition, they can have a powerful endorsement that encourages all doctors everywhere to prescribe their medication. Similarly, if a guideline is developed that argues for the increased use of medications for milder conditions, pharmaceutical companies stand to make a lot of money. Pharmaceutical companies, insurance companies and academic physicians are all striving to create treatment guidelines to shape how doctors treat patients. Moynihan and Cassels outline a number of instances where there appear to be conflicts of interest. Choudhry and colleagues report that almost 90% of clinical guideline authors have some relationship with pharmaceutical companies and they caution about the risk of conflict of interest between these groups.[56] Marcia Angell warns us of this same issue.[57,58]

There Is No Free Lunch: Banning Pharmaceutical Gifts
As the quote about conflicts of interest at the start of this section plainly states, there is an inherent conflict of interests between pharmaceutical companies' commitment to sell medications and the doctor's commitment to patient care. The article states that physicians' 'commitment to altruism ... scientific integrity, and an absence of bias in medical decision making now regularly come up against financial conflicts of interest.'[59]

This article by Brennan and a panel of academic physicians warns that no matter how small gifts and payments to physicians from the pharmaceutical industry are, they must be regulated. Gifts that cause potential conflicts of interest include:

> meals; payment for attendance at lectures and conferences, including on-line activities; CME ... for which physicians pay no fee; payment for time while attending meetings; payment for travel to meetings or scholarships to attend meetings; payment for participation in speakers' bureaus; the provision of ghost-writing services; provision of pharmaceutical samples; grants for research projects; and payment for consulting relationships.[60]

When I started my private practice, I decided that I would not have any branded information or items in my practice. I still chose to meet with pharmaceutical representatives, but I had to police the waiting room to remove items they would leave there. Personally, I think any meeting with a pharmaceutical representative must be done very cautiously, if at all, and all educational material they provide is suspect. Decisions around pharmaceutical agents are ethical issues, and the concept of self-serving bias shows that you may not always be the best judge of your intentions. For more information about the interaction between the pharmaceutical industry and doctors, see the 'No Free Lunch' website.[61]

Pharmacophilia (the love of pills) and Dehumanization
We have examined the various ways that the pharmaceutical industry tries and succeeds at influencing doctors' prescribing patterns. When this influence is combined with the pressure to see more patients to increase business revenues, it can be seen how prescribing more medication could be a compensation for spending less time with patients, particularly in the context of a

materialistic culture that values objects over less tangible human interactions. In this sense, *the pill has come to replace the doctor–patient relationship.* The physician gets to feel like they have done something (instead of just feeling like they should have spent more time actually listening to the patient). The patient feels like at least they 'got' something tangible from the brief visit with the physician.

Increased prescribing and decreased consultation time is a symptom of the materialization or objectification of the doctor–patient relationship. Instead of the relationship being viewed as a potentially healing interpersonal interaction, it becomes a transaction in which money is exchanged for an object: the pill. The patient views the doctor as a means for getting a pill and the doctor views the patient as a biochemical imbalance to be manipulated with a pill. Instead of a human being who is suffering and a human being who has learned how to alleviate suffering, there is a passive body whose health depends on taking a pill and a technician dispensing an object. The relationship does not matter and the technician becomes inter-changeable with other technicians because the mediating variable is the pill, not the relationship. Similarly, the human being of the patient becomes a 'consumer' in a line of consumers. If medicine becomes primarily about objects giving objects to other objects, it has become dehumanized.

In the psychotherapy literature, there is a word for the replacement of a relationship with an object: *fetishism.* In a fetish, there is an obsession with an object that replaces human inter-action. Psychoanalyst Robert Stoller, in his book, *Observing the Erotic Imagination,* describes the motivation behind reducing another person to a body part: 'we anatomize them … because we cannot stand the revelations of intimacy, we deprive others of their fullness.'[62] Stoller believes that reducing the other to a body part or replacing a relationship with an object is a psychological defense against the anxiety of relationship. The risk is that the process of dehumanization goes both ways. One cannot dehumanize someone and remain human oneself. It is not a human action to treat someone else as an object. The act of dehumanizing another 'dehumanizes the dehumanizer.'[63] Stoller is concerned not just with the physical aspect of human sexuality, but with sexuality as an expression of human intimacy and interpersonal connection.

The reduction of a human being to a body part is one of the primary complaints raised about contemporary medical practice. The contemporary physician, rather than relating to the complexity of a human being, focuses only on a body part or an organ system and then tries to find the right pill to fix that problem. If the physician can remember that they are using a reductionist model for a specific purpose and can then shift focus back to the whole person, this is the use of science at its best. However, if the physician forgets that they are using a reductionist model and comes to perceive that model as reality, they have become an impaired physician and an impaired human being; they have dehumanized themselves in the process of dehumanizing the patient.

Doctors can get stuck in this mode of interaction, or even worse, they can defensively hide behind it because the *intimacy* of genuine human interaction is too anxiety-provoking. The pill can serve as a fetish object that replaces or even represents genuine interpersonal relationship. Objectification is a very dangerous force in contemporary medicine and it is a major contributor to the dehumanization of all the human beings in the health care delivery system, patients and clinicians alike. This is not to say that doctors should not focus on body parts or prescribe pills, but that this should be one skill doctors have, while retaining their capacity to *be* human and compassionate in their clinical interactions.

The next section further explores aspects of objectification and dehumanization in medicine.

I–It Medicine and I–Thou Medicine

External forces such as the insurance industry, government regulation and the pharmaceutical industry would not shape physician behavior if there were not a corresponding internal representation of these forces within the physician. People have treated other people like objects throughout human history – this is not an invention of economic biomedicine. We could even say that dehumanization is part of what it means to be human, that we all have this potential within us.

Martin Buber speaks of the distinction between 'I–Thou' and 'I–It' relationships. *The Cambridge Dictionary of Philosophy* describes these different kinds of relationship:

> I-Thou is characterized by openness, reciprocity and a deep sense of personal involvement. The I confronts the Thou not as something to be studied, measured, or manipulated, but as a unique presence that responds to the I in its individuality. I-It is characterized by the tendency to treat something as an impersonal object governed by causal, social, or economic forces.[64]

This distinction between I–Thou and I–It resonates with our present discussion about human and professional relationships on the one hand and android and technician relationships on the other hand. Perhaps what makes a human being *human* is the necessity of choosing between the 'I' of humanization and the 'It' of dehumanization.

Physicians have actively and passively created the current health care delivery system, in cooperation with economic and social forces. Physicians share the same socio-cultural beliefs that shape economics and society, and thus can embrace the economic rationalist model. They are trained as scientists and taught concepts of 'clinical detachment,' 'objectivity' and 'neutrality,' that grow out of the biomedical model. There is a need to teach appropriate boundaries in medicine, otherwise physicians would be doing all the things that physicians do in soap operas, like having affairs with their patients and getting over-involved in their lives. However, a good boundary is different from detachment. A boundary is a lot like a cell membrane; it is an active process requiring energy in deciding what to let in and what to let out. The membrane does not keep everything out, nor does it keep everything in – it is a continual decision-making process. A boundary is still a connection, but it is a form of connection that is monitored and constantly re-evaluated with the aim of creating a therapeutic relationship.

Detachment[65] is a severing of human relationship. It is cold, disconnected, uncaring and it withholds the Self of the physician from the patient. It is not a positive goal to strive for. While it is true that a clinician sometimes needs some distance from human relationship in making important clinical decisions, he or she is still responsible for being a caring and compassionate human being who is emotionally available to the patient. It is also the responsibility of the physician to manage the professional boundary with the patient. Maintaining human connection and managing professional boundaries may seem like contradictory responsibilities, but that is the work of being a professional.

We, as physicians, should strive for scientific objectivity *and* human connection; these can be difficult tasks to juggle at the best of times, but even more so if we do not have a conceptual paradigm that has room for both. How do we integrate different conceptual paradigms so that we provide treatment that is technically safe and effective and also care that is humane and compassionate? The holistic framework that will be developed in this book addresses this dilemma.

What about Health Care Reform in the US?

Worldwide, governments are concerned about the cost of health care and want to make sure they are getting value for money. Arbuckle usefully points out in his book, *Humanizing Healthcare*

Reforms, that reforms will be structured according to the under-lying philosophical model used to understand health care. A biomedical model would lead to more objective and protocol-based treatments such as is found in evidence-based medicine. An economic rationalist model might also favor evidence-based medicine, but for slightly different reasons based on economic return on money spent. A foundational model would lead to reform that returns to the foundational values of medicine, such as compassion, social justice, equity and humanitarianism. Before we reform medicine, we should be clear about what our values are and how we define 'good medicine.' In later chapters, I will introduce a holistic framework that allows for the integration of many different models of medicine.

Contemporary medicine has become increasingly corpora-tized with CEOs and CFOs now making business decisions about how doctors will practice medicine. While we can blame the fragmentation and disconnection in medicine on the influence of pharmaceutical companies, insurance companies and the business side of medicine, it can be said that these are issues that are found in society as a whole. Technology that replaces or competes with face-to-face interactions; larger suburban homes with the corresponding loss of public meeting places; commuter culture – all contribute to fragmentation and disconnection in society. These factors are consequences of our current values of efficiency and speed over connection and quality.

One way of looking at the loss of compassion in contemporary medicine is as an expression of a larger societal problem, namely the general loss of authentic human interactions. This view suggests that the forces shaping medicine are larger than the health care system. This also means that if you, as a physician, choose to challenge disconnection and dehumanization in your own practice, you are also challenging a larger societal issue.

Many doctors have come to feel that they are powerless to change the way that they practice, let alone larger societal problems. Doctors I have met in the United States and in New Zealand are frustrated with the many forces impinging on their practice. As physician Peter Salgo states in his *New York Times* piece, 'The Doctor Will See You for Exactly Seven Minutes,' doctors 'have felt powerless to change things.'[66] He goes on to say that the power for change lies in patients demanding more time with their physicians and more genuine collaborative relationships. While I do think that people have a responsibility to advocate for themselves, I think that we, as physicians, need to challenge the sense of powerlessness that we have accepted as part of our daily practices. True health care reform will therefore require reform of society and reform of individuals. This book will look at ways of transforming the physician in order to reform the practice and culture of medicine; ultimately, this will have larger societal implications as well.

In *The Birth of the Clinic*, Foucault wrote that the 'first task of the doctor is therefore political: the struggle against disease must begin with a war against bad government.'[67] I have always taken this quote to mean that humanitarian ethics require the physician to challenge bad administrative policies that get in the way of good medicine.

In the United States, following President Obama's election to a second term, we are facing a new wave of health care reform under the Patient Protection and Affordable Care Act. There will be a natural tension in this reform between cost-cutting elements and elements supporting human connection, between a 'Quality Revolution' and a 'Compassion Revolution'. Using Arbuckle's terms, we could see this as an attempt to integrate the biomedical and economic rationalist models in terms of quality and the foundational model in terms of compassion. The difficulty lies in making sure that any reform encourages foundational values of compassion and client-centeredness.

The Quality Revolution

The Quality Revolution focuses on issues of safety, efficiency, technology and communication as ways to improve health care. The hope is that through a focus on quality, health care will be better and this will decrease costs in the long term. An important concept in terms of reform is the 'Patient-Centered Medical Home' (PCMH), to which the American Academy of Family Physicians (AAFP) devotes a web portal.[68] It illustrates five elements to the PCMH: a foundation in family medicine, quality care, practice organization, health information technology and patient-centered care. The element of *quality* consists of creating a 'culture of improvement,' updating care plans and risk assessments, using risk-stratified care management principles, incorporating patient safety into clinical practice and coordinating transitions in care. The element of *health information technology* includes having an Electronic Health Records (EHR) system and utilizing evidence-based clinical decision support tools. The element of *practice organization* has to do with financial planning, embracing a culture of change and creating a staffing model that supports a PCMH approach (team-based, defined roles, flexible schedules, health care coaching and care coordination and patient-friendly environments).[69] Some of these elements overlap with the concept of the micropractice (which we will discuss later in the book): low overhead, use of technology and eliminating layers of personnel between the patient and the doctor.

The Compassion Revolution

Some elements in the PCMH overlap with the Compassion Revolution. The element of *patient-centered care* fits with a focus on compassion as it creates a health care system that works around the patient, supports shared decision-making, empowers patient self-management and includes patient feedback and patient advisors on the structure and function of the health care delivery system. These principles are very similar to those of holistic medicine, as is the emphasis on a systems and whole-person focus. The AAFP adds a *family medicine foundation* to the Patient-Centered Medical Home. This includes a continuous healing relationship, whole person orientation, family and community context and comprehensive and coordinated care.[70]

Compassion is a large part of what this current book focuses on and it should be apparent that many of the PCMH concepts overlap with a holistic medical practice. The reason that I am calling a focus on compassion a *revolution* is that there is a growing focus on compassion in medicine that I believe is symptomatic of the degree of disconnection and dehumanization in contemporary practice. Many of the authors and organizations cited in this book could be considered part of the Compassion Revolution in medicine: Robin Youngson and the Hearts in Healthcare organization, Rama Thiruvengadam and Physician Heal Thyself Retreats™, Melanie Sears' book, *Humanizing Health Care*, Lee Lipsenthal's *Finding Balance in a Medical Life*, Allan Peterkin's *Staying Human During Residency Training*, the work of the American Holistic Medical Association and organizations like Heal Thy Practice, all focus on enhancing the whole person of the practitioner and the client. Parker Palmer's organization, Courage and Renewal, has a health care branch and has started an annual health care conference. Also, the influence of mindfulness has reinvigorated an interest in the well-being of physicians and health professionals. ALIA (Authentic Leadership In Action) grows out of the Buddhist Shambhala tradition and has run leadership programs specific to health care and medicine.

Disconnection in contemporary medicine is both costly (thus motivating the Quality Revolution) and dehumanizing. While there may be a tension between the Quality and Compassion Revolutions, they both stem from dissatisfaction with the same source: the current practice of contemporary medicine. For this reason, there is an inherent logic to combining compassion and quality as we move to reform and transform medicine. If health care in the US focuses only on quality, neglecting compassion, we will not be able to heal health care, but will only maim it further.

A recent article by Harding and Pincus states that, in the current health care system in the US, the 'problems are so widespread that trying harder within the current system is not enough. System-wide change is needed.'[71] Their call for system-wide change is similar, in many ways, to my argument for transforming the culture of medicine. The authors mention the Institute of Medicine's '10 Rules for Patient/Consumer Expectations of Their Health Care':

1. Continuous Healing Relationships beyond face-to-face encounters
2. Safety as a system property
3. Cooperation and Collaboration among clinicians and institutions
4. Evidence-based decisions
5. Individualization, care is customized to respond to individual patient circumstances and values
6. Patient as source of control, shared decisions between patients and clinicians
7. Shared knowledge, free flow of information
8. Anticipation of needs
9. Transparency in system performance
10. Value or continuous decrease in waste[72]

We can see that the focus of holistic and integrative medicine on individualized, patient-centered care, collaboration, preventative medicine, low-cost lifestyle modifications (compared to high-cost pharmaceutical interventions) and on the therapeutic value of a positive therapeutic relationship appears to have a prominent place in the new health care revolution, which the authors call a 'paradigm shift.' The call for a 'continuous healing relationship' is particularly relevant to our current book on enhancing healing through a transformation of the person of the clinician and the relationship between people and systems. While elements of the Quality Revolution focus on cost containment, it also provides motivation and a framework for redefining the role of physicians/clinicians and enhancing the therapeutic relationship. The call for quality therefore has substantial overlap with this book's argument for re-humanizing health care and for a whole-person focus.

Chapter 2

Health and Illness: Paradigms and Perspectives

Statistics cannot substitute for the human being before you; statistics embody averages, not individuals. Numbers can only complement a physician's personal experience with a drug or a procedure, as well as his knowledge of whether a 'best' therapy from a clinical trial fits a patient's particular needs and values.
Jerome Groopman[1]

Perspectives from Within Science

Let us look at a critique of contemporary medicine from the perspective of science itself. Science is a tool, a perspective or paradigm that can be used to understand the world and ourselves. It is very good at working with objective, material data. It is also good at drawing out relationships that are not easy to see on the surface. For instance, not everyone who smokes gets cancer, but science allows us to meaningfully compare large numbers of individuals who do smoke to those who do not, in order to reveal a correlation between smoking and cancer. Science is not so good at explaining non-material aspects of human being like spirituality, love, creativity, meaning and purpose. Science is the study of 'things.' There are many aspects of human experience that are 'thing-like.' However, there are many other aspects of human experience that are not reducible to the status of things. Thus, science is poor at understanding subjectivity and individuality.

The Limitations of Science and Scientism

> If modes of thinking, categorizing, and acting, long thought to be 'scientific,' are found not to optimally address the unique complexities and uncertainties of human behavior, then we must take another look at our basic assumptions and seek new ways to conceptualize our data base.
> John Beahrs[2]

> Not everything that can be counted counts, and not everything that counts can be counted.
> William Bruce Cameron[3]

John Beahrs provides a critique of the dominant biomedical paradigm used in medicine and psychiatry in his book, *The Limits of Scientific Psychiatry: The Role of Uncertainty in Mental Health*. (Another book that deals with similar issues is Rupert Sheldrake's *The Science Delusion: Freeing the Spirit of Enquiry*.[4]) Beahrs does not oppose the use of science, but recognizes that, like all tools, science has uses and limitations. According to Beahrs, science is a tool with which we can attempt to know reality. However, it is only a tool and not reality itself. When this is forgotten, science becomes a dogmatic system that excludes important aspects of reality. This dogma states that we can know everything we need to know about human beings and the world through the reductionist materialism of the biomedical model. To distinguish the use of science as a tool and the dogmatic over-application of science as a belief system, Beahrs uses the word 'scientism.' He contrasts science and scientism as follows:

> *Science* basically means knowing. Only more recently has the word become indelibly associated with that particular method known as the controlled experiment and its correlate, statistical dominance, both of which contribute to greater

certitude that we give those beliefs we call scientific. To assume that these are the only valid sources of scientific data is to embrace a dogma I refer to as *scientism*, whose definition of reality is that which can be measured and tested. According to the scientific dogmatist, for practical purposes anything that cannot be measured and tested does not exist.[5]

Science is one way to examine the components of life, whereas scientism mistakes what is perceived through the lens of science as the only reality. Scientism mistakes a detail for the whole of reality. In other words, it focuses on only one dimension of reality perceived and interpreted through science. In scientism, the tools that are used to perceive reality, such as numbers, statistics, protocols and test results, eclipse awareness of the whole person. Beahrs discusses the trade-off between having a precise explanatory model and a model that can be generalized. 'It is not hard to see that the more we attempt to make a model adequate – both precise and reliable within a given area – the fewer number of cases it will adequately describe.'[6] Beahrs comes to the conclusion that we need more than one paradigm for understanding human reality to give the best medical care possible to individuals. He embraces what science is good at and then recommends a multidimensional model of understanding health and illness that includes science as well as other modes of understanding. He concludes that 'increasing scientific precision and respecting human uniqueness are two processes that must coexist and that cannot be fully reconciled to one another. On the one hand, each limits the other's scope, but on the other hand, ensures that it will be employed only where most appropriate.'[7] What Beahrs' work provides is a lesson in the philosophy of science that allows us to contextualize science as one modality, among many, for understanding human experiences of health and illness.

Perception, Knowledge and Error in Contemporary Medicine

Medical education today is focused on imparting to doctors the latest evidence-based treatments embedded in the current scientific understanding of disease. Doctors are not encouraged to think philosophically and the curriculum does not include the history of medicine and science. Doctors are not taught to understand the role of beliefs and expectations in shaping perception and decision-making. Nor are doctors taught to the findings of cognitive science that demonstrates the limitations of observation and knowledge. Beahrs' critique, above, examines the biomedical model from a philosophy of science perspective. This section examines errors in perception and knowledge in contemporary medicine that result from the way we perceive and organize data and conceptual systems.

How Doctors Think

Jerome Groopman, in his book *How Doctors Think*, provides a critique of evidence-based medicine and examines cognitive errors in medicine. Groopman cautions us about the loss of depth and subtlety that he fears are the consequence of the current medical education system's over-emphasis on clinical guidelines and algorithms. He states that clinical 'algorithms can be useful for run-of-the-mill diagnosis and treatment ... (b)ut they quickly fall apart when a doctor needs to think outside their boxes, when symptoms are vague, or multiple and confusing.'[8] He goes on to say that 'algorithms discourage physicians from thinking independently and creatively. Instead of expanding a doctor's thinking, they can constrain it.'[9]

Groopman examines the kinds of errors, mistakes and misunderstandings that can arise from a lack of fit between doctors' thinking and clinical reality, such as: attribution error, affective error, confirmation bias, commission bias, satisfaction of search error, vertical line failure, false positive/negative, availability errors and cognitive errors.[10] Space does not permit a detailed discussion of each of these, but the fact that there are so many different kinds of cognitive errors should caution us, as physicians, about being overly certain of our perceptions and clinical formulations.[11] No matter how good the science and how solid the clinical protocol, these are only as good as the reasoning of the human being perceiving the data. Groopman shows that the human brain is fallible and takes many shortcuts to simplify incoming data, thus making the data more manageable and understandable. The cost of this simplification is the loss of accuracy.

Research on cognitive and perceptual errors points to the impossibility of certainty in medical diagnosis. Both false positive and false negative errors are possible. The first is thinking that a patient has a certain diagnosis when they do not (a Type I error in statistics). The second is thinking a patient does not have a certain diagnosis when they do (a Type II error). In both situations, the patient is given the wrong treatment because the doctor has made an error in diagnosis. We risk making one of these errors *every* time we make a diagnosis.

Diagnostic certainty becomes even more complicated when you realize that 'new' illnesses arise periodically. For instance, doctors were puzzled in the 1980s when some patients' immune systems began to fail. Eventually, in 1983, this cause was determined to be the human immunodeficiency virus or HIV. Similarly, Lyme disease presented doctors with a puzzling set of symptoms that were eventually linked, in 1982, to an infection by spirochetes spread through deer tick bites. Another example is posttraumatic stress disorder, which did not exist as a diagnostic entity until 1980. Many Vietnam veterans were initially misdiagnosed with schizophrenia because of the hallucination-like flashbacks and nightmares they had upon returning from military service.

New Ideas Do Not Fit in Old Bottles
It is very common in the history of medicine to find the 'expert testimony' of 'thought leader' scientists who did not believe new

ideas and theories because they did not fit with the contemporary scientific understanding of the day. Consider Nobel laureate Max von Laue's threat about the newly discovered field of quantum mechanics: 'If that turns out to be true, I'll quit physics.'[12] Ignaz Semmelweis faced ridicule by his fellow physicians when he proposed that little particles, invisible to the naked eye, were responsible for obstetric infections and that washing hands when going from dissecting in the morgue to delivering babies could reduce infection rates.[13] In both cases, discomfort with a new paradigm led to automatic rejection because it did not fit the contemporary belief system. This again calls to mind Beahrs' discussion of scientism as a belief system, rather than using science as a tool to understand reality.

In *The Body Electric*, Robert Becker discusses his life's work measuring electrical and electromagnetic systems in living beings. His discovery of the role of electrical and electromagnetic fields in bone and wound healing clashed with contemporary understanding. In his book, he discusses the constant resistance (which he calls 'political science') that he and his lab faced in pursuing ideas that did not fit into the dominant explanatory paradigm, even though they had solid scientific evidence.[15] Becker cautions that 'scientific medicine abandoned the central rule of science – revisions in the light of new data.'[16]

Looking at the work of Groopman and Becker, we can see that good medicine requires respect for the limitations of the human mind and the explanatory models we construct in order to understand the world. Cognitive errors, faulty memory and adherence to belief systems obscure doctors' ability to correctly perceive and know reality. People crave certainty. Beliefs, whether they are 'scientific,' political, economic, or spiritual, provide a false sense that we know reality. A belief system, whether it appeals to science (as scientism) or to religion, can become a fixed, closed view of reality, where the belief distorts any new contradictory data or perception (this is also the definition of a 'delusional disorder' in psychiatry). It seems to be part of our human nature that we mistake contemporary understanding of the world as *the* final and correct understanding.

What Science Reveals about Human Relationships

David N. Elkins provides another perspective on the limits of the biomedical paradigm in *Humanistic Psychology: A Clinical Manifesto*. Humanistic psychology is a formal discipline based on the work of figures such as Abraham Maslow, Carl Rogers and Rollo May who valued concepts like 'unconditional positive regard,' 'self-actualization,' and 'patient-centered' therapy. Humanistic psychology takes personal growth, human values and human relationship as the goal of psychotherapy. Oriented more towards healing than treatment, it provides a conceptual model distinct from the biomedical model.

Elkins states that a scientific, biomedical model has been misapplied to psychotherapy, replacing the healing nature of human relationship with the illusion of scientific objectivity. He convincingly argues that most people enter psychotherapy, not because they are mentally ill, but because they are having difficulty in life and wish to grow and learn. Thus, Elkins believes that the true focus of psychotherapy is 'listening to a person who is demoralized, experiencing emotional pain, or having difficulties in life and giving that person support and guidance based on our experience and psychological knowledge.'[17]

Elkins provides scientific support for his position, but he also appeals to a humanistic paradigm. Both science and humanism support the notion that human relationship variables contribute to healing in psychotherapy. Psychotherapy efficacy studies, he says, have 'determined that "contextual factors" – not modalities or techniques – were the major determinants of therapeutic effectiveness!'[18] More specifically, Elkins states that contextual factors found in all therapeutic approaches 'include such elements as the alliance, the relationship, the qualities of the therapist, client agency, allegiance, client expectations, and extra-therapeutic factors ... personal and interpersonal elements are major determinants of therapeutic outcome while techniques have little to do with therapeutic effectiveness.'[19]

Elkins argues that the rise of 'empirically supported therapies' in psychology is not just about science because there is a plethora of scientific evidence supporting the healing effect of human relationship. He cites former president of the American Psychological Association, Ronald Levant, on some of the difficulties in how the debate has been framed. In 2004, Levant wrote:

> Empirically-validated treatment is a difficult topic for a practitioner to discuss with clinical scientists. In my attempts to discuss this informally, I have found that some clinical scientists immediately assume that I am anti-science, and others emit a guffaw, asking incredulously: 'What, are you for empirically *unsupported* treatments?' McFall (1991, p. 76) reflects this perspective when he divides the world of clinical psychology into 'scientific and pseudoscientific clinical psychology,' and rhetorically asks 'what is the alternative (to scientific clinical psychology)? *Unscientific* clinical psychology' ... There are, thus, some ardent clinical scientists ... who appear to subscribe to scientific faith and believe that the superiority of the scientific approach is so marked that other approaches should be excluded. Since this is a matter of faith rather than reason, arguments would seem to be pointless ... Punctuating these interactions from the practitioner perspective, the controversy seems to stem from the attempts of some clinical scientists to dominate the discourse on acceptable practice, and impose very narrow views of both science and practice.[20]

Levant's comments recall Beahrs' discussion of scientism, and pick up elements of Groopman's concern that we are training clinicians to think like robots. Levant also exposes the dangers of language and dualistic thinking. Defining paradigms that are not based on scientific reductionism in the negative, as 'unscientific,' frames the debate in a prejudicial manner. Elkins appeals to humanism as an alternate paradigm for understanding human growth and relationship. Rather than scientific and unscientific approaches to psychotherapy, it is possible to define different paradigms, such as a biomedical paradigm and a humanistic paradigm. Rather than thinking in dualistic, black and white terms, we can have different tools and different ways of understanding. The challenge would then be in determining when it is most appropriate to use a biomedical approach or a humanistic approach.

Elkins writes that 'credibility, skill, empathic understanding, and affirmation of the patient, along with the ability to engage with the patient, to focus on the patient's problems, and to direct the patient's attention to the patient's affective experience, were highly related to successful treatment.'[21] I argue that these same qualities are important for good therapeutic outcomes in medical settings as a context for biomedical intervention. Therapist/doctor attributes determine the quality of the doctor–patient relationship and influence the quality of the 'data' that can be obtained from the patient. When doctors possess the attributes identified by Elkins, it helps both the doctor and patient to weather difficult times in the relationship, such as when the patient is not improving or treatments are not working. In the case of managing chronic medical conditions that have multiple contributors (mind, body, emotion, diet, exercise, lifestyle considerations), these qualities in the therapist or doctor may make it more likely that patients will make changes in their lives that can have far-reaching medical and health consequences, such as starting an exercise program or stopping smoking.

What Elkins proposes is that we need another paradigm, in addition to the biomedical, in order to understand the transformative power of human relationships in psychotherapy. From research on the healing elements in the psychotherapy relationship, we can extrapolate to all therapeutic interactions in medicine. There is a wealth of research on human connection, social networks and health.[22] Humanistic psychology is one more field of scientific study that shows how human relationship can be healing.

Consciousness is the Ground of Being

Physicist Amit Goswami has written a book called *The Quantum Doctor*, in which he develops the concept of 'Integral Medicine,' which he describes as 'the truly holistic medicine.'[23] His aim is to use concepts and insights from quantum physics to develop a unified understanding of different models of healing, including both contemporary as well as alternative perspectives, such as Ayurvedic and Traditional Chinese Medicine. The essence of his critique of contemporary medical science is that it mistakes matter (e.g. the body) as primary. Instead, Goswami argues that quantum physics shows that it is consciousness that determines matter, including the body. (In quantum language, matter exists in a wave form of energy and is in a state of possibility; the inter-action of consciousness 'chooses' or collapses the energy wave into a particle.) This concept is consistent with the age-old teachings of many spiritual healing traditions as well as with more modern versions of energy healing.

Goswami has developed a five-dimensional model of human experience, consisting of the physical, the vital, the mental, the supramental and the bliss body. As with many models of holistic medicine, Goswami argues that human beings consist of different dimensions of being and experience which interact, but can also be examined individually. According to Goswami, contemporary medicine primarily focuses on the physical body, and is 'true' when applied at that level. However, he adds that it is inadequate for understanding all of health and illness because it neglects or denies contributions from other dimensions of human experience. In other words, contemporary medicine is not the only 'truth' when applied to what Goswami calls the vital, mental, supramental and bliss dimensions.

Goswami's critique of contemporary medicine is based on his understanding of the difference between classical and quantum physics. He describes contemporary medicine as 'machine medicine' which views people as objects or things: '*machine medicine*, designed for machines (that is the picture of the patient in the classical worldview) and by machines (the physicians who are self-avowed machines).'[24] The classical worldview shapes what is understood as a logical intervention, for instance, 'if the world is a machine, mind is a machine, and even the soul is machine, as some observers contend, then how can anything but machine medicine have any validity?'[25] In contrast to machine medicine, Goswami offers 'conscious medicine,' a view that includes the machine aspects, but goes beyond it to other human dimensions as well. 'A quantum doctor practices conscious medicine designed for people not machines. What conscious medicine prescribes includes the mechanical, but extends also to the domains of vitality and meaning, even love.'[26]

From a classical physics perspective, it is difficult to understand how spirituality or thought can affect the physical body and play a role in health and illness. The concept of *upward causation* characterizes the classical view of reality in which consciousness is viewed as a *product* of the molecules of the body and the brain. This is the view that underpins contemporary medicine. In this paradigm, it is difficult to see how consciousness can have an effect on health because consciousness is viewed as a product of the body, not something that contributes to the body's creation. In contrast, the concept of *downward causation* views consciousness as shaping the form that matter takes. This explains a mechanism by which more subtle dimensions can affect the physical.[27]

Downward causation and upward causation are two principles

that are both true; the body can influence consciousness, but consciousness can also influence the physical body. Goswami takes this observation of quantum physics even further. He states that the science of quantum physics provides support for the view that consciousness is the ground of being. In other words, the body is a manifestation of consciousness rather than consciousness being a manifestation of the body. This leads Goswami to ask the question: 'Are we to apply downward causation to a world that is separate from us so that we do not have to be responsible for our action, or is the world us, and we have to accept responsibility along with our freedom of choice?'[28] Goswami states that we can be viewed as having two different modes of self-identity:

> In the classical mode, we are localized and determined; we can call it the particle mode of identity. In the quantum mode, we are nonlocal and free; we can recognize it as the wave mode. So balancing the modes of movement of the vital body means balancing classical and quantum modes – the conditioned and creative modes, if you will – of self-identity.[29]

Goswami proposes the term *Integral Medicine* to include both the 'particle identity' of contemporary medicine and the 'wave mode' of identity associated with holistic and healing traditions, in which spirit and consciousness can transform the expression of matter (the human body). Thus, his Integral Medicine includes the concepts of both upward and downward causation.

Goswami critiques conceptual confusion in alternative as well as contemporary medicine, describing five philosophical shortcomings of alternative healing practices:

1. They fail to distinguish between mind and consciousness.
2. The causal role of consciousness as the origin of downward causation is either missed or is obscured in ambiguity.

3. The distinctive role of mind as opposed to the brain is missed.

4. The distinctive role of the vital body compared to the physical body is also missed.

5. Neither consciousness, nor the mind, nor the vital body is acknowledged to be non-physical.[30]

Essentially, these critiques can all be related to the question of whether matter or consciousness is primary. Classical physics describes the world as being made out of bits of matter that interact in chemical and molecular pathways. However, a quantum view deconstructs matter until it starts to become less and less material and more and more a matter of energy. Goswami's shift in perspective is supported by the work of quantum physicist Niels Bohr, who stated that, 'Everything we call real is made of things that cannot be regarded as real.'[31] Another quantum physicist, Werner Heisenberg, said in his Nobel Prize speech that the atom has 'no physical properties at all.'[32] Deepak Chopra points out that 'if the atom isn't physical neither is the universe, and neither is the human body.'[33] This is Goswami's argument, that the human body is not primarily physical, but rather is a manifestation of consciousness. This provides a radical critique of contemporary medicine's assumption that only physical matter is needed to understand all health and illness.

One of the complaints that contemporary medicine has about alternative healing models and holistic medicine is that there is a chaotic array of different conceptual models and non-physical explanations for why certain techniques are healing. For instance, what is the 'chi' of Traditional Chinese Medicine? How can 'like cure like' in homeopathy, while allopathy (contemporary medicine) uses 'opposites' to cure? *The Quantum Doctor* goes a long way down the road of integrating contemporary and alter-native medicine into a logical conceptual framework that grows out of quantum physics.

The most radical aspect of Goswami's book is the proposition that consciousness is the ground of being and matter is an expression or manifestation of consciousness. This is truly a revolutionary paradigm from the perspective of contemporary medicine which is firmly entrenched in materialism (the philosophical position that only matter has meaning) and it opens the way for idealism (the position that ideas shape reality). This shift challenges contemporary medicine's assumption that matter is all that matters. Dimensions beyond the physical are also important in health.

Perspectives from Religion, Poetry and Mysticism

Contemporary medicine grew out of earlier eras of medicine in which religious, spiritual, mystical, narrative, poetic and symbolic elements were included in health care. We have 'advanced' in the sense of editing out superstitions in medicine, but we have lost something in regard to intrinsic aspects of human beings – the need for a connection to a larger sense of meaning and purpose as well as a symbolic and poetic mode of being and representation. We will now review this need.

Religion, Spirituality and Medicine

Michael Cohen, a lawyer interested in legal issues in Complementary, Alternative and Integrative Medicine (CAIM), has written several books, including *Healing at the Borderland of Medicine and Religion*, which examines the overlap between traditional models of spiritual healing, contemporary medical treatment and CAIM approaches to health and illness. He describes a 'new health care' model that operates by 'negotiating different world views, epistemologies, hermeneutics, and metaphors for health and healing ... harmonizing where possible, integrating where appropriate, and synthesizing where beneficial.'[34] *Negotiation* is a good word to represent the active work of balancing different paradigms. Negotiating implies that there is a dialogue between different models, rather than a struggle to establish the dominance of one model. Cohen states that this dialogue requires 'medical pluralism' to negotiate the 'borderland between medicine and religion, between the scientific and the mystical, between knowledge that is considered objective and publicly accessible and knowledge that is considered subjective and privately accessible, and between outer and inner, material and spiritual, overt and covert, and quantifiable and perhaps immeasurable.'[35]

In offering medical pluralism as a solution for the differences between various explanatory models of health and illness, Cohen speaks of integrating different views in a 'negotiated synthesis.' He suggests a multidimensional approach:

> (in) psychological terms, the synthesis might involve being able to operate on two levels simultaneously, the intellectual and the emotional/spiritual; negotiating an agreement, for example, while also attending to spiritual insights and personal feelings arising in the negotiation process; or listening outwardly to the patient's medical history with an ear for medically significant details while listening internally – intuitively – for the most appropriate therapeutic action. In spiritual terms, such a synthesis might be conceptualized as maintaining an interior, contemplative focus even while engaging in exterior activities 'in the world.'[36]

The argument for medical pluralism is one of tolerance, but Cohen does offer a critique of aspects of contemporary medicine as well. Particularly in the sense of contemporary medicine's assumption that it alone possesses the truth of human health and illness, Cohen cautions that scientific inquiry 'has a shadow aspect that manifests as dominance, exploitation, subjugation and arrogant imposition of authority.'[37] This is particularly true when examining medical traditions from other cultures. Western-trained scientists often assume they have a monopoly on truth. Past explanatory models and traditions are considered quaint, misguided and influenced by primitive or false beliefs. One-sided belief is the same thing as dogma.[38]

Cohen's arguments about integrating and synthesizing different approaches to health and healing echo those of Beahrs. They are also similar to the work of Larry Dossey who is a champion of bringing the spiritual dimension back into medicine. Dossey has written that, 'I used to believe that we must choose between science and reason on the one hand and spirituality on the other, as foundations for living our lives. Now I consider this a false choice, because in my own life I have found that science and spirituality can co-exist and even flourish.'[39] The challenge is not in choosing between paradigms, but rather how to integrate different paradigms to best address all human dimensions of health and illness.

Mysticism, Medicine and the Perception of Reality

(A) high understanding it is, inwardly to see and know that God, which is our maker, dwelleth in our soul; and an higher understanding it is inwardly to see and to know that our soul, that is made, dwelleth in God's substance: of which substance God, we are that we are.
Dame Julian of Norwich[40]

Mysticism is a holistic experience that transcends the ego to allow an experience of more dimensions than those of body, emotion and mind. Those who have mystical experiences often report a different perspective on life and may experience a unification of mind, body and spirit. The experience of these ineffable states has long been associated with physical, emotional and spiritual healing.

Mysticism can be defined as the approach to the divine or ultimate reality through direct experience, in contrast to experience mediated through the institutions of organized religion. Many different experiential practices grow out of mystical traditions, such as meditation, various mind–body practices, dietary practices, fasting, dancing, chanting and the induction of trance states. These practices have developed for the pursuit of self-knowledge and through self-knowledge, to commune with God, Spirit, or Nature. The experiential knowledge gained through these practices has a common theme – the mental dimension is limited in its ability to grasp reality. In this sense, mysticism points to the limitations of intellectual and logical theories of health and illness, such as the positivist approaches of the biomedical and economic rationalist models.

There is an inherent difficulty in teaching or writing about mysticism due to its transcendent quality that unifies reality rather than separating it into categories. This is what has famously led teachers of Zen Buddhism to reply to questions with all sorts of strange actions, like holding up one finger, putting their shoes on their head and walking out of the room, or replying with the question, 'What is the sound of one hand clapping?' Through these spontaneous and sometimes unusual responses, the teacher hopes to jolt the student out of their preconceived notions and mental categories.

Mysticism is common to most, if not all, religions, cultures and traditions. It points the way, no matter how indirect the pointing seems, to an experience of a larger reality than the everyday reality of the mind and ego. One mystical tradition is Taoism, which grew out of ancient Chinese culture. The yin/yang symbol expresses the essence of Taoism: the interrelatedness of light/dark, masculine/feminine and active/passive. Taoism is based on cultivating harmony between these pairs of opposites. The word 'Tao' is often translated as 'the way,' and it represents concepts such as: *path, universal life energy,* or *truth.* When one is in harmony with the Tao, health and balance is obtained. However, the definition of the Tao is open-ended; it can be alluded to, maybe even pointed at, but it can never be definitively defined.

Around 500 BCE, the Taoist sage Lao Tzu said that:

> The way that can be spoken of
> Is not the constant way;
> The name that can be named
> Is not the constant name.
> (Lao Tzu)[41]

Here Lao Tzu expresses at a metaphysical level the realization that a word is not the thing itself; it can only point to a concept. There is the symbol (the word) and what is represented by that symbol. That which is symbolized is greater than the word itself.

If there is a dimension of human experience that can be perceived, but not explained or put into words, this calls into question our ability to grasp the true nature of reality and to set up protocols and guidelines for dealing with reality. This gets into the whole field of epistemology, or the study of how we know what we know. Consider this fourth-century BCE quote by another Taoist sage, Chuang Tzu, about the difficulty of knowing what is 'right' and what is 'wrong.'

> Suppose you and I had an argument. If you have beaten me instead of my beating you, then are you necessarily right and am I necessarily wrong? Are both of us right or are both of us wrong? If you and I do not know the answer, then other people are bound to be even more in the dark. Whom shall we get to decide what is right? Shall we get someone who agrees with you to decide? But if he already agrees with you, how can he decide fairly? Shall we get someone who agrees with me? But if he already agrees with me, how can he decide?

Shall we get someone who disagrees with both of us? But if he already disagrees with both of us, how can he decide? Shall we get someone who agrees with both of us? But if he already agrees with both of us, how can he decide? Obviously, then, neither you nor I nor anyone else can know the answer.[42]

The difficulty of knowing what is 'right' and 'wrong' can be taken a step further beyond an argument to the perception of reality itself. Chuang Tzu does just this in his famous butterfly story:

Once Chuang Chou dreamt he was a butterfly, a butterfly flitting and fluttering around, happy with himself and doing as he pleased. He did not know he was Chuang Chou. Suddenly he woke up and there he was, solid and unmistakable Chuang Chou. But he did not know if he was Chuang Chou who had dreamt he was a butterfly, or a butterfly dreaming he was Chuang Chou. Between Chuang Chou and a butterfly there must be *some* distinction! This is called the Transformation of Things.[43]

Practitioners with a belief system of scientism forget that science is an approximation of reality, not reality itself. As can be readily appreciated by anyone who studies the history of and philosophy of science and medicine, intellectual concepts often influence which aspects of science and reality are accepted and which are rejected because they do not fit into the dominant explanatory paradigm. Any explanatory model has strengths and limitations (just as any tool has certain uses) and science is just one explanatory model, one way of approaching and defining the world. A mystical approach would caution that a scientific approach can never 'name' true reality. In other words, there are important and influential dimensions of human reality that cannot be reduced to words, let alone numbers or statistics.

Poetry and Medicine

Poetry shares similarities with mysticism in that it can evoke subtle dimensions of human experience that resist reductive quantification. It does so through a metaphorical and symbolic use of language, in contrast to the analytical language used by science. Poetry provides an alternative to the biomedical paradigm through integrating, rather than separating the body, emotions, thoughts and spirituality. This is a different perspective at attaining universal truth through integrative unity rather than reductive separation. Science abstracts from the individual and looks at the individual as one of many objects. Poetry goes deeper into the individual experience until universal aspects arise.

In Elkins' book, discussed above, he states: 'I believe that the personal, if plumbed deeply enough, has a strange way of touching the universal.'[44] Elkins tells his personal journey as a psychotherapist and also cites a number of poets, artists and psychotherapists. He ends one chapter with a poem called 'Healing,' by D.H. Lawrence:

I am not a mechanism, an
assembly of various sections
And it is not because the mechanism
is working wrongly that I am ill
I am ill because of wounds to the soul
to the deep emotional self
And the wounds to the soul
take a long, long time
Only time can help
and patience
And a certain difficult repentance,
Long, difficult repentance,
Realization of life's mistake,
And the freeing oneself of the mistake

Which mankind at large has
chosen to sanctify.
(D.H. Lawrence)[45]

Lawrence's poem stands as a critique of the common medical practice of looking for a broken mechanism to explain illness and suffering, a practice that could be called medicalization of the soul. Lawrence speaks back to this medicalization and insists that he has wounds of the soul that are a deeper cause of his physical illness. He is optimistic that these wounds can heal, not with applications of medication or the fixing of broken mechanisms, but through time, patience and work. To alleviate suffering by fixing what is broken is a noble task, but what is happening in contemporary medicine is that a biomedical fix is being habitually and reflexively offered for what used to be considered facts of life: shyness, restless legs, upset stomach, natural ageing, menopause, etc. This is the 'machine medicine' that Goswami spoke of, in which human beings are viewed as nothing but malfunctioning mechanisms that can be engineered and reprogrammed.

What Lawrence chooses is to look inward and attend to his wounds with attention rather than with a quick-fix intervention to end the suffering. Poetry is not about making things better, but observing what is. It trusts the reality of the subtle things in life, such as emotions, spirit and heart – the intangibles that get such short shrift in contemporary medicine, but which have limitless depths of meaning. In essence, acceptance can lead to transcendence.

Poetry serves a healing function as it addresses the whole of a person. Attention, observation and acceptance activate something deep within the person with poetry serving as the bridge between the external world and internal states. Poetry embraces those 'things' that are difficult to define yet are of utmost importance. The act of poetry begins with observation, but can end in transformation. Edmund Pellegrino writes that poetry 'nourishes the poet's soul and emboldens the poet to break the bonds of ordinary logic and language to fathom a little more of the mystery of human healing.'[46] Contrast this with contemporary medicine's war against disease which leads to the reduction of the human into an organic machine. Thus the goal of contemporary medicine is to 'normalize' anything that stands out. The goal of poetry is to attend to and honor that which stands out.

Some medical schools offer electives in 'Poetry and Medicine'. These courses expose students to the poetry about medicine and healing and also offer opportunities for the students to write their own poetry. There is something surprising that arises when one is writing from the depths of one's own self rather than from the technical mind of the trained physician. Things come together in a different way through the logic of emotion and the conflict of existential issues. Learning and growth can occur in a way that is not linear and not technical. Poetic self-expression reflects an experience of suffering, joy, humanity and even death that does not find its way into the medical chart or progress note. Without the opportunity to learn and process the difficult material that arises during medical training in a different way, dimensions of the student's humanity become obscured and diminished.

Johanna Shapiro has written a book specifically about medical student poetry: *The Inner World of Medical Students: Listening to Their Voices in Poetry*. She describes a number of different narratives of medical student poems and the functions that they can serve: chaos stories (crying for help), restitution stories (self-reassurance), journey stories (self-discovery and identity formation), witnessing stories (examining suffering) and transcendence stories (healing).[47] One of Shapiro's concerns is how the acculturation process in medical education affects the humanity of the student. She writes that students may 'internalize the message that actual parts of who they are – perhaps their sensitivity or their tender-heartedness – no longer have a place in their professional persona.'[48] Shapiro notes the restriction and distortion that medical education can have in regard to the whole person of the patient and the student. She sees a parallel process occurring in which the essential humanity of both the student and patient are molded to fit into a biomedical paradigm focused on the most superficial of human realities: observable symptoms and observable behaviors. She observes that medical training 'attempts to order the world by relying on knowledge that can be obtained by reductionism, objectivity and essentialism, as well as logical, rational thinking, and relationships that can be controlled by hierarchy, authority, and power. This leads to models of understanding and relationships that are excessively formulaic, rule-bound, and lacking in human connection.'[49]

I wrote poetry prior to medical school, but I had never published anything until I took a two-week 'Literature and Medicine' class that Dan Brauner and Suzanne Poirier developed at the University of Illinois at Chicago. The university published medical student writing in a journal called *Body Electric*. Having two of my poems published in this journal was formal recognition for my own efforts toward creating a counter-curriculum of re-humanization. My poem, 'I stare out,' has been republished in a number of places, including the journal *Hippocrates*, an academic article by Poirier, Ahrens and Brauner, and even in Johanna Shapiro's book *The Inner World of Medical Students*. This poem that I wrote as a medical student is a good example of the counter-curriculum. While it kind of popped out of me without much thought, it echoes throughout my career as a kind of counter-point to my clinical work. The poem's theme of disconnection and numbness apparently struck a chord for many people. It is available at:

http://davidkopacz.com/poetry-i-stare-out.php

An unpublished poem of my own, written during the depths of my internship year, illustrates the dehumanization that can take hold in the service of contemporary medical education. During this year, I was stressed, overwhelmed, sleep deprived, filled with self-doubt and was having stress-related physical symptoms. I felt myself losing touch with that part of myself that could feel and reflect on my experiences. Another way to say this is that I had developed the ability to observe myself objectively while not being in touch with my own subjective feeling. The background for the poem is that I was on vacation at my parents' house over Christmas break. I remember looking out the window, eating cereal in the morning, when I noticed tears flowing down my face without any subjective experience of emotion. This was even more disturbing because I had observed this same phenomenon in a Vietnam veteran I had interviewed in the ER. Without emotion, he had recounted a series of extreme losses and misfortunes in his life. I was struck by the disconnection this man had between his emotions and his words (and I wrote about that in another poem). I recognized this disconnection as disturbing and 'not normal' and then I observed this same disconnection in myself. If it had not been for the tears, I would not have noticed that there was any disconnection in myself, just numbness and a need to push harder and work more and then to try to recover on my 'break,' so that I could go back to the hospital and work some more.

Numbness and emotional disconnection is a dangerous state that occurs all too often in the medical education process. The medical acculturation process often teaches students to push emotions 'underground,' and to function as an objective scientific observer and heartless technician. My hope in including a personal poem is that it touches something universal in the medical education process and practice of medicine.

it is internship year
I cannot write any poetry.
I had a dream,
I wrote some poetry
at the bottom
of a progress note
and painted light grey around it
I had to tear it off
you cannot write poetry
In a patient's chart.

I had a dream
a patient
was trying to kill me
I beat his head against the ground
I ran away
I woke up
I had a nervous tic
in my left eye
for one week
even when I did not drink too much coffee.

I cannot write poetry this year
maybe if I could write
I wouldn't have gotten that tic
I wouldn't have had those dreams.
(David Kopacz, 1993)

As my poem from internship year shows, when medical education limits how doctors connect with the patient's human experience, it correspondingly limits the student's own human experience. Excessive objectification and reductionism is inculcated into the doctors of tomorrow through the medical education process today. The students' human experience becomes medicalized.

Shapiro speaks of 'preformulation' in medical thinking, a kind of conditioned response in which experience and human reality is objectified 'into predetermined categories and interpretations,'[50] for instance listening for diagnoses rather than listening to a person. The student learns to interact only through diagnoses, categories, and flow charts, and loses the more complex aspects of human interaction. Shapiro writes that experience 'becomes formulaic and loses its dynamism and organicity ... the *person* of both patient and student – is all too easily lost.'[51] Shapiro's critique of the medical student acculturation process dovetails with those of other authors who have been considered in this chapter. There is a common thread which cautions against the unopposed use of contemporary biomedicine. These perspectives also illustrate other essential dimensions of human being that cannot be understood through reductionist biomedical views of humanity.

Socio-Cultural Perspectives

Culture shapes our experience of our self, our relationships with others and how we view the world. Culture even influences how we think, how we conceptualize problems and what kinds of solutions seem relevant. In his book, *The Integrated Self*, Louis Kavar states that 'culture is fundamentally a way of thinking about and organizing life and all that it contains. An individual's way of thinking, which is manifested in speech and behavior, is rooted in the individual's culture.'[52]

Language, too, is a part of culture and influences our view of the world and how we conceptualize and solve problems, and we will now examine medicine from linguistic and cultural perspectives.

The Philosophy of Language and Power

The dream of reason did not take power into account.
Paul Starr[53]

Language is something we use every day but rarely consider how it shapes us as human beings. French philosopher Michel Foucault explored the alienating language and terminology which shaped the development of various professions, including mental health and medicine. Similarly, Austrian Catholic priest and cultural critic Ivan Illich has written about language and power in his critique of contemporary medicine. Taken together, Foucault's and Illich's work challenges physicians to be aware that, as a result of their acculturation to the medical profession, they may become blind to how medical language objectifies and disempowers people.

Foucault was concerned with the way that the development of jargon and professional language replaces the internal experience of human beings. He wrote that the doctor's 'gaze that sees is a gaze that dominates.'[54] This *dominating gaze* transforms the object of the gaze (the patient) into what Foucault calls a 'docile body (which) may be ... used, transformed, and improved.'[55] Foucault's critique of the medical and mental health professions can be summarized as: the creation of language by a class of experts leads to the alienation of an individual from their own thoughts, experience and body. Rather than being experts on their own internal experience, patients look to professionals to interpret and explain to them what is happening in their bodies. A person then loses subjectivity, as the subject of the patient becomes the object of the professional. The patient becomes a 'docile body' that is interpreted, manipulated and improved by the trained professional. Within this framework, power, as well as responsibility for health, shifts from the individual to the professional.

Ivan Illich has made similar investigations to Foucault into the role that language and professional class play in the creation of societal attitudes toward health and illness. Illich was concerned with what he calls the 'medicalization of life,'[56] in which subjective experience comes under the authority of a professional class of experts who interpret bodily experience through the lens of the medical model. Illich argues that this process alienates people from themselves. He takes a strong, critical stance toward contemporary medicine of the 1970s. He states that the medical system actually results in 'the paralysis of healthy responses to suffering, impairment, and death. It occurs when people accept health management designed on the engineering model, when they conspire in an attempt to produce, as if it were a commodity, something called "better health." This inevitably results in the managed maintenance of life.'[57] Illich warns that human beings become alienated from themselves when 'the language in which people could experience their bodies is turned into bureaucratic gobbledegook; or when suffering, mourning, and healing outside the patient role are labeled a form of deviance.'[58]

Like Foucault, Illich sees contemporary medicine concentrating power in the hands of professionals, with subsequent disempowerment of patients. It would be interesting to ask Foucault and Illich whether they thought that physicians are conscious of the 'nefarious' consequences of their actions in disempowering humanity through medical language. My feeling is that they would say the majority of physicians operate in a system that they do not understand. Indeed, some physicians may also be victims of a system in which they are encouraged to usurp others' power and authority (reminiscent of the *dehumanizing the dehumanizer* concept). I imagine that Foucault and Illich would make a distinction between the motive of helping others and the consequences of those motives. As history shows, people do not always understand the consequences of their actions; I am sure that many missionaries thought they were 'helping' others as they contributed to disempowerment and the destruction of traditional ways of life.

While a physician reading Foucault and Illich may become defensive and feel that these writers' view of reality is limited by their own philosophical belief systems (post-Marxist, post-structuralist deconstructions of the evils of industrial society's alienation of its workers), their arguments do provide another dimension of awareness for the practicing physician. A wise doctor will be aware of issues of language and power as they go about their daily practice of medicine. Illich states that 'medical bureaucracy creates ill-health by increasing stress, by multiplying disabling dependence, by generating new painful needs, by lowering levels of tolerance for discomfort or pain, by reducing the leeway that people are wont to concede to an individual when he suffers, and by abolishing even the right to self-care.'[59]

Illich's critique states that the 'medical and paramedical monopoly over hygienic methodology and technology is a glaring example of the political misuse of scientific achievement to strengthen industrial rather than personal growth.'[60] This critique is important in regard to rehumanizing medicine as a similar question arises as to whether contemporary medicine supports the personal growth of human beings or whether this goal has been subsumed by the operational needs of the health care delivery system and the profit motives of corporations.

Illich thinks that the negative effects of the medical system can only be reversed by individual change, not system change. He wrote, 'I believe that the reversal ... can come only from within man and not from yet another managed (heteronomous) source depending once again on presumptuous expertise and subsequent mystification.'[61] Illich argues that people will not become empowered by substituting a more politically correct language or establishing a watchdog agency. Instead, the empowerment has to come 'from within' the person themselves; this holds true for both doctors and patients. The reversal of dehumanization cannot be legislated, mandated or managed.

Reading Foucault and Illich challenges us to expand our assumptions about language, power and professionalism. Some have recognized the power differential in the language of contemporary medicine and have tried to remedy it by creating a new language without elements of a power hierarchy. In one example, patients become 'service-users' (SUs) and doctors become 'service-providers' (SPs). These changes stem from the influence of economic models of medicine as well as from consumer movements. We have to be careful with language, though. The desire to have a neutral and interchangeable terminology may lead to more neutral and interchangeable relationships, which may actually further erode the humanitarian and professional aspects of the doctor–patient relationship. Changing language without changing attitudes just makes people trickier, helping to conceal issues that actually require open scrutiny. The truth of the doctor–patient relationship is one of power imbalance, rather than a power-neutral exchange of goods or a reasoned purchase of services. Personally, I think these elements of professionalism and humanitarianism should be strengthened in medicine rather than diluted by changing terminology to a more generic, marketplace language. Rather than physicians having a technician role or entering into a relationship based solely on an exchange of services, they should embrace their role as professionals who have sworn to hold themselves accountable to a higher mode of ethics than that of the marketplace. This can still be consistent with a more collaborative style of medical decision-making. Perhaps the problem is not inherent in the power hierarchy, per se, but in physicians' abdication of their *foundational* professional values and ethics.

Cultural Perspectives on Human Experience

Authors Ethan Watters and Rebecca Solnit warn about the risk of biomedical explanations for human problems. Watters speaks of the dangers of exporting Western[62] views of mental health to other countries around the world. Whether it is the 'misguided' altruism of trauma therapists flocking to disasters or pharmaceutical companies trying to open up new markets and create demand for their products, he cautions that one culture's explanation of health is being imposed on another culture. Solnit argues against pathologizing human responses to trauma and points out that resilience and compassion often arise in individuals and communities after disaster strikes. Both authors present views of human nature and culture that are complex and nuanced in comparison to reductive biological explanations of human experience. This challenges contemporary medicine's view that it is a value-neutral observation of reality. Watters and Solnit argue that contemporary medicine is an explanatory system that grows out of a particular culture and that it shares and propagates the assumptions of that culture.

Ethan Watters, in his book, *Crazy Like Us: The Globalization of the American Psyche*, takes a critical look at the spread of American psychiatric concepts, terminology and diagnosis. In his view, this is less like the spread of scientific enlightenment, and more like a colonization process in which one culture imposes its views on other cultures. He warns that, if the only explanation of human behavior is a reductionist biomedical explanation, there is a risk of 'flattening the landscape of the human psyche itself.'[63] Watters does not just complain about the spread of American culture, but also provides a critique of some of the basic assumptions of science and the motivations of global companies.

He has two criticisms of American psychiatry: first, that through applying American psychiatric constructs, principles and approaches, one culture is imposing its beliefs on another culture (regardless of whether that view is scientifically 'true'), and second, that the science of American psychiatry really is not, in fact, more 'true' than other explanations of suffering, health, and illness. As he states, 'how a people in a culture think about mental illness – how they categorize and prioritize the symptoms, attempt to heal them, and set expectations for their course and outcome – influence(s) the diseases themselves.'[64] Watters quotes Harvard medical anthropologist Arthur Kleinman as saying that most 'disasters in the world happen outside of the

West ... Yet we come in and we pathologize their reactions. We say: "You do not know how to live with this situation." We take their cultural narratives away from them and impose ours. It is a terrible example of dehumanizing people.'[65]

In some ways, this process is similar to the imposition of a belief system, such as Christianity, on other cultures, except that the motivations are industry profit and scientific arrogance, rather than saving souls. When Christian missionaries sought to convert 'heathens', the motivation was based on one group of people feeling they had a better and truer view of reality than another. This is the classic 'end justifies the means' argument. The history of American and European cultures' interactions with indigenous cultures reveals many abuses and atrocities.[66] Is the export of American concepts and treatment of mental illness just another chapter of arrogant colonialism? A broader concern is to question the strain of scientism that is fashionable at the moment. Do evidence-based scientists possess the truth and have the right to impose their views of what is and is not a valid approach to health and illness?

As a way of understanding how American psychiatric models of posttraumatic stress disorder (PTSD) are exported today, let us look at one of Watters' chapters in more depth: 'The Wave That Brought PTSD to Sri Lanka.' While Watters recognizes the presumed good intentions of those who went to Sri Lanka to help after the 2004 tsunami, he questions the consequences. 'Although undertaken as humanitarian outreach, these efforts often look more like massive attempts at indoctrination. To accept the ideas of PTSD, other cultures first had to be "educated" in the appropriate symptoms of PTSD and modern modes of healing.'[67] He goes on to write that

these campaigns seemed to imply that the psychological consequences of trauma were similar to a newly discovered disease, and that local populations were utterly unaware of what happens to the human mind after terrible events. That implicit assumption often left anthropologists shaking their heads in disbelief. It takes a willful blindness to believe that other cultures lack a meaningful framework for understanding the human response to trauma.[68]

Watters examines cultural differences in understanding the source of traumatic disruption as either internal anxiety or external social disruption. It is worth considering how different cultures vary in regard to individualism and collectivism. This concept proposes that people vary in the extent that they view the self in terms of the individual or in terms of the social collective. American culture views the self as an isolated, separate individual who exists independently of the social context. The American and Western view that PTSD is an internal anxiety state may not make sense for a more collectivist culture in which the self is defined in terms of the group, and social relations and physical actions are given more value than individuals' internal psychological states.[69]

Watters also explores the possibility that PTSD may be a culture-bound syndrome, rather than a universal 'disease' or 'disorder.' For instance, PTSD may be more a product of American and Western cultural explanations of the role of suffering rather than a universal human reaction to suffering. Watters references Patrick Bracken's view that PTSD could be a symptom of a 'troubled postmodern world,' because in 'most Western societies there has been a move away from religious and other belief systems which offered individuals stable pathways through life, and meaningful frameworks with which to encounter suffering and death ... The meaningful connections of the social world are rendered fragile.'[70] Could it be that social disconnection is traumatic and this puts people in Western culture at higher risk of developing PTSD after a disaster or trauma?

Watters writes that without 'social mechanisms to cope, we

have become increasingly vulnerable and fearful. Indeed many have pointed out that we are now a culture that has a suspicion of resilience and emotional reserve.'[71] Rebecca Solnit picks up some of Watters' themes in her book exploring the positive aspects of human nature that are sparked by disaster, *A Paradise Built in Hell: The Extraordinary Communities That Arise in Disaster*. She argues that 'the prevalent human nature in disaster is resilient, resourceful, generous, empathic, and brave,' whereas the language of therapy 'speaks almost exclusively of the consequence of disaster as trauma, suggesting that humanity is unbearably fragile, a self that does not act but is acted upon, the most basic recipe of the victim.'[72]

Solnit challenges the underlying assumptions of assigning medical and psychiatric concepts to external events. It matters what the individual thinks about themselves: whether they are internally resourceful or vulnerable to external forces. If the individual is passive, dependent and susceptible to vulnerability without outside intervention, he or she can begin to feel incapable of maintaining basic human physiological and psychological functions. This view suggests that it may be American culture's untenable belief that suffering can be avoided (whether treated pharmacologically, solved through the court system, or negated through consumerism) and that this avoidance actually amplifies the posttraumatic response. As Solnit writes:

Contemporary language speaks of the effects of disaster entirely as trauma, or even more frequently as post-traumatic stress disorder, PTSD. The twin implications are that we are not supposed to suffer and that in our frailty we are not merely damaged, but *only* damaged by suffering. If suffering is a given, as it is for most religions, then the question is more what you make of it rather than how you are buffered from it altogether. The awareness of mortality that heightens a sense of life as an uncertain gift rather than a burdensome given also recalls religious teachings, and it is often shared by survivors of individual traumas.[73]

Watters and Solnit argue that our cultural beliefs about human nature and life events can create a sense of victimization or transformation. Culture shapes experience. Focusing on what we have lost creates victimization, while focusing on the opportunity for change creates resilience and personal growth. This distinguishes healing from contemporary medical treatment. It also distinguishes indigenous perspectives on health and illness from Western views.

Watters' and Solnit's concerns echo the philosophical and linguistic concerns of Foucault and Illich, that an educated, professional elite class will become an intervening and mediating force between individuals and their own experiences; and between a culture and its ability to define health and illness. The argument that scientists are replacing 'superstitious' and 'false' medicine with modern and 'true' medicine has to consider that science emerges from a culturally based belief system. It is sometimes easy to forget that *newer* is not always *better*. Watters notes that long-term outcomes for people with schizophrenia are better in non-industrialized countries than in the modern, contemporary psychiatric hospitals with the newest and most expensive psychiatric medications. (One possible explanation for this is that strong social networks may be more therapeutic for people with schizophrenia than the latest psychopharmacology.) Effective cross-cultural work requires open-mindedness, the willingness to be 'wrong,' and a pluralistic stance in which there are multiple ways of approaching truth. Effective medicine requires a similar approach.

A Maori[74] Perspective on Health and Illness

Mason Durie is a Maori psychiatrist from New Zealand who critiques Western biomedicine from the perspective of an indigenous culture. His framework is consistent with what Arbuckle calls the *traditional model* of health and illness. As someone trained in the scientific method and psychiatry who understands Maori spiritual and cultural beliefs from personal experience, Durie is uniquely situated to understand the benefits and limitations of a science-based medical system as it interacts with the indigenous Maori culture of New Zealand. Like Watters and Solnit, Durie recognizes that contemporary Western biomedicine contains cultural assumptions that do not make sense from the perspective of other cultures. He details a holistic model of health and illness, called *whare tapa wha*, which integrates the physical with emotional/mental, social and spiritual dimensions.

Durie's critique of contemporary medicine is that it overemphasizes certain dimensions of human experience and ignores dimensions that are extremely important to Maori people. For instance, a *biomedical model* does not understand the Maori view that good health cannot 'be gained by simple measures such as weight, blood pressure, or visual acuity.'[75] Durie explains that even though they are difficult to measure, spiritual and emotional factors are equally important. For Maori people, the biomedical view of health and illness just does not seem to make sense. Durie writes that, from a Maori perspective, contemporary medicine's 'interest in physical disease greatly outweighed an interest in the person as a whole within a sociological and ecological environment ... (and a) ... cellular focus no longer (seems) adequate for understanding the complexities of health.'[76]

The consequence of having a national medical system in New Zealand that does not make sense to a large segment of the population (Maori make up approximately 15% of New Zealanders)[77] is that Maori may be even less likely to seek out medical care, contributing to health disparities between Maori and other New Zealanders. If a system does not make sense or meet one's needs, there is little reason to engage in that system.

Like many Westerners, Maori may feel that contemporary medicine fails to adequately address their health needs. What is missing for Maori people is a focus on other aspects of human experience in addition to the biomedical science perspective. According to Durie,

> Maori thinking can be described as holistic. Understanding occurs less by division into smaller and smaller parts, the analytical approach, than by synthesis into wider contextual systems so that any recognition of similarities is based on comparisons at a higher level of organization ... Healthy thinking from a Maori perspective is integrative not analytical, explanations are sought from searching outwards rather than inwards, and poor health is typically regarded as a manifestation of breakdown in harmony between the individual and the wider environment.[78]

Maori belief, like that of many indigenous cultures, is collectivist in orientation; identity is found in relation to others and is intimately connected to the physical environment. This is difficult to fully appreciate for someone from an individualistic culture, in which identity is defined through the individual and is therefore portable. The loss of land and relation to specific spiritual places in the environment, for collectivist Maori people, seems equivalent to an 'identity crisis' for someone from an individualistic culture.

Durie does not argue for an abandonment of science, but rather an expansion of contemporary medicine to include emotional, spiritual and relational dimensions. He writes that, in order to acknowledge Maori perspectives on health and illness, there needs to be included

> another less readily defined dimension which takes into account spiritual values, not necessarily unique to Maori, but

more readily acknowledged by Maori as an essential part of human experience. In this regard Maori are more likely to link good or bad health with interpersonal and inter-generational concerns rather than with autoimmune systems or the impact of a raised blood pressure on renal functioning. Both perspectives may of course be equally valid.[79]

This is an important point – a holistic view is not in competition with contemporary biomedicine. A holistic view integrates many different explanations and experiences as contributing to health. Even where it is not possible to integrate certain perspectives, we can still move back and forth between different explanatory models and languages. In this regard, to have a holistic perspective is a little bit like being multilingual. An example that I heard in a workshop on Maori culture emphasized that, when encouraging a lifestyle change, appealing to a Maori grandmother's sense of individuality is likely to fail. If a physician were to say, 'If you exercise more and change your diet, your blood sugar will improve, you will lose weight, and you will be healthier and feel better,' this argument would not be effective. But saying, 'If you exercise more and change your diet, you will be able to live longer so that you can take care of your grandchildren better,' would have a much greater chance of making sense to her.

Mason Durie provides an understanding how Maori people conceptualize health in the model of *whare tapa wha* (or 'four-sided house'). It includes the physical dimension, which is such a large part of contemporary medicine, but it also includes spiritual, mental (which includes emotions) and social network dimensions to health. The spiritual dimension of health, *taha wairua*, is the 'capacity for faith and wider communion,' in which 'health is related to unseen and unspoken energies.' The mental dimension, *taha hinengaro*, is the 'capacity to communicate, to think, and to feel,' with mind and body being inseparable. The physical dimension, *taha tinana*, is the 'capacity for physical growth and development.' The dimension of the extended family and social connections, *taha whanau*, is the 'capacity to belong, to care and to share,' in which 'individuals are part of the wider social systems.'[80]

Whare tapa wha is a truly holistic model: it is not hierarchical, as each of the four dimensions is additive, and the whole is greater than the sum of its parts. It is somewhat similar to the biopsychosocial-spiritual model used in medical education. However, in practice, this model is not applied with equal weighting of each dimension; the biological is still predominant and the psychosocial-spiritual is tacked on at the end, if it is considered at all. The *whare tapa wha* model is equally balanced between dimensions.

A Maori view of health and illness values principles of interconnectedness and interrelatedness, and what Durie has called an 'integrative not analytical' perspective.[81] It serves as an example of an indigenous holistic, *traditional* model of health and psychology. In examining this view, there is also an inherent critique of the dominant, contemporary medical perspective. While Western science and culture tend to be dismissive of indigenous medicine as naive, simplistic, even primitive, it could be argued that Maori views of health and humanity are complex, nuanced and multidimensional. Perhaps it is our own view of biological reductionism that, while technologically complicated, is actually primitive and simplistic in the way it treats human beings.

Conclusion

Human experience is complex and nuanced. The ability to take on multiple perspectives, what Cohen calls *medical pluralism*, is a fundamental necessity for understanding human experience. Integrating these different perspectives is definitely a challenge that takes, time, energy and commitment.

The remainder of this book proposes a holistic framework

incorporating the views of contemporary biomedicine along with the dimensions of spirituality and culture discussed in this chapter. Its purpose is to create a medical practice that is not dehumanizing, into which doctors and patients can bring the whole of themselves.

Part II

HOLISTIC MEDICINE:
A FRAMEWORK FOR THE WHOLE
HUMAN BEING

Overview

Contemporary medicine faces a dilemma and is at a decision point. Proponents of the *biomedical model* recommend that medicine becomes more standardized and protocol-driven by only using evidence-based practices. Proponents of the *economic rationalist model* recommend that medicine becomes more cost-effective and more efficient (this is also part of the argument in health care reform and the Quality Revolution). Those from indigenous cultures, and even a great many Westerners who favor alternative and complementary medical techniques, recommend going back to the *traditional model*'s pre-biomedical and pre-economic models of health care. Many within medicine argue for a return to the *foundational model*'s values of compassion, social service and the view of health care as a right, not a commodity (this forms much of the basis for the Compassion Revolution in medicine). The confusing and passionate debate about the future of medicine stems from these different competing models of medicine that are sometimes contradictory. How can we choose between a healing balance with the environment, compassion and human service, evidence-based technology and economic viability?

There is another alternative: to recognize that all the different models of health care have their place in contemporary medicine; they are tools that have their own strengths and weaknesses in explaining human experience and in generating treatment techniques. If we know the assumptions and values of these different models, we can emphasize one or the other model when it is most appropriate. But to do this we need a meta-model, or a larger framework, that can hold together many perspectives of health and illness. In this way, we can move forward to reform medicine without having to regress to the past or attempt to force medical care into one explanatory model.

Many people (clients and health care professionals alike) are looking for this new kind of medicine. Called by various names –

such as alternative, complementary, integrative and holistic – the 'new' medical systems aim to provide health care without the dehumanization so common in contemporary medicine, and they are growing in popularity. A 2008 publication from the National Center for Complementary and Alternative Medicine (a branch of the National Institutes of Health in the US) documents that 38% of adults were using some form of Complementary and Alternative Medicine (CAM).[1] This is not just an American phenomenon. Up to 65% of adults in New Zealand,[2] an estimated 60% of the population in Australia[3] and approximately 45% of people in the UK use CAM.[4] One out of every three prescriptions written in Germany is for an herb.[5] The World Health Organization estimates that 65–80% of the world's population relies on some form of 'traditional' (i.e. holistic, alternative) medicine.[6] All these statistics point toward dissatisfaction with the practice of contemporary medicine.

The next part of the book proposes a holistic framework that can hold together multiple models and approaches to medicine. A holistic approach is based on the concept of healing. Healing involves bringing together into wholeness what has been separated. This may be bringing together the edges of a wound, bringing together mind and body, or bridging elements of the health care delivery system that have been fragmented and no longer communicate clearly. Healing ultimately arises from the underlying wholeness of the organism or system.

As a way of understanding what it means to be a whole person, I introduce a nine-dimensional framework that includes integral aspects of being human: body, emotions, mind, heart, self-expression, intuition, spirit, socio-environmental context and a temporal context of learning and growth. A truly holistic practice recognizes these aspects of humanity and their potential roles in contributing to health and illness.

Chapter 3

Redefining Medicine

The practice of medicine is essentially founded on the engagement between two human beings, the physician and the patient, and is not ultimately contingent upon technology or technicianship, although these clearly have had a huge impact on the way medicine is practised today.

Vincent Di Stefano[1]

Reflecting their burnout and frustration with aspects of the biomedical and economic rationalist models, many physicians are actively searching for new models of medicine that respect the human dignity of both doctor and patient. Patients are on the same quest, and if physicians do not offer what they want, they seek it from non-medical practitioners. The fields of *alternative, complementary, integrative* and *holistic* medicine have arisen as attempts to re-humanize medicine. They can be conceptualized as different models of medicine, just as we examined different models of contemporary medicine in chapter one: traditional, foundational, biomedical and economic rationalist. We will examine each of these redefinitions of medicine in turn.

The names and definitions of these models are still in flux as they are developing over time. This reflects both the ambivalence of adherents of new medical models toward biomedicine, and the ambivalence of adherents of biomedicine to these new medical models. For instance, the Office of Unconventional Medical Practices was formed in 1992 at the National Institutes of Health.[2] The use of the term 'unconventional' automatically puts the 'unconventional' practitioner at a disadvantage compared to a practitioner of 'conventional' medicine. The definitions used for different paradigms of medicine reveal a great deal about the power relationship with 'status quo' medicine. By defining something in negative terms, those who have power to name and define have the power to shape what is included and what is excluded in a debate. For instance, what if practitioners of alternative medicine started calling what they did 'new' medicine and called contemporary medicine 'old' medicine? Who would want to practice 'old' medicine?

There is considerable confusion (and emotion) about the definitions of *alternative, complementary, integrative* and *holistic* medicine. In fact, sometimes definitions of one include the names of the others. For instance, the Australasian Integrative Medical Association uses the word 'holistic' in defining what integrative medicine is. A large part of this confusion stems from a lack of clarity between specific therapeutic techniques and interventions (medication, surgery, acupuncture, herbs, etc.) and the underlying philosophical assumptions and values of these new fields.

Another significant source of confusion is that we are in a time of rapid change in medicine, both within the mainstream of contemporary medicine and on the fringes. In *Limits of Scientific Psychiatry*, Beahrs points out that there can be a mutually beneficial relationship between orthodox and fringe elements within medicine. The orthodox is conservative and provides stability and checks on the more extreme aspects of the fringe; the fringe provides enthusiasm and new ideas that can reinvigorate the orthodox and lead to evolution in medicine. Hermann Hesse presents a similar idea about the relationship between individuals and cultural change. In his book *Steppenwolf*, he argues that culture owes a great deal to those individuals who do not fit in, but exist on the periphery with one foot in the culture and one foot out of it.

We will now review the new medicine models and clarify their values as different approaches to re-humanizing medicine.

Alternative Medicine

The term 'alternative medicine' became popular in the 1960s and 1970s. As the name implies, it defines itself as a rejection of, or reaction to, contemporary medicine. The explosion of interest in the US in alternative medicine since the 1960s can be viewed in the context of the counter-cultural movements during that time. These rejected mainstream culture and often sought to create new cultures based on what were seen as more human values of compassion, sharing, social justice, protection of the environment, non-violence and a holistic, harmonious relationship between individuals, society and the Earth.

In alternative medicine, practitioners may spend more time with clients, in a more relaxed setting, and they often provide a more 'hands on' type of treatment with more care and nurturance. The downside is that there are all manner of people proclaiming 'alternative' cures, some reputable and some not. Working outside of the context of contemporary medicine allows freedom to provide services in a different model of care, but it creates challenges as far as regulation, licensure, safety and efficacy are concerned.

Alternative medicine is the 'opt out' option in regards to contemporary medicine. In the extreme caricature of alternative medicine, it would define orthodox contemporary medicine as 'bad' and fringe medicine as 'good'. Rather than seeking to reform contemporary medicine, it advocates the creation of separate systems of clinicians who have often received no orthodox training. Alternative medical practitioners sometimes devalue scientifically based treatments in favor of prioritizing human connection, intuition, spirituality or 'natural' modes of healing. Instead of seeing contemporary medicine as one tool with strengths and weaknesses, they may demonize it for its worst aspects, viewing it as dehumanizing, cold, objectifying and disempowering. It may also seem to represent a hubristic attempt by science and technology to exert total control over human life, like the 'terminator' – a hostile, inhuman machine bent only on destruction. From this perspective, the only option for survival of the human race is to either hide underground or to make periodic guerrilla attacks on the dominating purveyors of death. I admit, this is an extreme characterization, but when a group of alternative medical practitioners get together, there can be a mixture of anger and self-righteousness (almost a crusader mentality) toward contemporary biomedicine.

I do not mean to portray the motives of alternative medicine in a purely negative perspective. I myself have a streak of the *alternative* mentality. For instance, when I reached a point where I felt I could not practice the way I had wanted to within a medical model in which the only role of the psychiatrist was to prescribe medicine for 24 patients a day, I opted out of contemporary medicine and created my own practice. I still prescribed medicine, but I also provided psychotherapy, focused on longer appointment times and provided mind–body treatment interventions. I did not completely reject contemporary medicine, but I did de-emphasize the *economic rationalist* model's influence in my practice by basing appointment times on the needs of the client rather than on the financial needs of the health care delivery system.

Contemporary medicine's stereotype of alternative medical practitioners is that they are either hippies and quacks, or charlatans. The former are kind-hearted, but are ignorant of science and thus dangerous. The latter are uncaring opportunists and thus dangerous. Alternative medicine is viewed as an illogical hodgepodge of discredited concepts (vitalism and life energy) with smatterings of 'primitive' Eastern and indigenous concepts and practices.

Biomedicine's attitude toward alternative medicine has sometimes been based on economic and emotional fears – fear of losing control, patients and income – and sometimes on scientific principles – paternalistic and humanitarian concerns about patients' health, well-being and safety. When the American Medical Association (AMA) was first formed, it was created by a group of allopathic physicians who banded together to drive out any practice of medicine that was different from their own. They attempted to define 'good' medicine according to their model of medicine, thus marginalizing any practitioner with a different philosophy of healing (see Paul Starr[3] and Roberta Bivens[4]).

Complementary Medicine

Since the 1980s, there has been a gradual shift in the attitude of mainstream medicine in the US toward 'alternative' practices. At first, it seemed like the focus was on educating physicians as to what kind of 'quackery' their patients might 'fall victim to' so that they could warn patients and try to protect their health. Physicians were encouraged to ask whether a patient was taking supplements or herbs in order to counsel against their use (because of the lack of scientific evidence of these alternatives). There was reluctance to admit that some aspects of contemporary medicine were not working for everyone or that some people might want a different approach to healing from illness.

During this time, there was also a loss of appreciation of history; many proponents of the biomedical model forgot that modern pharmacology literally has its roots in herbal medicine. In their book, *Natural Remedies That Really Work*, Shaun Holt and Iona MacDonald state that a 'quarter of prescription drugs are taken directly from plants or are chemically modified versions of compounds that are taken directly from plants, and over half of pharmaceuticals are modified natural compounds.'[5]

Over time, the attitude of contemporary medicine seems to have shifted from *fear about harm* to interest in the *possibility of benefit* of some alternative treatments. In the 1980–90s, the term Complementary Medicine, or sometimes Complementary and Alternative Medicine (abbreviated 'CAM') became popular, reflecting this shift in attitude. *Complementary* reflects a shift from a dualistic 'either/or' choice to 'both/and' – adding in different approaches. Whereas alternative medicine was in opposition (or at least orthogonal) to contemporary medicine, CAM embodied the attitude that some alternatives might be beneficial. Contemporary biomedicine does not change in this model; the CAM model provides options which are added to it. The complementary approach could be provided by the physician, but usually it is provided by another practitioner.

As this shift occurred, mainstream health care organizations began to re-evaluate CAM. There is now more recognition that complementary approaches may either have an evidence base for treatment or add humanistic value to contemporary medicine. Many hospitals started offering different services added on to standard medical care: massage, energy work, acupuncture, meditation and yoga, to name just a few. In the complementary model, adding something creates a benefit and does not necessarily mean a choice between two different, incompatible options.

In a related development, some treatments that were once considered 'alternative,' and later 'complementary,' are now used by physicians practicing in the contemporary medical model. For instance, neurologists and cardiologists, who would not consider themselves holistic or CAM clinicians, are now prescribing fish oil (omega fatty acids) to reduce lipids.[6] This treatment is also becoming an evidence-based practice in psychiatry for adjunctive treatment of depression.[7]

In 1998, a branch of the US National Institutes of Health was created with the hybrid name, the National Center for Complementary and Alternative Medicine (NCCAM). The NCCAM website defines many different CAM treatment modalities and it reviews the research results of studies funded through NCCAM.[8] The Center started a project for the incorporation of CAM information into 14 health professional schools' curricula between 2000 and 2003. A 2007 issue of *Academic Medicine* featured articles reviewing different aspects of this project.[9] The incorporation of CAM education into medical education has created a great deal of controversy, with proponents hailing it as a major advance and opponents decrying it as teaching pseudo-science. Whatever one's perspective, it shows how medicine is always changing.

Integrative Medicine

Integrative medicine seeks to integrate aspects of CAM within contemporary medicine's evidence-based biomedical model. We can view newer models of medicine on a spectrum, with alternative medicine rejecting biomedicine, complementary medicine providing the optional add-on to contemporary medicine and integrative medicine combining select CAM principles and techniques with contemporary medicine. Integrative medicine is thus an expansion of biomedicine to include evidence-based CAM treatment techniques.

In the 1990s, the term 'integrative medicine' became popular in many countries around the world. In Australia and New Zealand, in 1992, the Australasian Integrative Medicine Association (AIMA) was formed. Their website defines the AIMA's philosophy and core values, including respect for patients' autonomy and participation in the healing process and:

– promoting models of health care which attend to a person's experience of illness, as well as their symptoms of disease via ethical, natural and wherever possible, evidence-based therapies.
– following the Declaration of Helsinki (of the World Health Organization) that maintains: that a physician must be free to use the most appropriate treatment if in his or her judgement it will result in the alleviation of suffering or the restoration of health or saving the life of a patient.
– encouraging a holistic attitude amongst doctors and medical students and enhancing skills in whole person medicine.

– encouraging the 'wellness' paradigm amongst medical practitioners by fostering an attitude of Prevention and Health Promotion as a fundamental cornerstone in primary care.[10]

In 1994, Andrew Weil and colleagues founded the Program for Integrative Medicine at the University of Arizona. This became the Arizona Center for Integrative Medicine (ACIM) in 2008, with the mission of leading 'the transformation of health care by creating, educating and actively supporting a community that embodies the philosophy and practice of healing-oriented medicine, addressing mind, body and spirit. Our commitment is to live the values of Integrative Medicine, thus creating a unique model for transforming medicine.'[11]

In 1999, the Consortium of Academic Health Centers for Integrative Medicine[12] was formed. It currently has 57 member universities throughout the US, Canada and Mexico. The consortium is funded through member dues, its biannual international research conference and the George Family Foundation.[13] Jon Kabat-Zinn, who has developed excellent programs in Mindfulness-Based Stress Reduction, played a key role in this organization's development.

The varied organizations formed under the rubric of integrative medicine show that it is a model of medicine that includes a great variety of values. Furthermore, the hybrid term Complementary, Alternative and Integrative Medicine (CAIM) has arisen, which contributes to confusion as to the distinctions between complementary, alternative and integrative medicine. Rather than delineating clear distinctions between these different models of medicine, CAIM lumps them all together. It is true that there are many areas of overlap between these models of medicine, but our focus here is on trying to tease out the different underlying assumptions and values of each model separately.

One way of understanding these different terms is through the historical shift that has occurred within the mainstream of contemporary medicine toward CAIM concepts. Along with the formation of new professional organizations that seek to promote a change in the way medicine is practiced, there have also been a number of books examining the scientific base of CAIM. The *Physician's Desk Reference for Herbal Medicine*[14] is a testament to physicians' changing attitudes toward integrating complementary and alternative medicine. This book reviews scientific studies for many herbs, including information on the active compounds, metabolism and drug–herb interactions (biomedical model). The book reports how traditional cultures and folk medicine have used different herbs (traditional and CAM models). The book then gives prescribing information for the evidence-based use of herbs (integrative model). This shows a truly integrated approach to the use of herbs in medicine. It makes sense to treat both pharmaceuticals and herbs as active biological compounds that have both beneficial uses and adverse effects.

Holistic Medicine

Holistic medicine is based on connection: connection to different dimensions within a person and between the whole of the doctor and the whole of the patient. Holistic medicine is the practice of seeing all the dimensions of the whole person, not just a state of illness or a disease, a diagnosis, or billing code. A holistic approach is to accept the person in their entirety, including their illness. The physical body, science, pharmaceuticals, surgical interventions, physical health and exercise are all aspects of the physical dimension of health. Holistic medicine does not stop there, but includes dimensions of emotion, thought, compassion, self-expression, intuition, spirituality, context and time – valuing each of these dimensions individually, but even more so the interrelationship of dimensions. What happens in one part of a person affects all other dimensions. Ultimately, holistic medicine is about doctors having a different relationship to their own humanity, which translates to a different relationship with their patients. Holistic medicine is, thus, a perfect prescription for dehumanization in contemporary medicine.[15]

Contemporary medicine divides the human body into nine major sub-systems: circulatory, digestive, endocrine, muscular, nervous, reproductive, respiratory, skeletal and urinary systems. There are specialists and subspecialists for all of these different systems. A holistic approach does not mean that intervening at a sub-system level does not have relevance, but that such intervention should always be considered within the larger context of the whole.

Holistic medicine recognizes that all things are made up of component parts, while at the same time they are part of a larger whole. For example, a rock is made up of molecules, which are made up of atoms, which are made up of all sorts of funny-sounding subatomic structures. The rock is on the beach, which is part of the coastline, which is the boundary of a continent, which is in a hemisphere of the Earth, and is on the Earth, which is in our solar system, in the Milky Way Galaxy, which is in the universe and there may be other universes. The study of the rock may seem to be only limited to the component parts of the rock itself, but the rock also has a larger context that it exists within. Depending on what you are studying, you may choose various levels to examine. A holistic approach would consider all the dimensions in which the rock exists. Similarly, the whole human being is composed of different, yet mutually interactive sub-systems. Individuals are also sub-systems within larger social, cultural, economic, political and environmental systems.

The term 'Integrative Medicine' is increasingly replacing 'Holistic Medicine.' Physicians first formed the American Board of Holistic Medicine (ABHM) in 1996, and first gave certification exams in the year 2000. They then added the term 'integrative,' to become the American Board of Integrative and Holistic Medicine (ABIHM) in 2008. In 2014, the ABIHM is offering its last board certification exam, this is largely due to the formation of the American Board of Integrative Medicine (ABoIM).[16] Diplomates of the ABIHM will, for a short time, be allowed to sit for the ABoIM exam without completing the residency training program that will be the future pathway to the exam. For the first time, a board exam in integrative medicine will be credentialed by one of the two primary board certification organizations in the US, in this case the American Board of Physician Specialties.[17] This gradual shift from 'holistic' to 'integrative' paralleled the efforts of the physicians to get recognition as a formal medical specialty. While the ABoIM will become the gold standard as far as credentialing for physicians in integrative medicine, the ABIHM will shift its focus to a larger field beyond physicians and toward an international membership as an international academy. There are exciting things happening in the field!

All this terminology of complementary, alternative, integrative and holistic medicine can be quite confusing. While the recognized terminology for physician board certification will be integrative medicine, the concept of holistic medicine continues to be relevant. The American Holistic Medical Association (AHMA) was founded in 1978 and has worked to expand the role of the physician to include humanistic elements as well as to bring scientific rigor to investigating alternative medical techniques. In many ways, this is similar to the idea of integrative medicine. An important distinction is that it is possible to consider holistic medicine as a philosophical framework that allows for the existence of many different models, whereas integrative medicine could be considered to be more concerned focused on integrating CAIM principles into a biomedical model. In this sense, integrative medicine brings CAM into contemporary medicine, whereas holistic medicine brings contemporary medicine and CAIM into a larger framework. I introduce this distinction between a framework and a model in an attempt to bring some clarity to this question. Holistic medicine has the benefit of being founded upon a philosophical systems model that allows for the understanding of multiple sub-systems and multiple models. These sub-systems may operate with different, even contradictory mechanisms. The following sections take a closer look at holistic medicine.

Clarifying the Values of New Medical Models

If you have found yourself confused at times in this chapter about what the actual difference is between alternative, complementary, CAM, integrative, CAIM and holistic models of medicine, I am not surprised; this is a confusing area with overlapping terminology. This section will review some of the different sources of confusion as well as some different ways of understanding these models in order to clarify the distinction between them and their relationship to contemporary medicine.

Well-being or Treatment?

Contemporary medicine views its role as the treatment of disease through therapeutic surgical or technological interventions that alter the anatomy and physiology of a human being in order to treat disease. However, CAIM and holistic medicine broaden their scope beyond treating disease to the promotion of wellness and well-being. It could be argued that everything that promotes well-being is also therapeutic in some way (for instance through the field of psychoneuroimmunology). It is also possible that some things may help people feel better, but that they are not strictly therapeutic.

Let us look at massage as an example of an intervention that can be either therapeutic to treat disease or simply promote well-being. People who are not sick with a disease often go for a massage in order to feel better. No one argues whether they actually feel better or if they just think they feel better (a placebo response). Other people get a massage because they have a disease and the massage is therapeutic in regard to that disease. We could consider massage to be therapeutic (changing the nature or severity of the disease) in conditions such as headaches, muscular dystonia, or sports injuries, for instance.

What if someone has major depression or cancer and they choose to combine a number of techniques in order to improve their well-being? Could all these things together be therapeutic and change the nature or severity of the disease process, even if individually none of them had a biomedical evidence base proving effectiveness? Or, should these be considered complementary treatments, add-ons to the *real* biomedical treatment? What if a person combined massage, exercise, diet change, aromatherapy, listening to relaxing music, taking a photography class and starting to paint with watercolors? They say that they feel better from doing these things. Is this a placebo effect (these things are not making them feel better – they just think that they should feel better because of them)? Could there be some additive effect on decreasing stress and improving well-being that through psychoneuroimmunology leads to a measurable biochemical and physiological effect?

How a doctor views their role as technician, healer or both determines how they will engage with patients. If doctors view their role as strictly limited to technical EBM interventions, they will be in a technician role in relation to patients. If doctors view their role as a technician plus a healer, they will seek to promote well-being in order to help people to be happier and healthier as well as providing EBM techniques to treat disease.

Technique and Philosophy as a Distinguishing Factor

The source of much of this confusion lies in two different aspects of these models: techniques and philosophy. There is a bewildering array of techniques to consider that are grouped under CAIM and holistic medicine. For instance, Traditional Chinese Medicine, Ayurvedic Medicine, homeopathy, herbal treatments, energy medicine, prayer, meditation, spiritual practices, the use of crystals or magnets, etc. There are also different philosophies that are combined in these models, such as humanistic, holistic, biomedical, as well as various Eastern and indigenous philosophical models. What is even more confusing and causes conceptual difficulty for both proponents and opponents of these new medical models is that the techniques grow out of different philosophical traditions that have different values and principles to each other and to the biomedical model. This is perhaps the greatest limitation of integrative medicine – deciding what can be integrated within a biomedical model. There may be techniques or philosophies that are very useful for re-humanizing medicine, but that are difficult to study from a biomedical model to determine whether or not a given treatment technique is evidence-based. Herbs are easy to study from a biomedical perspective with a pill and a placebo control, but how would you create a blinded study for aromatherapy where it is obvious to the subject whether or not they smell something, for instance? Also, where is the line between something that makes someone feel better (enhancing well-being which may positively influence health in the long run) and something that is therapeutic? Massage can help someone feel better and more relaxed and it can also have some therapeutic benefits for certain conditions, but can massage be considered an evidence-based treatment if we know it promotes wellness and does not have any harmful side effects? Or, to return to aromatherapy, if a person enjoys a scent, takes a deep breath and sighs and feels more relaxed, can that be considered therapeutic for conditions that are known to be made worse by stress, such as depression, anxiety, diabetes and headaches? Because holistic and CAIM techniques focus on inducing well-being, treating suffering and treating disease, there can be confusion as to where the line is between an intervention that promotes well-being and an intervention that is therapeutic for treating disease.

All of these new models of medicine also contain varying elements of different philosophies, such as holistic, humanistic, or those of other cultures. The humanistic element we can think of as an attempt to re-humanize medicine, and is present in all of these models. A holistic philosophy of interconnection, which is the opposite of a reductionist biomedical model, is also a part of many of these new models. CAIM and holistic medicine often borrow from other cultural traditions, not just including a technique like acupuncture, but also adopting aspects of the philosophical model of Traditional Chinese Medicine (TCM), such as concepts of *qi*, energy flow through the meridian system, the five element theory, etc. In China, medical students actually learn what we in the West would call a form of integrative or perhaps holistic medicine. Doctors are taught both systems of medicine: Western biomedicine and TCM. They then rely on their professional training to help them decide when one or the other model might be useful or in what way to combine the models. The two models exist side by side to each other and are allowed to have contradictions, but also usefulness independent of each other for specific clinical presentations. This leads us to another way of clarifying the difference between these new models of medicine: their relationship to biomedicine.

How Models Relate to Contemporary Medicine
One way to attempt to clarify the distinctions between these different models of medicine is to look at how they relate to contemporary medicine. Contemporary medicine is largely influenced by the biomedical model (which values science and evidence-based medicine) and the economic rationalist model (which values managing profit and loss). Alternative medicine rejects the biomedical model and opts out of contemporary medicine. Complementary medicine leaves biomedicine unaltered, but adds on complementary techniques/practices. Integrative medicine combines select CAM techniques/practices

(that are able to be shown to be evidence-based) with biomedicine. Holistic medicine provides a holistic framework or metamodel that recognizes the utility of integrative and biomedical models, but places these within a larger context that values nonobjective aspects of human being (subjectivity, meaning, love, spirituality, etc.).

We can look at how each model answers the question, 'Is evidence-based medicine the only legitimate model of medicine?' Biomedicine says *yes*. Alternative medicine says *no* and rejects the biomedical model. Complementary medicine, *yes, but* consider these other options, too, if they do not hurt anyone. Integrative medicine *largely says yes* (it includes other options, but subjects them to the evidence-based scrutiny of biomedicine). Holistic medicine says *no*, it is *not the only* legitimate model, *but yes it is one of many* legitimate models with which to treat human beings. Holistic medicine's answer is the most complex, the most inclusive, and yet also clearly contextualizes biomedicine as one model among many. In the following chapter we will examine the principles of holistic medicine.

Chapter 4

Principles of Holistic Medicine

Principles of Holistic Medicine

1. *Optimal Health*
2. *The Healing Power of Love*
3. *Whole Person*
4. *Prevention and Treatment*
5. *Innate Healing Power*
6. *Integration of Healing Systems*
7. *Relationship-centered Care*
8. *Individuality*
9. *Teaching by Example*
10. *Learning Opportunities*

The American Holistic Medical Association formed in 1978 and has developed ten principles of holistic medicine. As will be seen, these are not about specific treatment modalities, but encompass a new paradigm and philosophy of relationship. This creates an expanded scope of practice for holistic physicians concerned with the whole human being, not just the biomedical aspects of a person. These ten principles are: *optimum health, the healing power of love, the whole person, prevention and treatment, innate healing power, integration of healing systems, relationship-centered care, individuality, teaching by example* and *learning opportunities*. I will go through each of these principles below, quoting from the AHMA website descriptions and then elaborating as to how these principles are pertinent to this book.[1]

1. '**Optimal Health** *is the primary goal of holistic medical practice. It is the conscious pursuit of the highest level of functioning and balance*

of the physical, environmental, mental, emotional, social and spiritual aspects of human experience, resulting in a dynamic state of being fully alive. This creates a condition of wellbeing regardless of the presence or absence of disease.'

The principle of optimal health contrasts with a disease-focused model of health and illness, in which you either have health or you have illness. Through including other dimensions of human experience in health, such as emotional, social and spiritual, the scope of a physician's practice is extended beyond simply managing a person's biochemistry. Optimal health is an achievable goal for any person, no matter how ill they are. A person could be dying of terminal cancer, yet their physician could be working to enhance their optimal health from a psychological, social and spiritual sense.

The significance of an optimal health paradigm is that it broadens the view of a patient beyond their physical body and expands the role of the physician beyond the physical dimension of health and illness. Physicians will vary in their degree of comfort and expertise in addressing non-physical health issues, but they still should be able to identify and refer appropriately to other disciplines and specialties.

2. *'The Healing Power of Love. Holistic health care practitioners strive to meet the patient with grace, kindness, acceptance, and spirit without condition, as love is life's most powerful healer.'*

The focus on love rather than technology as the most powerful healer is another dramatic shift in holistic medicine. Evidence-based medicine and the service-provider/service-user model of health care are definitely not based on love. Economic exchange of payment for services, in which doctors are interchangeable units in a corporate or bureaucratic structure and all patients are interchangeable 'service-users', does not leave much place for love or connection. One way of looking at how evidence-based medicine is often used is that any patient with the same diagnosis gets the same treatment from any doctor. At the scientific level, this is laudable, but at the individual level it is a bit absurd. People are unique individuals and they are not interchangeable cogs.

The distinction between the doctor–patient relationship as an exchange of love versus an exchange of goods and services recalls Lewis Hyde's discussion of gift economies versus exchange commodities. In a gift economy, 'a circulation of gifts nourishes those parts of our spirit that are not entirely personal, parts that derive from nature, the group, the race, or the gods.'[2] In contrast, 'when we profit on exchange or convert "one man's gift to another man's capital" – we nourish the part of our being (or our group) which is distinct and separate from others.'[3] The distinction Hyde makes between gift and the exchange of capital is that with a gift a greater sense of interconnection is created, whereas capital increases the isolation and separation between people. I am obviously not arguing that physicians should give away their services (although most physicians, myself included, have written off debts and charged reduced fees, which are bad business practices from a purely capitalistic perspective), but I think that the idea of gift is part of the doctor–patient relationship. In a holistic paradigm, the physician develops their whole self in order to give of themselves to the patient. What the patient receives is more than a simple service or billing code, but the gift of attention and care from another human being. In healing, the patient gives back to the physician, who in return is nourished in seeing the vitality and life that comes from connection and caring. As Hyde writes, a 'gift that has the power to change us awakens a part of the soul.'[4] The gift of healing goes two ways and can awaken the souls of both the physician and the patient. Soul food nourishes both the giver and the receiver. Goods and services may exchange hands, but leave the soul unnourished.

If love is life's most powerful healer, we can ask the age-old question: what is love? Psychiatrist M. Scott Peck defines love as the 'will to extend one's self for the purpose of nurturing one's own or another's spiritual growth.'[5] This definition is quite suited to our discussion of the healing role of love in holistic medicine, particularly when spiritual growth is understood to encompass the growth of the whole or total human being. To use Peck's definition of love, a physician loves a client when he or she extends her or his self for the purpose of the healing and growth of the whole person of the client. Love is a gift that has a reciprocal nature. 'Love ... is invariably a two-way street, a reciprocal phenomenon whereby the receiver also gives and the giver also receives,' writes Peck.[6]

One last comment on love comes from Dr. Francis Weld Peabody, when he said that the 'secret of the care of the patient is in caring for the patient.'[7]

3. *'Whole Person. Holistic health care practitioners view people as the unity of body, mind, spirit and the systems in which they live.'*
This concept of treating the whole person is the fundamental basis of holistic medicine, as love, healing, relationship and individuality, and all the other principles of holistic medicine really grow out of the awareness of what a whole person is. The meeting of the whole of the physician and the whole patient is healing, in and of itself. The definition of what it means to be a whole person will be explored in more depth in the next chapter.

4. *'Prevention and Treatment. Holistic health care practitioners promote health, prevent illness and help raise awareness of dis-ease in our lives rather than merely managing symptoms. A holistic approach relieves symptoms, modifies contributing factors, and enhances the patient's life system to optimize future wellbeing.'*
This principle of holistic medicine should be very familiar to anyone who studies health care cost and efficacy. Disease prevention rather than disease treatment is less expensive and

creates a healthier population. In holistic medicine, preventative medicine would include more than physical health screening. A holistic physician would be concerned with a client's current well-being, recognizing that it is correlated with health. Hopelessness, demoralization, job dissatisfaction, troubled relationships, spiritual confusion, all contribute to future illness as do genetics, substance abuse and lifestyle factors. Holistic medicine recognizes that physical, emotional, psychological, social and spiritual dimensions can mutually reinforce one another in a positive or negative way.

5. *'Innate Healing Power. All people have innate powers of healing in their bodies, minds and spirits. Holistic health care practitioners evoke and help patients utilize these powers to affect the healing process.'*
What is healing? Where does the source of healing lie? These questions are not often asked or answered in medical school, and yet they are the most important questions. If the ultimate healing power is in the pill and the scalpel, then there is no sense in troubling oneself with all the complications and messiness of a patient's emotions, thoughts, dreams and disappointments. If the ultimate healing power is not in the pill and the scalpel, then these other factors and variables assume massive importance.

There are so many studies that demonstrate that a person who is isolated, lonely, disconnected, or depressed has a significantly poorer outcome from a serious procedure, no matter how well it is technically performed.[8,9] To flawlessly perform a complicated technical procedure and then to abandon emotional and spiritual responsibility for a patient is what is called winning the battle but losing the war. The field of psychoneuroimmunology is pertinent to the concept of innate healing power. Psychoneuroimmunology (or PNI as it is sometimes called) demonstrates the interconnection between thought, emotion, the nervous system, the immune system, health and illness. This field provides a theoretical model to explain the ample research evidence that demonstrates the linkage between physical health, emotion, thoughts, social support and environmental stress.

After years of clinical work with clients and searching for the location of healing, I have come to view the answer in terms of hope and faith. The belief that healing only resides outside of the individual contributes to a sense of hopelessness, powerlessness, isolation, disconnection and even nihilism. This belief dehumanizes clinician and patient, while reifying technology's ability to cure. If you tell someone that their biochemistry is so messed up that there is nothing more you can do for them, you are betraying your patient and contributing to the hopelessness and cynicism of our time. If you believe that a person has the ability within themselves to heal from anything (understanding that healing, illness and death are not mutually exclusive), then you are empowering your client by encouraging them to reconnect to their own innate healing ability. While you need not take this into a spiritual realm, it is easy to take the next step to say that each individual contains within themselves self-renewing life. A spiritual view of illness addresses loss of connection on many levels. Healing, in a spiritual sense, is a reconnection to Self, life energy, chi, prana, spirit, God, the universe, etc. Illness is not a punishment or a failure. Illness is an integral part of life's eternal change and balance. Carl Jung wrote that there 'is no illness that is not at the same time an unsuccessful attempt at cure.'[10] In this sense, illness can be seen as part of life.

To be able to tell someone, 'Yes, you can get through this,' or 'I know you have it within you to live with whatever it is that feels overwhelming to you,' requires having faith in every person's innate healing ability. Holistic medicine asks that you bring your heart and soul into your work with people. As a physician of the body, heart and soul, you will often be challenged to find hope and meaning in situations that seem hopeless and meaningless. This aspect of the work is much more difficult than looking up the correct combination of medications or even performing a difficult surgery, because it can activate your own hopelessness, your own sense of the seemingly meaningless struggle of life that ends in death. Physicians see what is left after a human being dies – a physical pile of meat. This knowledge of death and familiarity with physical remains exerts a powerful pull toward materialism, loss of hope and a deadening of the spirit for physicians.

To reawaken hope in others, you must be constantly reawakening hope within yourself. The experience of facing your own deep, inner hopelessness can allow you to connect to the hopelessness of your client. It is true that there are hopeless times in life and these must be lived through; simply attempting to deny or negate hopelessness is not the same thing as having hope.

I have long found Vaclav Havel's explication of hope to both describe as well as create hope. Havel was the first president of Czechoslovakia after the 1989 fall of the Iron Curtain. He was an artist, playwright, political activist and he was imprisoned for his political statements. Havel describes 'hope...above all as a state of mind, not a state of the world. Either we have hope within us or we do not; it is a dimension of the soul, and it's not essentially dependent on some particular observation of the world or estimate of the situation.'[11] In this sense hope is a state of being, not necessarily an intellectual analysis or a weighing of the chances for success. He goes on to write that hope 'is an orientation of the spirit, an orientation of the heart; it transcends the world that is immediately experienced, and it is anchored somewhere beyond its horizons.' Havel states that his understanding of hope is 'more than a conviction; it's an inner experience.'

This description of hope is pertinent to the topic of 'innate healing abilities,' because the physician must have hope in their own innate ability to have a positive influence on the client as well as hope that the client can connect to their own innate sense of healing. Havel describes hope as something akin to faith or trust and also as somewhat of an existential and moral choice as well as being a gift from 'elsewhere.' In the face of death, illness, misery, despair and suffering, there is choice and for the holistic physician that choice is to always hope.

6. *'Integration of Healing Systems. Holistic health care practitioners embrace a lifetime of learning about all safe and effective options in diagnosis and treatment. These options come from a variety of traditions, and are selected in order to best meet the unique needs of the patient. The realm of choices may include lifestyle modification and complementary approaches as well as conventional drugs and surgery.'* This principle of integrating healing systems is what is often mistakenly assumed as the only definition of 'holistic,' a physician who performs techniques outside of contemporary medicine, such as acupuncture, prescribing herbs or recommending dietary changes. As the AHMA principle reads, these systems are integrated into contemporary medical practice out of an understanding of the uniqueness of each individual who seeks treatment. A physician may be interested in different modalities, but what matters is what each particular patient needs. Understanding a person from a holistic, multidimensional perspective means that optimal care involves assessing and intervening at the all levels of the human being.

To work with each human being, a holistic physician needs to be flexible, creative, knowledgeable of scientific studies and also have multiple heuristic frameworks for understanding what could be going on with each client. In contemporary medical training, doctors are encouraged to make a differential diagnosis of several different possible causes for symptoms. I remember a psychotherapy instructor who encouraged his students to come up with five different possible explanations for understanding a client before offering a psychotherapeutic interpretation. A holistic physician can construct a differential diagnosis using multiple different explanatory models. The benefit of understanding contemporary as well as holistic explanatory models is that a physician can be more creative and flexible, rather than having a 'one size fits all' mentality.

7. *'Relationship-centered Care. The ideal practitioner–patient relationship is a partnership which encourages patient autonomy, and values the needs and insights of both parties. The quality of this relationship is an essential contributor to the healing process.'*
The principle of relationship-centered care is not just some touchy-feely process; studies on why doctors are sued reveal that the relationship can be more important than whether or not a procedure is successful or not.[12] Good medicine is relationship-centered care. People want to be included in important decisions, like those around health and illness. A focus on relationship-centered care also counterbalances the tendencies of contemporary medicine to be dehumanizing and technology-oriented. The relationship can also be a great source of reward and support for both the physician and the patient in dealing with the very emotionally challenging situations that daily arise in a medical practice. A sense of working together, or of sharing the burden, can be a relief for both the physician and the patient, neither of whom operate well in isolation. Relationships, in and of themselves, can be healing, as they are a form of connection. The relationship is also where you bring all of your humanity into play with your client. The process of becoming more connected to wholeness is healing for both the client and you.

8. *'Individuality. Holistic health care practitioners focus patient care on the unique needs and nature of the person who has an illness rather than the illness that has the person.'*

Both social connection and connection to one's self are components of health. Everyone has their own history, their own desires, their own beliefs, even if they have the same illness. Therefore, a truly holistic model of care would entail a dimension of valuing and encouraging the uniqueness of the individual in the pursuit of well-being.

One of the objections to an evidence-based model that is carried out in a totalitarian way (fitting the patient to the illness) is that it leaves out the principle of individuality. Swiss psychiatrist Carl Jung felt that the central concept of his psychology was the process of 'individuation,' through which a person moves toward wholeness as an individual. For Jung, this was more than ego-consciousness; 'the self comprises infinitely more than a mere ego ... Individuation does not shut out the world, but gathers the world to oneself.'[13] Jung thus viewed individuation as not just an interior developmental process, but the process through which an individual can relate to the world. Diminishing individuality inhibits human connection and connection to the world. To diminish individuality is to objectify human beings and to diminish psychological and spiritual reality.

In Western culture, individuality is both valued and maligned. In chapter two, we discussed the concepts of individualism and collectivism in cultures. An individualistic culture is one that values individual rights over those of the group. A collectivistic culture is one that values group cohesion and group rights over the individual. An individualistic culture views the individual as the fundamental unit of life, or reference point, whereas a collectivistic culture views the group as the fundamental unit of life, or reference point. You may think at first that these are two completely opposite ends of a spectrum. However, these dimensions are actually orthogonal: they can vary independently. A culture can value the individual in some instances and the group in others. For instance, the United States is a very individualistic culture, but it is also influenced a great deal by Christianity, which has many collectivistic concepts and beliefs (do unto others as you would have them do unto you, treat strangers as your brothers and sisters, do not put yourself before others). It is possible to be both individual-oriented and group-oriented. Many of the cultural and religious debates about the individual and the group would be simplified if the truth was seen that people are unique individuals (one dimension) who are embedded in a social matrix (another dimension).

What I think Jung and many others would argue is that, through developing one's own unique individuality, one becomes better able to also participate within the group. The best citizen is one who possesses self-knowledge and has the capacity to connect to others. Another way to say this is that the best citizen is capable of love. As the old saying goes, you can only love another to the extent that you can love yourself. Returning to M. Scott Peck's quote on love, it is the 'will to extend oneself for the purpose of nurturing one's own or another's spiritual growth.'[14] Love of self and love of others are two mutually inter-dependent abilities that reinforce each other.

I had mentioned that the principle of the individual touches on powerful psychological and spiritual issues. Christianity tends to have more of a community focus than an individual focus. Some denominations may actually discourage a focus on individual personal growth, because this is considered to be sinful or proud. However, this is largely due to a misunder-standing of seeing the self only as the ego (without heart or spirit as part of Self). It is true that from a religious perspective, the ego could be considered 'evil' or 'sinful, or at the very least, 'selfish.' This is because the ego is separate from God or Spirit. However, if one considers that Self is a larger concept than ego, personal growth would include spiritual growth and would not be 'selfish.' Thus, individuation – the development of a sense of Self – leads to a greater ability to connect to others. There are many traditions of religion that view the individual as the place of contact with the divine. Most strands of mysticism teach that the place to find God or Spirit is within. In this way, a focus on individuality is not just an issue of psychological development, but also of spiritual and community development as well.

9. *'Teaching by Example. Holistic health care practitioners continually work toward the personal incorporation of the principles of holistic health, which then profoundly influence the quality of the healing relationship.'*
Teaching by example means that the physician does not just talk the talk, but also walks the walk. You cannot treat a whole person if you do not know, yourself, what it is to be a whole person. Similar to the way that psychoanalysts first needed to undergo analysis themselves, a holistic physician needs to do some personal work. The American Board of Integrative and Holistic Medicine requires the physician to undertake personal growth activities for recertification.[15] You can think of this as a different kind of continuing medical education – the counter-curriculum! Personal growth work is anything that you undertake to learn more about yourself, such as meditation, yoga, physical exercise, journaling, creative/expressive arts, psychotherapy, spiritual exploration, prayer, or any kind of mind–body–spirit work.

This principle of teaching by example not only exposes patients to healthy behaviors and attitudes; it also puts the physician and patient on the same level, as two human beings who periodically struggle with challenges as they go through their lives. Rather than an all-knowing professional and ignorant patient, teaching by example creates a situation in which two human beings can learn from each other. The doctor and patient are both on a journey of self-exploration.

Clinical detachment is taught as a skill and is emblematic, in some circles, of what it means to be a professional. However, most people do not respond to a cold, detached, aloof person who is unaffected by interpersonal interaction. Every human being does respond to human warmth, openness, accessibility, honesty and integrity. The principle of teaching by example is a good reminder not to lose your humanity through striving for pseudo-professionalism.

Personally, I think that any professional, not just those in the health care field, needs to be aware of their humanity as they go through professional training and education. I consciously undertook a program of re-humanization as I went through my training. In medical school, my friend Darin and I would go to the Art Institute café in Chicago (Tuesdays were free day at the museum) to study stacks of notes and medical tomes. After drinking free refills on coffee and studying for hours, Darin and I would stash our stuffed backpacks into a locker, and walk around taking in the artwork. In the café, we would eavesdrop on a group of artists who were regulars. While we never actually met them, I remember overhearing that my favorite of this group, an old guy with a Polish accent, was named Joseph. One time Joseph said to his companions, 'We *are* light, it is what we are; how could we be otherwise!' I scribbled Joseph's wisdom into my notes about anatomy and physiology. This hopeful statement and the shift from the intellectual study of reductionist biomedicine to the visual contemplation of art and beauty helped me maintain a human identity during the acculturation process of medical school.

I painted, journaled (a word my spell check does not like and suggests, helpfully, 'journeyed'), wrote poetry, meditated and made sure I always had handy a novel and a book on meditation, poetry, or philosophy. Professional training can be dehuman- izing. Luckily, there are lots of things that you can do to 'rehumanize yourself' to quote a song by The Police.[16] Through being aware of dehumanization and having gone through periods of re-humanization, we, as health professionals, can serve as a guides and role models.

10. *'Learning Opportunities. All life experiences including birth, joy, suffering and the dying process are profound learning opportunities for both patients and health care practitioners.'*

This is another profound principle that in some ways turns contemporary medicine on its head. Human beings go through all sorts of archetypal or universal experiences, such as birth, love, loss, growing to the fullness of physical maturity and then growing past or through that into old age. Everyone has hopes and dreams, likes and dislikes, successes and disappointments. Eventually, everyone dies, some slowly, some quickly, some 'when it is time,' others seemingly too early, some maybe even too late. These are all universal human experiences that are part of life.

Sometimes, we doctors forget what life is all about, about what is really important, about the fact that illness and death are as much a part of the human condition as birth and health. A technical, 'professional,' evidence-based way of viewing people who are sick focuses on what can be done to get them back to how they were. As Illich wrote, medical 'civilization ... tends to turn pain into a technical matter and thereby deprives suffering of its inherent personal meaning.'[17] To counterbalance this technical and interventionist tendency, we can also develop a sense of the journey of the human experience and that anything that happens in life has the potential to be a learning experience. Too much focus on 'curing' illness leads to a loss of perspective of the inescapable fact that illness and death are part of life. A physician is in a very unique position in society. The physician possesses tremendous technical knowledge that can be the difference between life and death, and yet at other times all this knowledge is 'useless' when in the face of chronic suffering and death. Where knowledge ceases to be important, wisdom can be helpful.

Everything that seems 'bad' in life can be learned from and can be a source of wisdom. People dramatically change their lives after a brush with death or illness. They may change careers or take a dramatically new perspective after a personal encounter with illness. In her book, *A Blessing in Disguise*, Andrea Joy Cohen writes about how people can grow from life events that seem the darkest and most potentially destructive.[18] The book contains essays from 39 different teachers, artists and healers who learned from difficult times in their lives and grew from them. If you are open to the concept of growing through adversity in your own life, you will be able to teach clients this concept as well. There are a number of growing fields that look at the concept of resiliency and posttraumatic growth, moving the concept of trauma as pathology to trauma as a potential opportunity for growth.

I will give a very small example from my own life of how something that seems 'bad' can turn out to be 'good' in the long run. I often use this example with clients, particularly around academic or work struggles. When I went to college, I had dreams of becoming an astronomical/aeronautical engineer and wanted to design spacecraft for NASA. Unfortunately, math was not my strong point and I failed my five-hour calculus class in my first semester at university. Sure, I did a lot of the typical Freshman rites of passage, and probably could have studied more. But it was the first time in my life that I put effort into something and just could not 'get it.' Usually I could do a practice problem and look at the answer and say, 'Oh, I see how it works.' However, with calculus, I just did not get it. This terrified me. What if I did not have what it takes to get through college? I considered alternate career options, which included becoming an alcoholic (it somehow seemed like a career option at the time) or becoming a subsistence farmer, living alone, somewhere in Canada where there would be fantastic snowfalls and I would sit inside a cozy cabin reading all winter and then working in the field all summer.

I went through a dark night of the soul, questioning my life, my future, my past. I thought about who I was, who I might be and about what was really important in life. I felt, within myself, the tremendous impulse that I *needed* to do something. I spent a lot of time the next semester staring at things, staring out my window in the dorm at the cold, Midwestern winter sunsets and darkness that followed; staring at my books and papers on my desk; staring into a drink; staring at others and generally looking for some meaning or purpose in my life (I just now realized that this was also the time when I met my future wife, although we were not dating at that particular time). One day I had an epiphany. I was staring at the books on my shelf wondering what I wanted to do, who I was and what was important to me. I picked up a book by M. Scott Peck, *The Road Less Travelled*, and flipped it over to read about who he was, about what he did and how he got to be so wise as to write a book about the challenges and rewards of facing the difficult realities of life. 'Hmm, a psychiatrist,' I thought, 'I don't know much about psychiatrists.' I put the book back and stared some more. I picked up another book off the shelf: *Modern Man in Search of a Soul*,[19] by Carl Jung ... another psychiatrist! I looked at some of my other books: literature, existential short stories, Richard Bach's *Illusions*,[20] and ethnographies about different cultures from my Anthropology class. I realized that what I was interested in was the human condition and it looked to me like psychiatrists could study just about any aspect of it: biochemistry, genetics, physiology, psychology, culture, spirituality, symbolism, art, religion, philosophy, literature, consciousness, *everything*, basically. The rest is history, as they say.

Looking back, I think I would have been a miserable astronautical/aeronautical engineer. Many family members and my school counselor encouraged me to pursue engineering. They saw an aspect of my personality that was a strength: technically oriented, patient, spending a lot of time alone drawing with the help of a ruler and circular templates, interested in how things work (although not very mechanically inclined), restrained, prone to think about something rather than impulsively act on it. All these are and were strengths, but I think it would have probably been a living death for me if I had chosen a career that only empha- sized these aspects. I needed to develop my 'inferior functions,' to quote Jung's concept of individuation.[21] A little later in college, I considered alternate career paths, such as becoming a marine biologist and studying dolphin language or getting a PhD in philosophy or religious studies. In the end, I felt that I needed to do what made me uncomfortable in order to be challenged and to grow. I needed to work with people, not animals, not ideas, not books. So, I went off to medical school, which tried to squeeze all the poetry and humanity out of me (here I am being only slightly dramatic).

To return to Havel's earlier quote on hope, teaching by example is about being able to find this sense of hope and purpose and meaning in oneself during the dark times of life and to offer the chance that this light might help another to kindle their own light that is buffeted by the winds of suffering, illness, trauma and hopelessness. To be able to be search for hope and find it in one's own life can be the most powerful force of healing for those who you work with.

In this chapter, we have reviewed the AHMA's ten principles for holistic medicine. It should be apparent that the purpose of these principles is to define the role of the doctor as more than just a biomedical technician, but as a human being who is on their own personal life journey and who accompanies patients on their own journeys through pain, illness, suffering, healing and sometimes death. The goal of holistic medicine is that the whole person of the physician meets the whole person of the patient. What does this mean – to be a 'whole' person? We will examine this question in the next chapters.

Chapter 5

A Holistic Framework for Being Human

The human impulse toward wholeness is evident in both ancient and modern transformative disciplines
Michael Murphy[1]

The ten principles of holistic medicine, discussed in the previous chapter, are all reminders to bring all of yourself to the encounter with the whole person with whom you are working. They are reminders to strive to be fully human in your interactions with people. But it is fair to ask, what does it mean to be fully human?

Paradigms of Human Being

There are many different ways to understand what a whole human being is, such as the biopsychosocial model from medicine or the mind–body–spirit model from New Age and personal growth models. Various models arise from the fields of medicine, psychology, business, education and religion. We will look at several of these, and note that it is common practice to conceptualize a human being as consisting of separate, but inter-related, dimensions of experience.

The Human Being as Defined by Contemporary Medicine

We have discussed Arbuckle's models of medicine: traditional, foundational, biomedical and economic rationalist, each with their different values and priorities. While the traditional and foundational models have conceptions of human being that are complex and nuanced and value the doctor–patient relationship, the biomedical and economic rationalist models are more focused on objective measures of human being through the fields of science, management and business. In this section, we will look at the biological reductionist view of human beings, which is an extreme application of the biomedical model, and also Engel's biopsychosocial model, which was an attempt to re-humanize medicine.

The Whole Human Being in Traditional and Foundational Models of Medicine

These models of medicine respect human beings through preservation of traditional cultural views and spiritual views of what it means to be a human being. In the traditional model, human beings have an important place in the world and there is a strong sense of moral and ethical behavior that maintains this place. Rituals are designed to bring human beings into harmony with the physical, social and spiritual realms. In the foundational model, there is a basic respect for human beings with strong values of compassion and social service. Both the traditional and foundational models have a more holistic view of what it means to be a human being than either the biomedical or economic rationalist models.

A Biological Reductionist View of Human Being

The basic understanding of a human being in contemporary medicine comes from the biomedical model. In biological reductionist terms, the physician is a technician focused on rebalancing or repairing the machinery of the body of the patient. In this view, the body has physical parts and these parts sometimes require repair in order to function correctly. As the body ages, systems break down and can no longer maintain homeostasis, thus, lifelong pharmaceutical intervention is necessary in order to regulate blood pressure, blood sugar and cholesterol, for instance. This is a scientific and reductionist approach to human beings – non-physical, non-objective aspects of humanity that cannot be measured or counted are ignored or considered ephemeral, such as consciousness, spirituality and compassion.

The physical body of human beings can be subdivided into different sub-systems in order to identify malfunction. For instance there are nine major sub-systems: circulatory, digestive, endocrine, muscular, nervous, reproductive, respiratory, skeletal and urinary.

The Biopsychosocial Model

Concern about the objectifying and dehumanizing trends in medicine through the influence of the predominance of the biomedical model is not new. In 1977, George Engel published 'The Need for a New Medical Model: A Challenge for Biomedicine,' in *Science*.[2] In this article, he wrote, 'I contend that all medicine is in crisis and, further, that medicine's crisis derives from the same basic fault as psychiatry's, namely, adherence to a model of disease no longer adequate for the scientific tasks and social responsibilities of either medicine or psychiatry.'[3] In place of a reductionist biomedical model, Engel proposed a model of human being that included the biological level, but also added psychological and social dimensions. This model is widely used in medical education and it has its supporters and detractors. Supporters point out that the model includes highly pertinent psychological and social factors in understanding health and illness. Some critics say the biopsychosocial model adds too much 'soft science' and dilutes the biomedical model.[4] Others say that it does not go far enough and would like to add other dimensions to the model, such as a dimension of spirituality.[5,6]

While the biopsychosocial model's intention is to re-humanize medicine by considering additional dimensions, it has a difficult time holding its own against the biomedical and economic rationalist models that dominate in many workplaces. Partly, this may be due to the fact that it is still a model based on science: biomedical science, psychological science and social science. It expands the domain of what are considered valid scientific conceptualizations of human beings, but it is still not a very satisfactory explanation for what constitutes a whole human being. It is a somewhat sterile conceptualization of a whole human being, and it is not a very inspirational model. Also, the biopsychosocial model is primarily a tool to understand, diagnose and contextualize *others*, i.e. patients, rather than a framework that is useful for doctors to understand themselves as well as patients.

Perspectives on the Whole Human Being from Other Fields

Many fields strive to define what comprises a whole human being. Different models of human being grow out of fields of education, business, personal growth and philosophy. This section will examine some different conceptualizations of a whole human being.

The Whole Human Being in Education

Parker Palmer's book, *To Know As We Are Known: Education as a Spiritual Journey*, faces philosophical and spiritual questions around wholeness as they pertain to education. Palmer sees the purpose of education as not just the acquisition of knowledge, but the transformation of the whole student. He sees that this is not possible without the transformation of a whole teacher. He writes that only 'as we see whole can we and our world be whole,'[7] adding that the 'way we interact with the world in knowing it becomes the way we interact with the world as we live in it.'[8] Thus, how we view ourselves determines how we act in the world. If we want to *act* in wholeness, we must be *whole* first.

The Whole Human Being in the New Age

One conceptualization of human being that has become popular since the 1960s is the mind–body–spirit model. This model is commonly used in alternative and complementary disciplines. It does not necessarily eliminate the scientific study of the body, or the psychological study of the mind, but it expands the idea of human being to include a third dimension of spirituality (broadly defined and often including concepts of personal growth). This model preceded the scientific field of psychoneuroimmunology, which gives empirical validation to the idea that the mind and consciousness can affect physical health.

Eastern Conceptualizations of the Whole Human Being

A seven-dimensional model can be found in the chakra system from ancient Hindu thought. It includes physical, emotional, mental, and spiritual dimensions, plus adds dimensions of heart (love and compassion), self-expression and intuition. It postulates the flow of vital energy through different dimensions, or chakras (which means 'wheel' in Sanskrit). The model explains how unseen, universal life energy can manifest in different dimensions. This example of a traditional model of medicine continues to influence many in the West who are interested in a holistic, multidimensional model of human being.

The chakra model has been studied by Carl Jung in *The Psychology of Kundalini Yoga*. In this model, Jung saw 'symbols for human levels of consciousness in general.'[9] He believed that the complexity of the 'self,' which includes many different aspects and dimensions, could be best represented in symbols rather than in linguistic, verbal descriptions (this echoes the section on mysticism in which absolute truth cannot be spoken in words). For Jung, the chakras (spelled 'cakras' in his book)

> symbolize highly complex psychic facts which at the present moment we could not possibly express except in images. The cakras are therefore of great value to us because they represent a real effort to give a symbolic theory of the psyche. The psyche is something so highly complicated, so vast in extent, and so rich in elements unknown to us, and its aspects overlap and interweave with one another in such an amazing

degree, that we always turn to symbols in order to try to represent what we know about it. Any theory would be premature because it would become entangled in particularities and would lose sight of the totality we set out to envisage ... The cakras, then, become a valuable guide for us in this obscure field because in the East, and India especially, has always tried to understand the psyche as a whole.[10]

In the spiritual traditions of the East, the chakras are associated with particular locations within the physical body. Jung at times gives some credence to this in his discussion of common language that references different parts of the body for particular thoughts and emotions. He generally says, though, that the chakras refer more to 'psychical locations'[11] than to physical ones.

The seven-dimensional chakra model has also been adapted by contemporary psychologist Anodea Judith in her book, *Eastern Body, Western Mind*. She describes it as a 'systemic model' that can be used as 'a lens through which we can view the complex problems of the soul's evolution, both individually and collectively.'[12] Judith draws on Jung's work and presents the chakra model as a way of understanding different human dimensions. She sees the chakras as representing 'the organizational structure we create to cope with the world.'[13] She blends Western psychology's view of psychological defenses with the Eastern view of the body to create a holistic mind–body–spirit model.

The seven-dimension model based on the chakra system is also popular in the field of energy healing, as discussed in Barbara Brennan's *Hands of Light*,[14] Susan Matz's series, *The Art of Energy Healing*,[15] and in Richard Gerber's book, *Vibrational Medicine*.[16]

Physicist Amit Goswami discusses the chakra system from a quantum physics perspective in his book, *The Quantum Doctor*. Goswami explains how the concept of universal life energy corresponds to the quantum wave state. A specific dimensional manifestation, like a particular chakra, corresponds to the 'collapse' of the wave function into a particle state. This state, i.e. a particular chakra, is in turn a manifestation of the universal in the form of a particular, boundaried dimensional expression.[17] He states that the chakras 'are those places in the physical body where consciousness simultaneously collapses the vital and the physical in the process of which the representation of the former is made in the latter.'[18] In other words, the chakra system is a mind–body–spirit model that provides a theoretical and conceptual model for how spirit, thoughts, emotion and body can mutually influence each other and interact.

The Whole Human Being in Business

Rick Jarow applies the seven dimensions of the chakra system to creating fulfilling work in his book, *Creating the Work You Love*.[19] Jarow defines fulfilling work as that which a person can bring their whole human being into. Looking at the chakra model, this means that there would have to be physical, emotional, mental, heart, self-expressive, intuitive, and spiritual aspects to work in order for the whole person to be engaged.

I have also used the chakra system as a useful framework for understanding personal growth and clinical work in a class I taught to health professional students, for which I developed an unpublished text called *Finding Your Self*.[20]

Schwartz, Gomes, and McCarthy use a four-dimensional model of physical, emotional, mental, spiritual in *The Way We're Working Isn't Working*.[21] This model has been able to add the spiritual dimension while remaining grounded and practical. The book is not 'new age' (in the negative sense) at all, but rather gives examples using this model in work with international companies such as Google and Sony. The aim of this book is to create a mainstream approach for incorporating dimensions that are often dismissed by the mainstream as irrelevant. There is a growing awareness in business that a sustainable and profitable company must invest in and develop human beings and not just look at human resources as a means to the end of increased short-term productivity.

The Whole Person in Humanistic Psychology

Some models for understanding human experience take a developmental approach, meaning that as a person grows or evolves, their focus shifts from lower dimensions to higher dimensions. For instance, humanistic psychologist Abraham Maslow's 'hierarchy of needs' starts with the dimension of *physiological* needs, such as food, water, and sleep. Once a human being has met these needs, their focus shifts to a different dimension, that of *safety*. Once needs at this dimension are satisfied, a person's focus naturally shifts to *love and belonging*, where the maintenance of relationships, in and of themselves, becomes important. Maslow's next level is *esteem*, in which the focus is on self-esteem and mutual respect with others. Maslow's last level is the one that his work is best known for, *self-actualization*, in which the focus shifts from the material, emotional, and relational needs to morality, creativity, and spiritual needs. What was revolutionary about Maslow's theory was that human beings have basic needs that must be met before being able to focus on 'higher' levels of development. His concept of self-actualization fueled the human potential movement's focus on different modes of spiritual development, such as meditation, yoga, various forms of expressive therapies, body work, and humanistic psychotherapy.[22]

The Whole Human Being from a Philosophy of Consciousness Perspective

Another developmental model can be found in philosopher Ken Wilber's work. He has also proposed a nine-dimensional model of levels or spheres of consciousness. Similar to Maslow's hierarchy of needs, this model presupposes that one must first pass through 'lower' levels in order to be able to develop 'higher' levels. Wilber's levels progress through matter, the body, the mind, the soul, and then spirit. He has broken these levels down further into specific spheres: sensoriphysical (sensation and perception); phantasmaic-emotional (impulse and image); representative mind (symbols and concepts); rule/role-oriented mind (concrete operational); formal reflexive mind; vision-logic (integrative); psychic; subtle; and causal. Wilber has described these levels as a ladder and the climber is the 'self,' who progresses through these stages. He has also suggested that these stages can be viewed as a series of nested spheres in an 'actualization holarchy, each stage of which unfolds and then enfolds its predecessors in a nested fashion.'[23] Wilber has described the relationship between dimensions in his discussions with Tony Schwartz (cited in the above section on business):

> the higher stage always has access to those below it ... Each succeeding level has all the capacities of the previous level, and then it adds something extra. That something extra is what makes it transcending in relation to the previous one. What's negated is not the previous stage but its limitations. Each stage transcends *and* includes.[24]

Wilber further develops this model to include a correspondence between these internal stages within the individual with stages occurring in the physical body, culture, and social worlds.[25] This creates a very complex, holistic system that maps out the growth of consciousness as it interrelates sense of self, physical body, culture, and society.

The Whole Human Being

As can be seen, there are many different models of what it means to be a whole human being that have arisen from the fields of medicine, philosophy, religion, education and business. For the purpose of this book to re-humanize medicine, we need to come to some agreement on how we will define what it means to be a whole human being. This model needs to be broad enough to include important human dimensions, but not so broad as to be unwieldy in clinical practice. The model also needs to be useful for physicians to understand themselves for their own personal growth and to understand their patients' health, illness and personal growth.

The biopsychosocial model is a good start, but it is hard to get too enthusiastic about it as a model for re-humanizing medicine. It does not really include the aspects of human being that are non-scientific and non-rational (for instance, spirituality and compassion). Adding spirituality to this model to get the biopsychosocial-spiritual model is another step in the right direction.

I have chosen in this book to build on the seven-dimensional model from the chakra system that Jung, Judith and others have adapted to Western audiences. This model has great flexibility and utility and has been developed over 4,000 years as a way of describing what it means to be a whole human being. My choice in using this model is based more on the utility of the conceptual model than on any argument about the scientific or metaphysical existence of chakras. In this regard, I follow Jung's precedent of focusing on the psychical and symbolic (or we could say human) aspects of this model, rather than on the metaphysical.

I add to this seven-dimensional model two more dimensions, those of *context* and *time*. The dimension of context allows for inclusion of familial, social, cultural and environmental factors, which are of crucial importance in understanding what it means to be human. The dimension of time reminds us that people grow and change over the course of their lifetimes. This allows for a developmental aspect of human being. This is important if we want to include an aspect of personal growth in medicine. The addition of time and context brings us to a nine-dimensional model.

A nine-dimensional model has a lot of variables to remember, but it gives us a lot of latitude to explore the whole person in medicine. It seems like a nice counterpart to the nine sub-systems of the physical body. It also includes within it the biopsychosocial-spiritual dimensions, as well as the mind–body–spirit dimensions.

I by no means propose that this is the only valid model of what it means to be a whole human being, but I maintain that it is a useful model for medicine. Each dimension could be subdivided further, which is in keeping with a holistic model that is comprised of separate, but interrelated dimensions, in which each part can also be viewed as a whole sub-system. For instance, an anthropologist or sociologist may find that one dimension for context is too limiting and could easily find five or six subdivisions of context. Similarly, a Buddhist monk may find that one dimension for the heart and compassion is too limiting, and could propose that there are multiple dimensions of compassion.

One last important point in understanding the use of a multi-dimensional holistic framework for human being is that each dimension may have different kinds of realities that hold true at its level that may not hold true at another level. This allows for biomedical truth, poetic truth, the truth of compassion and spiritual truth to all simultaneously exist in different dimensions. Rather than trying to reduce all truth to one dimension (such as a reductionist biomedical approach) we can have what Cohen called 'medical pluralism,' the ability to bring multiple models of understanding to the complex issues around human health and illness. It is important to remember in the following discussions that each dimension has its own rules and truths, but is also in interrelationship with all other dimensions. It is a bit like understanding that the chemical and hormonal micro-environment of the kidney is in interrelationship with the rest of the body and that changes could occur in the heart and brain related to changes in the kidney. What is different is that we are not simply looking at chemicals affecting other chemicals, but rather we are looking at how thoughts influence the physical body and how spirituality influences emotions and how the heart influences relationships. Just because the truth and language of one dimension cannot be translated into a biochemical language does not invalidate that dimension as a valid realm to consider in medicine. Human beings deserve a model of medicine that strives for a complex understanding of what it means to be a whole person.

Nine Dimensions of Human Being and Experience

This book will use a holistic framework of human being having nine different but interconnected dimensions:

Physical
Emotional
Mental
Heart and Compassion
Creative Self-Expression
Intuition
Spirituality
Context
Time

The Physical Dimension

The physical body is the aspect of human being that contemporary medicine primarily focuses on. The physical body is a material, observable and very concretely delineated dimension. Contemporary medicine is 'physical body' medicine and it is materialistic. Holistic medicine distinguishes itself from contemporary medicine by recognizing the interconnectedness of the physical body with other human dimensions. Holistic medicine is not materialistic, but includes the material dimension as one of many dimensions, thus it is multidimensional. The more discrete and visible a dimension is, like the physical, the more easily it can be broken down into a taxonomy of visible parts and structures. This is what we have in contemporary medicine with its division of the body into different organs and sub-systems.

The physical body interacts with all the other dimensions, in what Goswami would call upward and downward causation. In other words, dimensions such as mind, body, spirit and emotions mutually influence each other. Research from the social sciences and psychoneuroimmunology show the interrelationship of emotion,[26,27] psychology,[28] social connection,[29,30] creativity,[31] and spirituality[32,33,34] on physical health. Science is beginning to show that non-material human aspects affect the health of the physical, material body. A medical practice that only looks at the observable, physical dimension of human reality is an impoverished practice that ignores many important determinants of health.

The Emotional Dimension

The emotional dimension is much more subjective than the physical dimension. Emotions indicate how people subjectively feel about things rather than an intellectual or objective analysis. Emotions flow between people; they are contagious. They are less 'thing-like' than, say, a liver or an arm, but they are no less real. Emotions have their own language and logic. Psychologist Daniel Goleman has popularized the concept of 'emotional intelligence' to differentiate the realm of emotion from the analytical reasoning that traditional IQ tests measure. Our earlier discussion of poetry and its uses in humanizing medicine speak to the development of emotional intelligence in addition to technical intelligence.

Emotions are fluid, internal experiences generated by a complex multidimensional feedback-mechanism. They are created through the interaction of external events, people's past experiences, conditioning and personality variables such as temperament. We know that the experience of emotions corresponds to changes at the microphysical level through hormones and neurotransmitters. This is not to say that the emotional dimension can be reduced to the physical dimension. Emotions serve as a bridge from the body to the social world of others. While emotions are sometimes broken down into 'positive' and 'negative,' all emotions are part of life and give people feedback about their likes and dislikes, as well as about interactions between internal and external environments.

Patterns of emotional expression can be implicated in illness, both mental and physical. However, emotional expression is also mediated by the context of people's cultural and family upbringings. While emotional expression may vary across cultures, there is a growing body of literature around emotion, social connection and mental and physical health.[26,27,28,29,30]

Sexuality is often considered in discussions of emotion. For instance, in her book, *Eastern Body, Western Mind* Anodea Judith describes the second dimension as that of sexuality, rather than emotion.[35] Emotions are part of sexuality, but so are all the other human dimensions. I do not break sexuality out as a separate dimension, but see it as an expression of the total human being. More specifically, sexuality can be examined in the context of physical relationships and practices, patterns of emotional relatedness, the perspective of love and the heart, spiritual beliefs and social relationships.

The Mental Dimension and the Ego

The mental dimension is even less 'physical' or material than emotions. There is a lot of current research mapping brain images and how they relate to various activities, emotions and cognitive functions. While it is important to study the physical correlates of thoughts and emotions in the brain, we should not forget that each dimension has its own lived experience. If we only try to understand thoughts and emotions from an outer, objective perspective, we miss the truth of inner human experience (e.g. reducing emotional or intellectual experience to what can be seen and measured physically through neurochemistry and brain imaging).

The mind is an interaction of the uniqueness of the individual, with the past experiences and conditioning of that person, along with social and cultural beliefs. The mind is a structured dimension and works to create categories of experience, dividing the world into comparisons and contrasts. It could even be said that the mental dimension tends to divide, whereas the emotional dimension tends to connect. Integrating these two dimensions allows a person to both differentiate oneself from others as well as to be part of a social web of relationships.

Taking this integration even further, the physical, emotional and mental dimensions can be integrated into the ego. The ego is thus a three-dimensional structure that is concerned with the general day-to-day operations of the human organism, but does not understand the 'bigger picture.' It is like a middle manager who runs the day-to-day business, but has no larger appreciation or understanding of the greater economic, social and international perspective of the company, or the reason why the company exists and what its purpose is. The ego is a necessary foundation, but can cause trouble if it is not counterbalanced by a larger perspective. The function of the ego is to optimize the physical, emotional and mental comfort level of the human being. An equally important function of the ego is to maintain open communication; relaying information to the 'upper level management' of the other dimensions whose job it is to understand the 'big picture.'

The Dimension of the Heart, Love and Compassion
The dimension of the heart (we are now discussing the metaphorical heart, not the physical heart muscle) goes beyond the dualistic gain/loss, pleasure/pain orientation of the ego. This level is important in medicine as it is the dimension that allows for the humanitarian action of putting another person's well-

being before one's own. Also, as the principles of holistic medicine remind us, love has an innate healing power. While the emotional dimension connects people with their environment, emotions can have a personal, perhaps even selfish nature. Emotions are more concerned with the feelings a person has about the world than they are with how one's actions affect others and the larger world. In this way, the function of the heart dimension is to provide a larger context beyond the ego and to give feedback and information about interconnection. At the level of the heart, a person is able to 'transcend' the ego, but as Wilber reminds us, this means it 'transcends *and* includes.'[36]

The Dimension of Creative Self-Expression

This level of human being is concerned with creative interaction of the individual with the world. While some might think of self-expression as a 'self-help' issue or artistic function, people are constantly engaged in expressing who they are. Similarly, people can also suppress themselves because of various psychological or social distortions. All human beings are unique and find fulfillment through letting what is within intermingle with the outside world, as they actively create the structure of their lives.

Creativity is an aspect of self-expression. I use 'creativity' in a very broad sense, not just in terms of creating artistic objects, but as a way of describing how people navigate the inspirations of their inner lives and the demands of their outer lives. Dreams, desires, passions and motivations are universal, but how individuals choose to express these inner currents is self-expression. Self-expression is reflected in choice of clothing, hairstyle, decorating sensibility, choice of hobbies and pastimes, choice of friends and partners, choice of career or even how one responds to loss or traumatic events. When life is lived in a creative way, there is a constant balance and interplay between the inner aspects of individuality and the outer aspects of situational context.

In clinical work, this dimension is important for determining whether or not clients are actively engaged in doing what they want to do in their lives, or if they are doing what other people want them to do. A lack of self-expression can often build up into a feeling of being weighed down, being unfulfilled, or even being depressed. Thus, fulfillment in life is a function of this dimension, as is the feeling of lack of fulfillment and depression.

The Intuitive Dimension

Intuition can be thought of as direct knowing without the use of the five senses. Betty Edwards, author of *Drawing on the Artist Within*, defines intuition as 'the power or faculty of attaining direct knowledge or cognition without rational thought.'[37] This dimension provides an understanding of time through instantly connecting past, present and future. Everyone has intuitive ability, although they may or may not listen to it. In both research and clinical practice there are many stories about how intuition can lead to sudden scientific breakthroughs or clinical insight. The dimension of the intellectual mind is largely a function of what is put into it, like a computer. Intuition helps a person connect information in creative new ways.

Intuition is an important aspect of clinical work. Does something just not feel right with a particular client? It is important to be aware of this sense. Also, clients' intuition can be honored by encouraging them to share their own hunches as to what is happening in their bodies and lives, no matter how small or insignificant it might seem to them. This is a great way to expand outside of the clinician's own clinical 'box' by adding new ways of conceptualizing a situation or illness.

The Spiritual Dimension

Spirituality is not the same as religion. Spirituality is a sense of connection with the larger whole of the universe. Meaning and purpose are found through this connection. The current scientific perspective of contemporary medicine does not consider the meaning of why someone gets sick or what one can learn from illness, but a spiritual evaluation of the meaning and purpose of sickness is often quite helpful and profound. For instance, David Tacey writes from a Jungian perspective that, in illness, 'Something "spiritual" wants to manifest in our lives, but it cannot do so. An energy or force is present, but if it cannot be expressed in a spiritual form it gets trapped in the body and leads to sickness.'[38]

Everyone has a spiritual dimension, even atheists. Meaning, understanding and purpose are functions of the spiritual dimension. Similarly, the drive to connect with others, to be part of society, or to have a relationship with the physical world, can all be seen as aspects of spirituality. Many of the issues of existentialism or existential psychology, such as the questions 'Why am I alive?' or 'What is the purpose of my life?', are in the domain of spirituality. Connecting to the spiritual dimension can be done in many different ways, such as playing with kids or pets, walking in nature, discussing life issues with someone, or in specific practices like meditating or engaging in ritual. Some people find spirituality in the context of a living religious practice, although religion is not always inherently spiritual. We can turn again to Tacey, who provides a working definition of spirituality:

We are forever trying to put things into formulas and rules. But I believe the seeking of the spiritual is a personal choice, and we cannot pin it down to any one tradition or code. It is best that we are not too prescriptive about it, and that our definitions are general and broad. For me, spirituality is not merely something we do when we are being self-consciously spiritual. It is the pursuit at all times – and not just in meditation or prayer times – of a particular attitude towards ourselves, the world and others. The attitude is one of reverence, awe, and openness to mystery. The spiritual attitude impels us to search for connectedness, and this search intensifies when we live in disconnected times such as now. There are many kinds of connection, but spiritual connection seeks relationship with something greater than ourselves, something that links us to the cosmos, but also to what is most genuine and true in ourselves.[39]

Tacey's definition of spirituality is actually quite like the definition of holistic medicine used in this book, in that it refers to a state of being and attitude, rather than to a particular practice or technique. The spiritual is about *connection*, as is holistic medicine. In some ways, it could be argued that holistic medicine is the spiritual counterpart to the biological reductionist approach of contemporary medicine. Contemporary medicine is the search for something smaller than the individual, a malfunctioning organ, a chemical imbalance, or a gene, whereas holistic medicine is the search for something larger than these things: for a larger context and meaning for illness in an individual's life. While the philosophy of biological reductionism ignores or invalidates a spiritual approach to health and illness, a holistic approach can include biological reductionism as one dimension among many different ways of understanding. The spiritual dimension can be seen as one pole of the spectrum ranging from physical to spiritual.

The Contextual Dimension

No human being lives outside of context, but the nature and impact of these contexts can vary greatly. The contextual dimension refers to all external influences that act upon and are acted upon by individuals. Elements of the contextual dimension include physical, family, social and cultural environments. These contexts influence the way that individuals express themselves, and can be supportive of or inhibit individuals' health and growth. Finally, all of these dimensions influence individuals and are, in turn, influenced by individuals.

The *physical environment* is important for many reasons. The physical environment influences activity and exercise levels, the kinds of food available, toxic or infectious exposures, and also if there is the risk of trauma, such as war, accidents and abuse. The physical environment is the milieu in which individuals grow. Some environments are more supportive and some are less supportive. Also, just like plants, different individuals may thrive in different environments. What may be traumatizing and overwhelming to one person could be inspiring to another. So, in examining the physical environment, the interactions between individuals and their environments are perhaps more important than simply looking at the environment itself.

The *family environment* is another important context to consider, as it shapes a person's expectations, beliefs, possibilities and expressions. These are important in all fields of medicine in which the goal is to change behavior. Quitting smoking, taking a medicine, exercising, or challenging an abusive or masochistic way of interacting with others all require understanding the context of the behavior. If doctors do not understand the context in which a behavior is occurring, they really do not understand the behavior. For the most part, there is logic to every behavior – once the perceptions, motivations, beliefs and contextual history of a person are understood.

The *social environment* shapes people's expectations and opportunities. A woman growing up in the United States has many more possibilities for her life in terms of profession than a woman who grows up in a society in which women are not allowed to drive and cannot choose their profession (or possibly even have a profession). Most societies are made up of different cultures or subcultures, although in some societies the line between society and culture is more blurred. Social context includes issues like poverty, education, jobs, discrimination, voting rights and the extent to which individuals are able to choose the course of their own lives.

The *cultural environment* is the composite of the collective of many individuals and families who share some commonality. It can be defined as a shared system of meaning. Culture influences expressions of emotion, communication style, gender roles, etc. One major research dimension in studying cultures is that of individualism–collectivism, which we have touched upon in earlier chapters. This dimension is a measure of the extent to which a culture encourages the development of the individual or encourages the development and cohesion of the group. This is not necessarily a dichotomous relationship, as some cultures value individualism in certain contexts and collectivism in other contexts. Understanding the extent to which an individual's cultural context is individualist or collectivist can help a doctor tailor their interventions accordingly. For example, a doctor may meet individually with a client from an individualist culture, whereas it is more appropriate to meet with a larger family unit for a client from a collectivist culture.

Together, physical, family, social and cultural contexts create a complex set of influences on the individual. The focus of medicine is generally on the health of the individual, but these contextual factors greatly influence health. Doctors do not have to be experts in family therapy, or anthropologists in order to take the contextual dimension into account. Doctors who are good and patient listeners and observers will appreciate the influence of the contextual dimension.

The Temporal Dimension

It may seem a bit strange to consider time as a human dimension, but I include it because it challenges physicians to see patients not just as the 'snapshot' of the moment, but as people who have developed over time. Being aware of the dimension of time allows physicians to develop a view of a person's current behavior and situation, and how these may be influenced by past life experiences. We know in psychiatry and mental health that this is extremely important, but it is important any time doctors are confronted with someone whose behavior is difficult to understand or who does not want to follow logical or reasonable medical advice.

The dimension of time works through all dimensions in different ways. There are pathologies, or challenges, of time. For instance posttraumatic stress states result from past (physical/emotional/mental/heart/expressive/intuitive/spiritual/contextual) events, which repetitively ricochet throughout the dimensions of a person, creating patterns of illness. The entire field of psychosomatic medicine can be viewed through such a lens of 'a pathology of time' in which past events manifest as present-day physical sensations caused by echoes of traumatic or overwhelming emotions.

Time is also an important dimension because to have a holistic practice means that you must take time to understand the complex dimensional interactions of your client. Building a relationship takes time. Trust, compassion and mutual understanding take time to build and they are not just aspects of holistic medicine. Spending less time with patients may be correlated with an increase in malpractice lawsuits.[40]

A human being exists in the moment, but is influenced by past life events. Personal growth and development are dimensions that occur over time. Since holistic medicine is not as concerned with returning someone back to who they were in the past (rather it focuses on supporting a person to grow and develop), time is a very important variable. In fact, you cannot have a concept like personal growth without an appreciation of the dimension of time. Similarly, a sense of hope is connected with time, in order to make sense of the past and to envision a future. A dramatically successful intervention for some clients can be simply reminding them of the dimension of time.

Someone who has had many different traumas and abuses may feel stuck in the past and feel that the future will never be any different. It can be life changing when a person understands how the context of the past has influenced their beliefs and actions, and that they can make a different choice in the present.

The Self

The term 'Self,' with a capital 'S,' is often used to denote some degree of wholeness beyond that of the small 's' self, or the ego. This term can be found in the work of Swiss psychiatrist Carl Jung (although he did not capitalize the word),[41] as well as in many other works on personal growth. In this book I will use the term *Self* to denote the aggregate of all human dimensions and their interactions. Self refers to wholeness, the sum total of the individual, not just the contents of the ego, but all aspects, conscious and unconscious, material and sublime. The Self includes each separate, individual dimension, but is also the sum total and synergistic interaction of each of these separate dimensions.

Many authors have written about the concept of *true self* and *false self*. It is beyond the scope of this book to exhaustively review those works, but the concept of Self is definitely valid for my discussion. The concept of Self is as important in examinations of health and illness as it is in discussing personal growth. Disconnection from one's physical body and emotions can lead to illness, and connection can be correlated with health. Disconnection from other people, one's heart, or a sense of spiritual connection can lead to mental and physical morbidity and mortality. Connection is correlated with health. From a holistic perspective, an integrated sense of wholeness in the form of the Self can be seen as innately healing, both for the physician and for the client.

In summary, the nine-dimensional model discussed here will serve in this book as a framework with which to understand a holistic perspective on what it means to be a 'whole' human being. This model applies to the physician or health care professional, as well as the patient. There is nothing particularly magical about choosing nine dimensions for the framework. Some may feel that there should be more or less than nine; others may subdivide the dimensions in different ways.

We have examined many different models of medicine in this book. I feel that this holistic model serves as an excellent framework that includes the best aspects of models commonly used in contemporary medicine (such as the biopsychosocial-spiritual) as well as the best aspects of models from alternative medicine (such as mind–body–spirit, or the chakra model). We will first focus on how this model applies to you, the physician or clinician, as a human being. Then we will use this model as a framework for developing a holistic medical practice in order to re-humanize medicine.

Part III

RE-HUMANIZING YOUR SELF

Overview

As a physician or health professional, you need to be a whole person before you can treat a whole person. Holistic medicine requires *you* to change in order to encourage healing and transformation in your client. This is somewhat similar to the archetype of the wounded healer: it is through healing one's own suffering that one learns the skill of healing.

In contemporary medicine, the person or self of the physician is not considered important, since the power of the treatment is found within the technique. (For the same reason, the person or self of the client is not considered important, either.) In holistic medicine, the self of the physician is the tool through which all techniques and interventions pass. What is considered therapeutic is not just prescribing a medication to change body chemistry, but the actual interaction between the doctor and the patient. This reorientation from an emphasis on technique to an emphasis on people and the healing power of human interaction is a hallmark of holistic medicine.

The following chapters are 'self-help'. The aim is to increase physicians' awareness of how their education and work environments can interfere with their ability to connect with the 'whole' of themselves and their patients. We take up the theme of conditioning and its counterpart, openness to new learning, and I provide a series of re-humanizing exercises. I will at times shift to addressing the reader directly as 'you,' as it is *you* as an individual physician or health care professional who must develop *your own humanity* and interact with the specific humanity of the individual patient with whom you are working. Please do not assume that I am the authority on you, but I have found this framework helpful for my own understanding and practice.

Chapter 6

Physician, Know Thyself

Physician, help yourself: thus you help your patient too. Let this be his best help that he may behold with his eyes the man who heals himself.

Friedrich Nietzsche[1]

Holistic medicine is not just about doing different complementary or alternative techniques; rather holistic medicine is a different perspective and form of connection that you, the physician, bring to clinical work. To practice holistically, we must be more than evidence-based medicine (EBM) technicians. Although technical skills are one dimension of physicians' work, we must approach the full humanity of the person we are working with from the full humanity of ourselves.

Much of medical education (and continuing medical education) focuses on teaching doctors how to perform techniques, such as drawing blood, starting an IV, or how to prescribe a medicine. Techniques such as these are procedures that can be easily taught and replicated, largely through a form of learning called 'conditioning.' Conditioning is a simple form of learning involving the formation, strengthening, or weakening of an association between a stimulus and response. In medical training, a patient with a symptom can be seen as a stimulus and prescribing a medication can be seen as a response.

Techniques are impersonal and objectified ways of interacting. A technique is inherently not holistic, meaning a technique is a procedure that can be applied again and again, regardless of the uniqueness of the client. To re-humanize medicine, a physician needs to be able to perform many different techniques, but care must be taken that this technical dimension is always seen in the larger, holistic context. *Technical training, by conditioning, narrows a person's focus. The narrowly focused thinking associated with technique has a place in medical care, but the practice of medicine is much more than developing a narrow focus.* Every inter-action you have with a client is an opportunity for both of you to grow personally and to develop new modes of connection and ways of working. Perhaps this all seems like common sense, but contemporary medicine has placed such a high value on 'evidence-based medicine' that many other dimensions of human experience are in danger of being ignored or even denigrated by the contemporary scientific and technical mind.

Conditioning and the Medical Technician

Conditioning is a type of learning that creates an automatic, fixed response to a given stimulus or situation. It is the kind of training that is most often used in medical training; however, condi-tioning can impair the physician's ability to function holistically as it creates sub-routines that are performed automatically, without reflective thought.

The earliest studies of conditioning were conducted by Ivan Pavlov, a Russian physiologist. Pavlov conditioned dogs to salivate by ringing a bell each time food was given to them. The dogs eventually salivated when the bell was rung, even if no food was present.[2] The bell became the stimulus and salivation the conditioned response. Another, more recent study done with rats showed that an organism's immune system could be conditioned to respond to a taste. In this case, an immune-suppressant medication was paired with the taste of saccharin. When saccharin alone was given (without the drug), the rats' immune systems still showed suppression.[3]

In this case, saccharin was the stimulus and immune suppression the conditioned response. This is an important study in understanding psychoneuroimmunology and how the brain, mind and immune system influence one another.

Conditioning is a very powerful and valuable method of learning, but like Pavlov's dogs – salivating regardless of whether or not food was present – it can lead to acting without thinking or reflecting on what one is doing. In other words, it is action that is done without conscious awareness.

There are medical emergencies where doctors need to function automatically and unemotionally. For instance, in a 'code' there is a set protocol to follow in order to resuscitate a patient. However, this mode of being does not suit the more complex interpersonal situations in outpatient medicine, which is where the vast majority of medical treatment occurs. Conditioned learning is one of the primary reasons that patients do not feel seen or heard by their doctors. This is because the doctor has already categorized the patient's concerns into a medical algorithm and has lost human connection. The physician really is not seeing or hearing the person in front of them; they are activating a reflex sub-routine to process the situation. This is what Jerome Groopman warns about when he cautions that an over-reliance on evidence-based medicine could be training a generation of doctors to act like machines.

Doctors and professionals are taught many 'facts' during their education. The majority of medical education is based on memorizing rather than on awareness and this knowledge becomes a conditioned belief system. But how can you sort out what you have been taught and what is true in reality? A frequent saying (attributed to a number of different sources – which shows the appeal of the concept) is that half of what is taught in medical school is true and half of it is false; the problem is that we do not know which half is which![4] If we only act in a conditioned way, repeating what we have been trained to think and do, we do not ask ourselves what is true and what is false; we act literally without thinking. Conditioning simplifies awareness of complex issues. It is a reflex arc, a response to a stimulus in which you act automatically, without consideration of the complexities of the situation. Conditioning interferes with your ability to know your Self or to know your client.

Physician, Know Thyself

Human conditioning is pervasive and physicians are an extensively trained and conditioned group of people. This is another way of looking at EBM; it is a conditioning protocol whose goal is uniformity and standardization of physicians' thought and action. The more trained and conditioned someone is, the more they respond the same way in a certain situation. This is a good thing if you are performing a cardiac catheterization by the book. However, if you are only following a conditioned protocol and the person on whom you are doing a surgical intervention has a variation of 'textbook' anatomy you may do the 'right' thing and kill your patient. *You want to be able to balance knowing how to do a 'routine' procedure with routinely being aware of what you are actually doing.* Compared to a non-conditioned behavior, a conditioned behavior can be done automatically, with less conscious awareness. This saves time and energy in 'routine' situations, but it can be dehumanizing if you begin to treat human beings only according to protocol.

Much of medical education is focused on objectivity, which generally means eliminating or ignoring subjectivity. However, to only think and interact from a state of objectivity disconnects a person from a great deal of human experience and human reality. Educator Parker Palmer states, 'we know reality only by being in community with it ourselves.'[5] This is why Palmer argues for respecting and valuing the subjectivity of both students and teacher in searching for truth and in the process of learning. He states that there has been too much emphasis on disconnected objectivity and not enough emphasis on connected subjectivity. Palmer sees subjectivity as the first step in knowing Self, and he sees knowing Self as necessary before being able to connect to others, as well as to community, institutions and society. In the chapter, 'Divided No More,' in his book, *The Courage to Teach*, Palmer explores how choosing to live, learn and teach from a position of wholeness leads to transformation of Self, relationships and even of society. 'We may discover that if one is on an inner journey, one is on the threshold of real power – the power of personal authenticity that, manifested in social movements, has driven real change in our time.'[6]

Education and health care delivery rarely address the development of a unique person with a unique path in life. Most education is training in what is right and wrong, how and how not to act, what to think and what not to think. (Hyman Muslin, one of my psychotherapy teachers, used to complain that students should be *educated*, not *trained*). All this training and conditioning can interfere with knowing who you are. If you do not know who you are, you really cannot be a whole person, and you really cannot practice holistic medicine, but you will be practicing dehumanized medicine.

Most of what people know of themselves and most of what they do is secondary to conditioning. Conditioning is what you are taught to think and do, by your parents, your religion, your friends, your culture and your profession. When you are acting out of a conditioned state, you are not truly expressing your Self; you are simply repeating what you have been told or taught. Conditioned learning and behavior is what Palmer would consider living a divided life, as human consciousness and action are not in relationship with each other.

Rats are conditioned to press a bar to get food. Even after they are no longer getting food, they will continue to press the bar for a long time. All organisms are capable of this type of learning, to pair a stimulus with a response and a behavior with a reward. Human beings learn this way, too. In certain situations, conditioning is not a bad thing. If your Driver's Education teacher did a good job and you paid attention, you will automatically use your turn signal before changing lanes. However, if you automatically prescribe a medicine every time you see a certain symptom, you are not doing your job of evaluating the context of the symptom and whether non-medication options might be more appropriate.

A good physician knows when to let go of conditioning. If we think of conditioning as a way of narrowing focus, we can see that it is useful in some situations, such as performing procedures. However, there are also times when a narrow focus is not appropriate and a physician needs to widen focus.

Conditioned thinking and behavior is not conducive to widening focus. To do this, a physician needs to move beyond conditioning. The narrow focus of conditioning (through EBM and biomedical models) is complemented by the use of a wider, holistic focus that takes into account the complexity of human being. *This is a balance between the certainty of knowing and the uncertainty of learning.*

Conditioning helps doctors to become self-confident; however, one can be overly confident. Over-confidence often takes the form of dismissing the concerns and symptoms of the patient that do not fit into the scientific framework and conditioned theoretical models. Confidence is counterbalanced by curiosity, which is a function of uncertainty. In a state of curiosity, there is a realization that you are venturing into the unknown. In a state of confidence, attained through conditioning, you are always in the realm of the known.

Like the yin/yang balance of Traditional Chinese Medicine, conditioned confidence and unconditioned curiosity work together. The skilled physician is able to move fluidly between these two modes of being. The physician who thinks he or she knows everything is not a good physician. The physician who fears they know nothing is not a good physician. When confidence and curiosity are balanced in good measure, you have an adaptable and capable clinician.

Conditioning can lead to action without awareness. Without

awareness, the physician loses the ability to take in novel information by connecting with the client to get accurate information. It can be said that to practice exclusively on the basis of conditioning and algorithm is to practice disconnected, excessively objective, cold and detached medicine. In other words, to practice solely from conditioning is to live a divided life. But since conditioning is an accepted and necessary part of medical training, how can one get beyond it to live an undivided, fully human life?

Beyond Conditioning:
The Foundations of Being a Whole Person

The spiritual teacher, philosopher and questioner, Krishnamurti, wrote a great deal about what it is to be a whole person. He saw that human beings are conditioned by society, family, culture, knowledge and ideas. This conditioning is always based upon other people's past experiences and is imposed upon and subsequently taken up by the individual in that family, society or culture. Learning that is conditioned in this way shapes individuals. Krishnamurti was concerned with how a human being can become free from social and ideological conditioning, and even free from the conditioning of past experiences. As he wrote, anything 'that is the result of memory is old and, therefore, never free … (t)hought is never new, for thought is the response of memory, experience, and knowledge.'[7] Krishnamurti's words reinforce the idea that conditioning in medicine can limit human engagement.

Krishnamurti often wrote about 'creative thinking,'[8] which he sees as the mind's true nature, its ability to be in the present rather than trying to fit the present into the past. He contrasts this function of creative thinking with knowledge, which is a fixed function of the past. He goes so far to say that 'where the known is, love is not.'[9] This statement is quite appropriate when looking at the way contemporary medicine is practiced. If the only goal of contemporary medicine is *knowing* in the form of diagnosis and intervention, then there is no room for love in this way of practicing. While this is no big loss within the context of contemporary medicine, it is a major loss from the perspective of holistic medicine. *Love as a source of healing* is one of the principles of holistic medicine and there is no chance of truly human connection without love.

The task of being fully human, for Krishnamurti, entails becoming aware that we are conditioned, that we crave the security of the known, that we crave connection to the certainty of the past and that we crave repetition of the past over new experience. Understanding how one is conditioned opens the possibility for creative thinking and true freedom.

Being Open to New Learning

Krishnamurti poses quite a conundrum when we begin to think about how his ideas could apply to medicine and medical education. On the one hand, people go to medical school to learn how to become doctors, but Krishnamurti writes that *where the known is, love is not*. Does that mean that a student learning medicine is losing the ability to love? That argument can be made when we remember the loss of idealism that students experience in medical training.

Samuel Shem's book, *The House of God*, can be read as one young doctor's journey of losing the ability to love through the course of medical training and his re-humanization process to love again. Shem's character, Roy, struggles to live in a hospital environment that promotes numbing, disconnection and dehumanization. Roy gradually becomes an agent of dehumanization. At first this occurs as he strives to learn how to be a doctor in that system, but eventually it is reinforced by his efforts to save himself. By using dehumanization as a tool to save himself, he loses himself – he loses his own humanity. He truly regains his Self by rejecting the cold-hearted approach to patient care and by reconnecting to his whole Self and reconnecting with other people.[10] In contrast to the 'laws of the House of God,' which are algorithms of dehumanization, Shem later developed 'rules for staying human.' Some of these include: 'choose teachers and models who are human; be with patients; and be open to the forces of compassion in the world.'[11]

The dilemma for physicians is that they need to learn what is necessary to be good technically, while also being able to 'set aside' this learning in order to truly connect with their own and their patients' humanity. In this way, they can retain their ability to love and remain open to interact in a way that is not a conditioned response.

Seeing the Forest and the Trees

If Krishnamurti's thoughts seem too philosophical, let's look at a more practical application of learning in terms of decision-making in life and death situations in the wilderness. Laurence Gonzales, author of *Deep Survival: Who Lives, Who Dies, and Why*, describes how the brain works to simplify reality by generalizing from past situations. He argues that simplified and misapplied past learning causes many people to die in crisis situations. Highly trained people with many skills and techniques for survival can do the 'right' thing at the 'wrong' time and die, because they become trapped by their conditioned mental paradigm. In a truly new situation, conditioned learning and action arising from over-reliance on past experience can become a liability. Through the study of wilderness survival stories along with an understanding of cognitive neural science, Gonzales comes to conclusions that echo those of Krishnamurti. Gonzales writes that knowledge 'of the sort you need does not begin with information, it begins with experience and perception. But there is a dark and twisty road from experience and perception to correct action. Unable to understand the forces they engage, unaware of their own position and condition, people can blunder blindly into harm's way.'[12]

Gonzales translates the philosophical question of how we can know ourselves and reality into the practical question of wilderness survival. He states that everyone,

> to one degree or another, sees not the real world but the ever-changing state of the self in an ever-changing invention of the world. We live in a continuous reinterpretation of sensory input and memories, and they are contained in presets that can, at any given moment, light up neural networks in a shifting kaleidoscope of energy, which we come to think of as reality.[13]

In medicine, as well as in the wilderness, life and death decisions are made on the basis of our perception of reality, but this perception is filtered through our 'presets' or conditioning.

Drawing on Your Whole Self

Another perspective on conditioning comes from Betty Edwards and her books *Drawing on the Artist Within* and *Drawing on the Right Side of the Brain*. Based on neuroscience research, her own experience as an artist and her experience as an art teacher, Edwards has come to see that people have two complementary but contradictory modes of perception and functioning. She contrasts *L-mode* (left hemisphere thinking) and *R-mode* (right hemisphere thinking). *L-mode* specializes in naming and categorizing in a linear system of thought that tends to 'rely on general rules to reduce experience to concepts that are compatible with its style of cognition ... uncomplicated by paradox or ambiguity.'[14] In contrast, she describes *R-mode* as a

> style of processing that is nonlinear and nonsequential, relying instead on simultaneous processing of incoming information – looking at the whole thing, all at once. It tends to

seek relationships between parts and searches for the ways that parts fit together to form wholes ... It seems undaunted by ambiguity, complexity, or paradox, perhaps because it lacks the 'reducing glass' of L-mode, which opts for general rules ... R-mode thinking is, almost by definition, difficult to put into words.[15]

There is similarity between the focus of contemporary, evidence-based medicine and the *L-mode*, and holistic medicine and the *R-mode*. Many of the criticisms of holistic medicine by contemporary medicine can be seen as *L-mode* critiques of *R-mode* functions, and vice versa. In this light, a physician must have highly conditioned techniques as well as the ability to set aside this mode of thinking in order to appreciate the complex, creative and paradoxical aspects of human life. In fact, if we listen to Edwards speak about drawing as if she was talking about medical practice, the following quote seems quite appropriate:

The ideal role of the right hemisphere ... is to provide access to the deepest levels of one's true experience and to serve as a reality check against the left hemisphere's tendency to make up stories when it does not really know the answers. The ideal role for the left hemisphere is to be an articulate spokesperson for all the information that comes up from the right and to discriminate between what's important and what is merely trivial. Each mode of thinking is incomplete without the other. You need access to both hemispheres to be whole.[16]

Edwards argues that the right and left hemisphere of the brain need to work together in order to have a balanced and complex view of reality. She describes the two modes as being able 'to work in a cooperative, complementary way while at the same time retaining their individual styles of thinking,' nevertheless, 'these styles of thinking are fundamentally different and can ... (each) view reality in its own way ... (having) ... different or even conflicting responses to the same event.'[17] So it is with contemporary and holistic medicine; both are necessary to understand and interact with the whole human being of the patient, but there can be times when holistic and contemporary views seem to conflict. If we look at the tension between contemporary and holistic medicine from Edwards' viewpoint, the challenge becomes more of balance than a fixed choice of 'one' versus the 'other.' Just as there has long been a tension between the art and science of medicine, Edwards reminds us of the harmonious tradition of two opposing systems of knowledge co-existing throughout human history, through 'the intellect or through the emotions; through logical analysis or through metaphorical synthesis ... Yin and Yang, rational and poetic, abstract and concrete, scientific and imaginative.'[18]

Conclusion

It seems that a big part of being a whole person is being aware that your perceptions and your knowledge are conditioned. In recognizing the limitations conditioning places upon you, you can start to free your mind for creative thinking which allows for continually constructing new mental maps of your Self and reality. This will help you to have a deeper and fuller experience of your Self and a more accurate experience of reality. This, in turn, will make you a better doctor. As an added benefit, your drawing might improve and you will have a better chance of surviving in the wilderness.

Chapter 7

Transforming Your Self

Holistic medicine accepts that we are multidimensional beings whose health resides in more than the state of our biochemistry and organ systems ... Its essential aim is transformational; both practitioner and patient are changed in the process.
Vincent Di Stefano[1]

The most important tool that you have in medicine is you, your Self. From the solid base of your whole Self, you can work with the whole Self of individual patients. In a holistic framework the same rules for healing and transformation apply to you, the physician, as well as the patient.

Previous chapters have warned about contemporary medicine's potential for dehumanization of doctors and patients alike. We will now focus on re-humanization through a *counter-curriculum* to promote and maintain all dimensions of your Self.

For thousands of years, many spiritual, philosophical and psychological traditions have focused on the central question of self-transformation. Although not developed specifically for medical practitioners (their wisdom is for anyone and everyone), they do suggest a way forward within the context of contemporary medicine.

Historically, in medicine, professionalism (as opposed to learning the role of technician) has always been part of medical education. Professionalism is concerned with the transformation of the Self of the practitioner to a different mode of being from that of the lay person or business person. With a focus only on technical skill and knowledge, we risk losing the transformative work of professionalism.

This chapter examines self-transformation through different disciplines and traditions. It then suggests exercises and approaches that can be used for transforming and developing the nine dimensions of human being.

A History of Self-Transformation

Many spiritual, psychological and philosophical traditions speak of the concept of 'Self' compared to 'self.' While the terminology may differ, the core concept is similar across all these traditions, both ancient and modern. The focus is to grow from a limited experience of 'self' to an expanded experience of 'Self.' In the context of this book we can think of 'self' as the dehumanized version of 'Self.'

Hinduism and Buddhism both promote the growth of the individual's consciousness from identification with the ego to a more expanded sense of Self. This occurs over the course of multiple lifetimes through reincarnation. In Hinduism there is the concept of 'Atman,' or a larger, world soul. For instance, the teaching 'thou art that' promotes an identification of the self with larger reality (in other words, Self). Buddhism similarly emphasizes moving beyond the orientation of seeking pleasure/avoiding pain to a more compassionate perspective and experience of Self as something larger than ego. It is believed in Buddhism that the pursuit of pleasure and the avoidance of pain creates suffering through craving and attachment. Through understanding the causes of suffering, it is believed that one can transcend suffering by obtaining a larger perspective.

Christianity also teaches moving beyond the selfishness of the ego to a more open-hearted and loving perspective. The *foundational* model described by Arbuckle draws on Christian tenets such as care for the poor and sick, humanitarianism and social justice. In fact, Arbuckle cites the story of the Good Samaritan as the central myth or archetype of the foundational model.

In chapter one, we examined a quote by Jewish theologian and philosopher Martin Buber, and his concept of I–Thou compared to I–It relationships could be seen in this same light of moving from the smaller I–It relationship to the larger and more complex I–Thou relationship.

Like many mystical traditions, Sufism, a branch of Islam, focuses on unity with the divine. This entails moving beyond the confines of the ego or more narrow self until there is no separation between the individual and God.[2]

The training of Native American shamans and traditional African healers has been described as overcoming 'ego-centrism' through 'ego sublimation.'[3] Thus, we can see that many world religions value this concept of moving from an egocentric to a more expanded spiritual perspective.

In psychoanalysis and psychotherapy, it is common to speak of different aspects or dimensions of self. Freud viewed the ego as having to balance between the instincts of the id and the admonishments of the super-ego or conscience. In Freudian terms, the neurotic self could be viewed as the limited 'self' and the psychoanalyzed 'Self' as an expanded awareness of one's unconscious motivations. Donald Winnicott, a British psychoanalyst, wrote about 'false self' constructions of defensive 'as if' personalities compared to a 'true self.'[4]

Swiss psychiatrist Carl Jung's description of the limited self and the expanded Self are similar to many religious and spiritual perspectives, which is not surprising as he had his own mystical experiences and drew from religion, philosophy and psychology in developing his theories. Jung viewed the limited self as that of the conscious ego and claimed that the expanded Self could come about through an activation of the unconscious in the ego, postulating an open line of communication between the limited perspective of ego consciousness and the activation of symbols and archetypes of the collective unconscious. Jung actually felt that the purpose of illness and psychotherapy was to facilitate individuation, which he defined as the process of enlarging one's consciousness from a limited to a more expanded perspective. In fact, from a Jungian perspective, it could be said that the purpose of life is the process of individuation: the movement toward the greater awareness and wholeness of the Self.

Many New Age philosophies also speak of this distinction between a small self and a larger Self. Transpersonal psychology has one foot in psychology and one foot in the spiritual and seeks to encourage the growth of limited individuality into expanded Self-awareness.[5] Different forms of energy healing modalities integrate spirituality and mysticism with concepts of psychological self-understanding, with the goal of expansion of consciousness and personal growth.[6,7] Many of these different disciplines and perspectives speak of psychological/energetic defenses as the *False Self*, a misidentification of consciousness with the limited or distorted aspects of self. In contrast, there is the concept of a *True*, or *Higher Self*, which is one's ability to balance an awareness of multiple dimensions of Self beyond those of the ego.

The conceptual framework used in this book is consistent with the conceptualization common to many religious, spiritual, philosophical and psychological perspectives, that there is a limited form of self and a more expanded experience of Self and that the movement from self to Self is transformative and healing. The movement of self to Self also provides a way of understanding dehumanization and re-humanization. *Dehumanization narrows the experience of Self to self. Re-humanization is the process of expanding self to Self.*

The concept of Self introduces several issues. The self/Self distinction is consistent with the scientific findings of social psychology, cognitive neural science and various traditions of mysticism: what we are conscious of is a limited version of reality.[6,8,9,10,11] 'Limited' consciousness is not 'bad,' but is rather a starting point to grow into the greater awareness of the Self. So the first issue in transforming self to Self is to be aware that we have a tendency to distort and limit our experience of Self – we limit our full humanity. This, in turn, limits our ability to fully experience our own true nature, the true nature of another person and ultimately the true nature of the world and reality. When one is operating from the self, the ability to have empathy, compassion and a sense of connection with the larger whole of humanity and the larger context of the Earth is limited. One transcends limitation by adding awareness, not by negating limited awareness. This is the root of the holistic paradigm, that there are multiple dimensions and that each dimension taken in isolation is limited. Each dimension has different rules and laws and strengths. Strength becomes weakness when it is not counterbalanced by the strengths of other dimensions.

The ego, described earlier in this book, forms the core experience of identity for most people in their everyday lives. It is a limited, three-dimensional experience of reality consisting of physical, emotional and mental awareness. The ego also is the source of many of the psychological defenses that are used to distort experiences of other dimensions into the language of personal pleasure, comfort and gain through seeking pleasure and avoiding pain. The ego could be considered an example of limited 'self,' in that it consists of an experience of a limited experience of Self. Many spiritual traditions speak of *transcending the ego*, but a holistic view would be to integrate the other human dimensions with those of the ego – as Wilber described a process that 'transcends *and* includes.'[12]

Everyone has the ongoing choice to approach Self (and through Self, reality) from a perspective of either limitation or openness. A reductionist approach would be to experience reality from one-dimensional materialism or a limited-dimensional perspective, such as the three-dimensional approach of the ego of body-emotion-mind. A holistic approach to reality would be to recognize the tendency toward limitation and to choose openness and multidimensional inclusiveness. Limited, narrow, scientific focus would still be useful for specific tasks, but it would be used strategically, with awareness that using a scientific lens blinds one to many human dimensions. Science and evidence-based medicine would be tools that are picked up, used and then set down again until next needed. It is the ability to be aware of one's potential for regressing to a limited perspective, as well as to be aware of one's potential of opening to a multidimensional perspective that forms the template for transforming self to Self.

How Can the Knower Be the Known?

The ongoing transformation of self to Self occurs through learning about your blind spots, limitations and distortions. However, how do you become aware of that of which you are unaware? How can you be aware of yourself as a perceiving subject when the object you are trying to perceive is yourself? 'How can the knower be the known?'[13] This ancient Hindu question from the *Brihad-Aranyaka Upanishad* illustrates the difficulty of the perceiver's attempts to perceive itself and the conundrum of self-knowledge.

Many traditions that have recognized this dilemma of knower and known have also proposed various solutions. One can receive feedback from outside the ego. Context is known through the organs of perception and the mind, and both are subject to distortion through the limitations of the physical organs or the psychological defenses of the ego. However, the Self is a larger perspective than the ego. It can thus provide a larger context and provide feedback to illuminate the blind spots, limitations and distortions of the ego. This requires engagement with the world in a continuous feedback loop. Some form of a mirror is needed to reflect the internal back to you through the external. Spiritual and contemplative traditions include many techniques for developing a deeper awareness of Self, such as meditation, prayer, communing with nature, or even the Native American vision quest.

Contemporary methods of reflection can be found in many forms of psychotherapy or self-help groups, which all have various systems of thought that are used for giving you a reflection of who you are and why you do what you do. Also, you can work to develop a conscious attitude using life, itself, as a mirror that reflects back to you your recurrent and repetitive blind spots, limitations and distortions.

The Buddhists often use the analogy of a mirror for your consciousness. However, this mirror requires constant polishing to reflect without bias. To transform (or 'know') one's Self requires both an inward mirror (observing your inner world) and an outward mirror (observing your external actions).[14] I suppose you could then say you would need a third mirror to observe interactions between inner and outer, but where would it end? How many mirrors would you need in order to fully observe and know your Self? It is a profoundly humbling experience to come to the understanding that one's perspective and knowledge can never be beyond the taint of ego-distortion or varying shades of misperception and misunderstanding of reality. It is for this reason that a wise person is constantly seeking feedback from inner and outer sources and reference points. Stephen Hall, in his book on wisdom, traces back to Socrates 'an essential and indeed profound aspect of true wisdom: recognizing the limits of one's own knowledge.'[15] For this reason, the wise person is always suspicious of claims of absolute knowledge.

Be Careful What You Wish For

A major caveat is necessary here. Many people start on self-improvement only to become trapped in another limited and restrictive belief system. It is possible to set off on the path to Self, only to end up creating a new version of limited self that is egoistic, disconnected and based on the dualism of superiority/inferiority. The attempt to make one's self 'better' can end up creating another limitation. People easily fall victim to thinking that they are more 'evolved,' 'better,' more 'developed,' even more 'human' than other people. Self-improvement schemes, whether on an individual or a group level, can lead to the creation of a new, narrow, fixed and rigid self-concept.

In 1962, Michael Murphy co-founded Esalen, an educational and experiential community dedicated to exploring multidisciplinary methods for promoting personal growth. Tony Schwartz writes that 'Esalen has served for thirty years as the primary testing ground for new approaches to the search for wisdom in America.'[16] And writing of Murphy's influence in the US: 'More than any single person, Murphy is responsible for the birth of the human potential movement.'[17] Murphy has written a tome on human transformation called *The Future of the Body*. He understands the risk involved in self-development and cautions that all 'programs for human betterment can be undermined by ignorance, incompetence, or moral perversity.'[18] He lists four destructive effects of any transformative practice, whether it is based on religion, spirituality, psychology, martial arts, exercise program or any therapeutic discipline, stating:

1. A practice can reinforce limiting traits, preventing their removal or transformation.
2. A practice can support limiting beliefs, giving them greater power in the life of an individual or culture.
3. A practice can subvert balanced growth by emphasizing some virtues at the expense of others.
4. A practice can limit integral development when it focuses on partial though authentic experiences of supraordinate reality.[19]

Murphy's warning is helpful to remember given our goal of transforming Self, practice, and medical culture. We can view medical education as a transformative and therapeutic endeavor that aims to change a lay person into someone who thinks and acts like a doctor. In fact, we can even use Murphy's critique of self-development programs for understanding how medicine can be dehumanizing, particularly his point that a *'practice can subvert balanced growth by emphasizing some virtues at the expense of others.'* Just as contemporary medicine emphasizes the physical body, science and objectivity at the expense of subjectivity, interconnection and the non-material reality, any educational or therapeutic endeavor whose goal is to change the way people think, act, or treat others runs the risk of leading to imbalanced development, which broadly speaking can be considered dehumanization.

It is with this awareness that I have been reluctant to include a 'list of things to do to be holistic,' as that seems very un-holistic. However, I do feel it is necessary to give some examples of things that you can do to develop awareness of different dimensions of the wholeness of your Self. While awareness is transformative, I want to caution against getting too caught up in self-improvement schemes, as those often quickly devolve into the all-too-human feelings of 'If I can make myself do this, I will be a better, healthier, more whole person.' Action should grow out of awareness and love, not out of a mental belief or technique imposed upon you or any other human being to reach some mental ideal. Science fiction author Philip K. Dick cautioned about the risks of trying to make a human being comply with some fixed concept:

> The reduction of humans to mere use – men made into machines, serving a purpose that although 'good' in the abstract sense has … employed what I regard as the greatest evil imaginable: the placing on what was a free man who laughed and cried and made mistakes and wandered off into foolishness and play, a restriction that limits him … to the fulfilling of an aim outside of his own personal – however puny – destiny.[20]

Dick writes that this restriction is engineered by men who are 'ideologically oriented' and trained in 'the use of technique' and 'armed with devices' and 'the use of these devices strikes them as a necessary ... method of bringing about some ultimately desired goal.'[20] While Philip K. Dick was often concerned with dystopias of social, political, psychological and even perceptual control, his words are relevant for any form of self-improvement scheme that has 'good' intentions. Transformative concepts and techniques should ideally assist in the individual developing greater Self-awareness, not in them becoming copies of someone else's idea of what the 'Self' should be. Philip K. Dick's writing often includes psychiatrists and physicians who are sometimes forces of humanization and other times forces of dehumanization. The distinction seems to be determined by whether the physician shows compassion and encourages people to become unique, self-determined individuals, or whether the physician seeks to turn patients into passive, controlled objects – in Dick's terminology, 'androids.' According to Philip K. Dick, the important point is whether an individual is pursuing and fulfilling a personal destiny or has taken on someone else's idea of what his or her destiny *should* be.

In the following sections, we will review a nine-dimensional model of human being, looking at each level in more depth. Please bear in mind that any true transformation will affect multiple dimensions, as each dimension is in relationship with all other dimensions. You may find that you prefer certain dimensions to others. It is natural to have some dimensions with which you are more comfortable.

I offer examples and exercises as suggestions for how you, as a physician or clinician, can develop a holistic awareness of Self. These are meant in the spirit of self-exploration and not as a list of rules to be followed. These exercises are in italics in the text.

Please do not take the following discussions to be a list of things you *must* do or as a specific path you must impose upon yourself. Rather, consider the examples and exercises as a set of concepts and possibilities to explore. Acceptance of who you are is a major part of implementing any change. This may sound paradoxical – that you have to accept what it is that you wish to change. However, the goal of holistic medicine is to develop the ability to see the whole reality of your client, and you can do this only by experiencing the whole reality of your Self. You can learn to use your Self as a tool for reflecting the reality of your client, but as with any mirror, it requires periodic cleaning and polishing to give a true reflection.

Transforming the Body

Your body is the physical manifestation of your Self. There are a variety of ways that you can support your body and deepen your connection to it. These include physical exercise, mindfulness and meditative practices, somatic therapies and awareness of nutrition. Adequate sleep, rest and relaxation are also necessary for the health of the physical body.

Everyone needs physical movement to maintain the body. Muscles maintain their strength and grow through use. A lack of use leads to atrophy and loss of strength and stamina. A holistic practice would always include some form of regular physical exercise. This could be going to the gym, walking, swimming, playing outdoor games with the kids, or engaging in various sports.

It is good to have a balance of different kinds of exercise. Anaerobic exercise, like weight lifting, builds muscle and bone strength. Aerobic exercise strengthens the cardiovascular system and tones the body. Body awareness and stretching exercises, like yoga, tai chi and mindfulness, develop flexibility and balance, and promote a sense of mind–body connection. As you begin to think in a holistic way, you can see that any intervention, technique, or activity that you undertake at one level will also affect other dimensions. Exercise can even be considered a form of treatment of obesity, diabetes, high blood pressure, high cholesterol and pain conditions. Weight-bearing exercises, like weight lifting, help strengthen bones and may help prevent osteoporosis. There are numerous studies that show the benefit of exercise on seemingly non-physical dimensions of emotion and mind, such as dementia, anxiety, depression and even attention deficit disorder. The book *Spark*, by John Ratey and Eric Hagerman, describes how exercise has a beneficial impact on medical and psychiatric conditions, as well as on basic processes like learning, memory and academic performance.[21] The body is a base for all of your other dimensions and taking care of your body provides a stronger platform for your emotions, mind and whole Self.

There are a number of exercises that are more meditative in nature, as well as being practices of physical activity. Yoga and tai chi not only bring your focus to your physical body, but also slow down your mind and promote a sense of integration. While in the West yoga is often practiced as a physical exercise, its original purpose was more than simple calisthenics and included development and integration of the mind, body, emotions, heart and spirit.

Yoga was developed by mystics in ancient India who found that their bodies would atrophy after prolonged bouts of seated meditation. In order to keep up their physical strength while they pursued spiritual enlightenment, hatha yoga was developed. Physicist turned 'quantum activist' Amit Goswami states that the 'Sanskrit word yoga means "union" or "integration,"' and he describes how yoga is a holistic paradigm that has many dimensions, such as *hatha yoga* (sequences of different physical postures), *jnana yoga* (the development of wisdom), *karma yoga* (action in the world), *bhakti yoga* (the cultivation of love) and *pranayama yoga* (breathing exercises).[22]

Tai chi is another physical and meditative discipline that combines physical movement, energetic awareness and meditation. Many martial arts have an emphasis on meditation and calming the mind in order to develop clearer awareness of the physical realm in conflict. There is a distinction between internal and external martial arts. Internal martial arts focus on conflict and resistance within consciousness and the Self. External martial arts focus more on managing conflict and resistance of physical bodies in space. Ultimately, to develop fluid and strong physical movement requires open and flexible consciousness. The combination of internal and external martial arts leads to the most effective physical action. Physicians can learn from this balance of inner and outer development to support effective management of physical bodies. We are trained to engage in external action, but little attention is given to the inner medicine of the Self.

There are many different somatic therapies that incorporate moving the body in different ways or of developing body awareness for therapeutic purposes. Massage therapies, chiropractic, osteopathic, somatic psychotherapy and various energy therapies are all examples of therapies that are aimed not only at aligning, balancing, or relaxing the physical body, but also at balancing the relationship of the body to emotional, intellectual and other dimensions.

Meditation and mindfulness practices, even seated ones in which you are not moving your physical body, have a strong physical awareness component. Physical breathing is the starting point of many meditative practices. Mindfulness is a relatively 'new' term for an old tradition of shifting and balancing consciousness. The field of mindfulness grows out of ancient meditative, mind–body–spirit traditions, but has merged with Western psychology and is now a well-researched intervention for a number of disorders, as well as a tool for enhancing well-being. Jon Kabat-Zinn's classic book, *Full Catastrophe Living*, discusses studies documenting numerous health benefits and includes an eight-week program in mindfulness.[23] Lee

Lipsenthal's book *Finding Balance in a Medical Life* has a chapter summarizing research on mindfulness that has used doctors, students and residents as subjects. Findings include improved immune function, decreased depression and anxiety, increased spirituality and empathy, improved knowledge of the effects of stress and greater positive coping skills.[24]

Dietary and lifestyle modification can have a tremendous impact on well-being and disease processes, such as obesity, diabetes, hyperlipidemia, heart disease, depression and anxiety, just to name a few. Yet, diet and lifestyle changes are notoriously difficult for patients to follow through with, as most doctors know. Nevertheless, every physician should have the skills to explain basic diet and nutritional information to clients, such as a diabetic diet or a diet to lower lipids. They should also know how to counsel on basic weight loss (increase exercise, decrease calories, shift from empty calories to nutritive calories, decrease intake of certain foods, but do not create a sense of deprivation through over-restricting as this leads to rebound bingeing). Unfortunately, not all physicians are trained in even basic nutrition and need to learn this on their own. Also, there are so many fad diets that it is difficult to know where to start. People also may vary in what balance of foods are right for their particular body, stage of life, and activity and stress level. Balance, moderation and high-quality food are probably the most important. Two authors whose work I have found useful are Dean Ornish's work on low-fat diets for reversing heart disease and Barry Sears 'Zone Diet' which might be better for blood sugar issues.

Personally, I learned a lot about nutrition from 10 years of following an ovo-lacto vegetarian diet. I started reading about nutrition prior to going to medical school, so I was already learning about nutrition and health prior to becoming a doctor. I was shocked when a medical student I was teaching (a future surgeon) told me that she did not need to learn anything about nutrition. 'I'll just refer to a dietician,' she said. It seemed that she felt learning about nutrition would compete with the 'important stuff' of learning about surgery. I wondered whether there might have also been a degree of superiority that surgery was more important than counseling about diet and nutrition.

Everyone has a body and patients will look to physicians for advice in maintaining the health of their body. If you have not had any formal training on nutrition during your medical education, you can still learn a lot even if you took a month of your spare time and looked through a book or two, or surfed the web for a few hours. Personal experience is even better. If you really want to learn about nutrition, try a couple of different diets yourself for a few months and see how you feel (the Mediterranean diet is quite nice). You will also have a lot more compassion and patience with your patients when they struggle with lifestyle changes.

While this discussion has mostly been about working with lifestyle modification, a physical approach would also include the majority of contemporary biomedical techniques of surgery and pharmaceuticals that aim at restoring the structure and function of the body at the organ or chemical level. Even contemporary psychiatry, which is generally thought to focus on the dimensions of emotion and thought, is predominantly concerned with the physical 'machinery' of neurotransmitters in the body and their correlation with emotions and thoughts. In this sense, contemporary, biological psychiatry really is more an approach to working with the physical body than working with the dimension of emotion or mind.

Physical Awareness Exercise

Begin by sitting in a comfortable place. Start by bringing your awareness to your breathing, the steady in-and-out of air through your lungs. You may just sit, noticing your breath, for several minutes.

When you are ready, allow your focus to gradually expand. You can allow your awareness to move through your body, noticing places of tensions and relaxation. With your mind's eye you can 'visit' each part of your body, even internal organs. Generally just allow your awareness to expand to your whole body. Do not let yourself get caught up in worrying about pain and discomfort; those are part of body awareness. Just notice where you have pain, stiffness or discomfort. This exercise is not causing those sensations; it is just bringing these sensations that were already there to your awareness. Also, do not fight your mind if it wanders; just gently bring your awareness back to your physical body (the purpose of the mind is to wander and wonder).

After visiting each part, individually, allow yourself to develop an awareness of how all the different parts of your body fit together into a whole. Feel the weight of your whole body on the chair. See if you can imagine your body feeling more and more connected, more and more solid, and more and more heavy. Return back to your breath and see if you can bring a sensation of your breath moving throughout your entire body, spreading outward from the center of your body to the top of your head, the tips of your fingers, and the tips of your toes. Allow your breath rate to find a comfortable rhythm and enjoy the sensation of being alive and in your body.

Transforming the Emotions

Emotions are a source of information about yourself, the world and the interaction of yourself and the world. You can get into difficulties in your life by relying only on emotion as your source of information and you can get into difficulties by blocking out this level of information about yourself and the world.

Emotions tend to arise quickly and to abate quickly. It is generally your own resistance to feeling emotions that causes them to linger. Grasping after positive emotions and trying not to feel negative emotions actually starts to interfere with the arising and abating of emotion. Sometimes I think of emotion as a wave that peaks and then subsides. Disorders of anxiety and depression, as well as more subtle difficulties with accepting internal and external reality, can be seen as an imbalance in this natural process of receiving a signal and then cleaning off the message board so that the next signal can come through clearly.

Psychotherapy, including self-help groups like the many 'anonymous' groups, mindfulness, meditation and the expressive arts can all help to point out where you get stuck by either clinging to or avoiding emotions. These practices can help you to develop emotional awareness. By practicing acceptance of your emotions through emotional awareness, it gets easier to feel emotions, to gather emotional information and to move on to the next experience in your life.

Psychotherapy is the classic, therapeutic way of working with emotions in contemporary Western society. One of the hallmarks of this approach is that it teaches you that your emotions are just one part of your larger Self. Psychotherapy helps you to feel your emotions and in doing so to allow your emotions to be part of the larger context of your Self. Many forms of psychotherapy will focus on balancing the extremes of people's psychological defenses which either over-value emotion (relating only through emotion) or under-value emotion (denying emotional reality). Talking with a trusted friend can also help you to connect to your emotions. The difference between talking to a friend and psychotherapy is that therapy intensively focuses on learning and personal growth. This is often a part of friendship, but it is not often the sole focus.

Like psychotherapy, many types of meditation and mindfulness work to develop a larger perspective of Self from which to observe emotions and thoughts as transient states. Meditation creates space for the unconscious emotions to come to consciousness. It also allows an experience of Self that is more than the compulsive associations of thoughts.

The expressive arts and even art therapy can be ways of

getting in touch with your emotions. Activities like painting, journaling, writing, sculpture, dance and drawing create space in your life for your emotions to be felt and recognized. As physicians, we can be so busy all day long managing other people's emotions that we do not really know how we feel about something unless we slow down, stop 'managing,' and give ourselves the time and space to connect to our own emotions.

There are many different techniques and exercises to connect to your emotional dimension. The main point is to use emotional awareness to engage in the world, to live your life and to be in relationship with other people. It is a real skill to be able to discriminate between when you need to go more deeply into an emotion to experience it and when you are actually clinging to an emotion. Many of the methods reviewed in this section can help you to distinguish between experiencing and clinging. When you feel stuck, you can always utilize the dimensions on either side of the emotional dimension to get perspective. Physical exercise can help you metabolize emotions and get a clearer picture of what you feel. Using mental logic can also give you a different perspective on your emotions.

Emotional Awareness Exercise

Start by sitting in a comfortable place and taking a few deep breaths to settle in. Now, focus on the level of your feelings and emotions. As you create a space for your emotions, you may notice sadness, happiness, peacefulness, stress, tension, or even fear that you will not be able to do this exercise 'correctly.' The challenge in this exercise is to allow your emotions to move and change, to swell and ebb. Sometimes it can even be helpful to name the emotion as you feel it: 'Oh, now I am feeling sad for some reason ... now I am remembering someone I miss very much ... now I am remembering a happy time with that person ... now I am feeling tense because I am aware of a stressful meeting I have tomorrow.' Remind yourself that emotions are natural forms of connection and information about yourself and your environment. You are meant to feel all emotions.

If you feel like you are getting stuck on one particular situation or emotion, that may be an important emotion and you may wish to return to it at a later point. Having a few different emotional 'stretching' exercises you can do, like running through the full range of emotions, can be quite helpful when you get stuck. For instance, imagine a time you felt very happy. Let yourself sink deeper and deeper into that situation and emotion; feel the different variations of emotion that arise. Then, imagine something you found very funny. Imagine a time you felt very angry ... Imagine a time you were very sad ... Imagine a time that you were scared ... Imagine a time that you were very excited about something ... Imagine a time when you felt at great peace. Once you have run through a series of emotions, you might feel you have a broader emotional context and this might help you have a new perspective on whatever it was that you felt stuck in.

Transforming the Mind

Western culture is a very mental culture. This is why many books on meditation will focus on taming, or quieting the mind, rather than on strengthening it. While contemporary medicine tends to glorify the mind through science and 'evidence-based' techniques, many personal growth and spiritual perspectives tend to demonize the mind as the 'problem' that holds back awareness and growth. The goal is the middle path of balance: to fully utilize the mental dimension, but not to let it dominate other ways of being.

Developing the faculties of the mind leads to the development of a sense of one's individual identity separate from family, culture and society. Also, the practice of science largely grows out of the mind's ability to separate variables, to break a whole into its component parts and to develop objectivity. Organization, policy, procedure, protocol – all these qualities arise from the mental dimension. Yet, there is an optimal balance of structure and organization with flexibility and flow. The goal of transforming your mind, therefore, is in achieving a balance of mental activity with physical, emotional, heart, self-expression, intuition and spirit.

Meditation is also a great way to contextualize emotions and thoughts in relation to the larger Self. Fluctuating thoughts are the primary reason that people say they 'cannot' meditate. However, a chattering mind is a universal reality. That is the purpose of the mind – to make mental connections between anything and everything. Meditation teaches the ability to accept the chatter of the mind and then to develop a larger perspective in which one's identity is not at the level of the mind, or ego. Instead, thoughts are part of the larger Self, which includes the ego while also expanding beyond it. Thoughts are constantly happening and the Self's job is to employ thoughts when they are useful and to allow them to go about their business in the background when other dimensional awareness is more useful.

Thinking can go awry, though. The field of Cognitive Behavioral Therapy (CBT) is a form of psychotherapy that focuses on examining how people's thoughts influence their feelings and behavior. CBT focuses on identifying irrational thoughts, such as negative thinking, predicting the future and over-generalizing from one situation to another. Unlike psycho-dynamic or psychoanalytic psychotherapy, which focus on the role of unconscious emotions, CBT focuses on addressing patterns of thinking that lead to distortions of reality, which in turn contribute to depression, anxiety and other forms of unhappiness. Mark Epstein, a psychiatrist and Buddhist practitioner, has an interesting book called, *Thoughts without a Thinker: Psychotherapy from a Buddhist Perspective*, which looks at some of the ways that Buddhist meditation parallels CBT and other forms of psychotherapy.[25]

You do not need to be in psychotherapy or formally study meditation in order to understand the nature of your thoughts and mental dimension. You can develop this ability through many informal processes as well. For instance daydreaming, journal writing, walking in nature and watching your thoughts, contemplating, or any activity that allows your thoughts to flow freely helps to clarify the mental dimension.

Mental Awareness Exercise

Sit in a comfortable place and take a few deep breaths. Focus your awareness on your thinking. Notice what it is like to think. Watch how your thoughts form and how one thought leads to another. Notice how your thinking has a tendency to turn on itself and starts to judge your thoughts or attach to them. (You may notice that certain thoughts also bring a swell of emotion or that at times you become aware of different physical sensations, but for now gently bring your focus back to your thinking.) Practice observing your mind at work. Do you focus more on the 'positive' or 'negative' thoughts that arise in your mind? What is the nature of your thoughts? Notice how your thoughts build and accumulate. Notice how your responses to your thoughts affect the thoughts themselves.

Remember that the primary reason people say they cannot meditate is that they have too many thoughts. It is not the thoughts that are the issue, but your attitude toward your thoughts. Watching how your thoughts arise and construct themselves gives you a valuable perspective in understanding your mental dimension. The goal of meditation is not to extinguish thinking, but rather to accept that you are always thinking and also to understand that there are deeper levels to you than thought. You can imagine that thoughts and emotions are like the waves of the ego and the Self is the deeper water underneath.

Transforming the Heart

It can be difficult to know how to balance the strengths of the ego (body–emotion–mind) with connection to others, but the dimension of the heart does exactly that. The mind and the ego specialize in developing a sense of self separate from the world. In the structure of the ego, the primary concern is what affects the individual. The dimension of the heart adds the ability of connection and compassion to the skills of the ego, so that the focus of concern shifts from the individual to include other people and the world. This allows you to have the experience of separateness as well as the experience of connectedness.

The heart is the source of the ability to love, which is one of the important principles of holistic medicine. The heart is also the source of humanitarianism, the ability to work for the benefit of others, which is a key aspect of the *foundational model* of medicine. The heart provides a context that is larger than ego. The ego gives to others while calculating what it might get back in return. The heart gives without a second thought as to personal benefit as the whole is considered more important than the part. The paradox is that the individual is part of the whole, so that in putting the whole first, the individual still benefits, but in a different way than the self-centered benefit the ego seeks. Without the added dimension of the heart, physicians may be excellent technicians, who are in control of their emotions and keep up on all the latest literature, but who cannot connect to clients at a deep, human level.

Many doctors enter medical school wishing to serve humanity. However, the technical training and learning how to be 'clinically detached and objective' can result in doctors losing their hearts in the process. We have already considered burnout, dissatisfaction and loss of idealism in students and physicians in earlier chapters, which could all be considered losing heart.[26,27] With so much emphasis on technical mastery, the importance of caring for another human being can get lost. The heart is a very tender place and must be continually tended and cared for.

Tending to the heart is what keeps doctors human and this is the subject of Robin Youngson's book, *Time to Care: How to Love Your Patients and Your Job*. Youngson is a UK-born anesthesiologist, who has worked in New Zealand for the past 20 years. His book's focus on strengthening compassion in medicine is an excellent reference for getting physicians' hearts pumping again. Youngson reviews the scientific, economic and humanitarian reasons why we need to focus more on the heart and compassion in medicine.

Similarly, Krasner and colleagues have examined how mindfulness training can improve physician well-being and promote a change in attitudes consistent with patient-centered care. They state that mindfulness-based programs could improve the quality of care, physicians' quality of life, physician empathy and decrease medical errors.[28]

Any form of caring develops the heart. This includes caring for yourself, your patients, your family, a pet, or even for a house-plant. Playing with kids or animals is a good way to open your heart. One of the tremendous benefits of having a pet is learning unconditional love. You can get mad at your dog for something that he or she may have done that you did not like, and two minutes later, your dog is your best friend again. One way to get in touch with your heart is to just sit with your pet and to feel how much they love you. Love tends to awaken love. If you can find love within your heart, it can often soften a situation that otherwise may not go so well.

Many people think having an open heart means you have to be like 'Mother Teresa' or 'Mahatma Gandhi' – a perfect, all-loving, self-sacrificing person who never feels fear, anxiety or anger. Gandhi actually had so much anxiety that the first time he tried to argue a case in court as a lawyer, he could not say a word and had to give the case to someone else.[29] Even as he pursued *Ahimsa* (non-violence),[30] he was jealous and quarrelsome and even aggressive with his wife.[31] Reading his autobiography, one quickly gets the sense of how strict and even harsh he was with himself. The amazing thing about Gandhi is not that he was free of anxiety, jealousy, anger or violence, but that he continually sought to open his heart to recognize and overcome these instincts.

Having an open heart is not just about being loving, but being connected. Love supports the pain that actually comes with connection. Having an open heart means that you are able to feel angry about injustice, angry enough to do something loving to address it. Not very many people close their heart because they do not want joy; most close their heart because they want to avoid pain. The ego's job is to maximize pleasure and avoid pain. The heart's job is to do what is right, not out of calculation, but out of love. The heart adds another dimension to the ego. Love and compassion arise through an open heart.

One last aspect of transforming your heart is to practice giving and receiving. Many people have a distorted idea that an open heart means you are a selfless giver, but it also means you continually receive back, which supports the expansion of giving. Without giving and receiving, you stay the same – isolated, detached, separate and you might even shrink with time, to become smaller, harder, meaner, more calculating. Giving expands your sense of Self. Receiving supports this expanded Self. To only give without receiving means eventually you will collapse, like an empty balloon. The heart gives and receives; that is what it does. Just remember the physical heart and its role in receiving deoxygenated blood, giving this to the lungs, receiving oxygenated blood and then giving this away to the body. A healthy heart is constantly giving and receiving.

Loving Kindness Meditation
Meditation is another route for getting a feeling for your heart. Buddhist 'loving kindness' meditation has been described by Pema Chodron in her many books.[32] In this practice, you begin with opening your heart to yourself and giving yourself loving kindness. You then imagine others to whom you are close, such as your children, your dog, your cat, your spouse, giving to them loving

kindness. Gradually you move the circle of love out from there to family, friends, acquaintances, strangers, expanding to include even those whom you do not like, such as enemies and antagonists. You can even move this circle of love out to the whole Earth or to the whole universe. If this practice seems easy, you probably are not being completely honest with yourself. Love can be hard work when you try to find it for those whom you do not like or who actively dislike you.

The mind leads with thinking, analysis and calculation. The heart leads with connection and care. Connection means that when someone else hurts, you hurt too. This is one of the primary reasons that people close their hearts; they do not want to feel others' pain. Another reason is that they have been hurt and they do not want to hurt again, so they close off their hearts. Actually, working with these questions could be a form of heart meditation:

Facing the Pain Exercise
What was one of the biggest hurts in your life? Notice how your heart felt that pain and also how you pulled back to try and cover and protect your heart. Can you let your heart unfold and open up, even if it means feeling pain like that again? Can you find within yourself love for yourself? How would you respond to a small child if they were feeling the kind of pain that you are feeling? Maybe you can comfort yourself as you would a small child. Watch out for your mind and all its rationalizations about why you do not need or deserve love. Allow yourself to release waves of love from your heart to your hurt. Know that your heart always has the capacity and innate ability to love that which has been hurt or feels unlovable in you.

To extend this meditation you may want to identify the pain that hurts you the most. What do you avoid because it hurts too much? Is it love, closeness, vulnerability, or even watching the news on television? In order to grow, you must go toward that which you would rather avoid. Practice gradually extending waves of love from your heart to the places that hurt the most.

Transforming Creative Self-Expression

Creative self-expression builds the structure of your life, like a scaffold or a blueprint. By stringing together things that you like and that you are drawn to, you gradually create an individual life that has certain recurrent elements. Do you like being out in nature? Do you like animals, math, reading, writing, working with people, working with intellectual problems? In following what you like and expressing it in the world, you gradually create a larger and larger life that has more room for you – more room for expressing who you are.

Creative self-expression takes the momentary impulse of emotional expression and begins to create something larger, made up of multiple emotional expressions. Emotional expression could be something like, 'I *want* that new toy!' Creative self-expression would then be, 'I am going to *make* a new toy to satisfy my emotional needs, but also something that everyone can enjoy!' To look at it from an arts perspective, emotional expression may be a splash of color on a canvas, but it is creative self-expression that directs a series of emotional expressions into the coherent form of a painting. From there, creative self-expression may channel emotional expression into a series of paintings that explore a certain theme. This series of paintings is a metaphor for the life you are creating.

Life patterns are of particular importance in exploring the dimension of creative self-expression. Looking at the patterns of your life reveals your conscious and unconscious motivations. What happens when you start out with an idea, or with starting a project? Do you get past the idea stage? Does the project get bogged down? Does it start off as a joy and then become a chore to finish? Or, how often do you start a project, work diligently on it as long as is required, bring it to completion and then experience both a tremendous sense of accomplishment as well as, eventually, a connection to a new, different or larger project? When you are in the flow of creative self-expression, you are active in your life, you are engaged, you are doing what you want to be doing and these activities give you space to connect to your Self and the larger world.

Your dreams and desires are the building blocks of creative self-expression. I have always liked Martia Nelson's description of embracing and empowering one's desires. In her book, *Coming Home: The Return to True Self*, she describes a way to extract the deeper meaning of desires that might on the surface seem one-dimensional, for instance wanting a new car. Nelson describes four levels of any desire: the *superficial*, the *essence*, the *internalized desire* and the *desire for True Self*. You may actually need a new car (superficial level), but the car that you desire and how you go about desiring reveal different needs and desires of a deeper level (essence desire). Nelson writes that 'you always really want the essence more than the thing.'[33] You may still actually acquire the thing, but if you understand the essence, this brings you closer to your True Self. If you can make the shift from what you want in the material world to what it is that you desire to manifest within your Self (internalized desire), you can start to work at creative self-expression internally and externally, which will be even more rewarding. Nelson goes on to say that beneath 'the desire for all things and all qualities of experience, inner and outer, lies the desire to discover your true nature.'[34]

Nelson's 'True Self' level is analogous to the term 'Self,' identified by many religious, spiritual and philosophical systems and corresponds to the use of the word 'Self' in this book. Rather than putting spirit, ego and matter into opposition, Nelson looks at the current that runs through each of these and manifests in different ways at different levels. This is the core feature of holistic understanding.

Another book about desire and fulfillment in work is Rick Jarow's *Creating the Work You Love*. He asks the questions, 'Is it possible to be who we are in our work, rather than veiling our authenticity in order to survive in the job market? Can we create forms of work that will allow us to offer the fullness of ourselves to the world?'[35] These themes are pertinent to this book as a holistic practice encourages the authentic, whole self of the physician to be developed in order to provide care to the whole of the patient. Jarow uses a seven-dimensional model based on the chakra system to examine different dimensions of work that engages the whole person.

Jarow sees a connection between individual change and societal change. He states that it is possible for anyone 'who is willing to challenge the life-negating suppositions of the current workplace ... to become a force in the transformation of the world.'[36] Self-expression is thus not just a concern for the well-being of the individual, but benefits all of society.

Another book that I have used for myself and that many of my clients have found helpful is Julia Cameron's, *The Artist's Way*. It provides a series of chapters on weekly topics that address the issue of 'artist's block.' Cameron applies the term 'artist' quite broadly to anyone who is stuck or 'blocked' in their life.

Interestingly, I have come to see what Cameron calls 'the morning pages' to be one of the most important aspects of the book, particularly in treating feelings of loss of vitality and depression.[37] The assignment is to write three pages every day. The pages do not have to be something big, like a novel; they are just three pages of whatever comes to your mind. This exercise trains you to develop the connection between inner self and outer world. The morning pages are like a kind of CPR (cardiopulmonary respiration) for creative living, as they get the current of creativity flowing from self to world and back again. At times, writing them can feel like some kind of tedious activity (like the manual chest compressions of CPR), but if you are patient and compassionate with yourself, eventually creativity will start pumping on its own.

Creative Self-Expression Exercise

Close your eyes and sit in a quiet, comfortable spot. Take a few deep breaths, connecting your heart, your mind, your emotions and your body.

To connect to your creative self-expression, you can start by looking at what you have already created in your life: your career, your studies, your relationships, your hobbies and your home. Look at your life over time; are there themes that recur, are there abrupt shifts, do you see a steady development, what aspects of your Self come in and out of focus over time?

Next, look at your dreams – not your sleeping dreams – your waking dreams about what you would like to do in your life. Take some time to look at your dreams. Set aside, for a moment, the idea of reaching the specific form of your literal dream; instead, look at the symbolism and the meaning of your dream. This can be a challenge because everyone puts a lot of energy into their dreams and they can hold them tightly. Give your dream a little space, a little air; let yourself look at it afresh. You can even use some form of imagery for this, setting your dream in a place in the sun, or on some particularly fertile ground, or imaging a large work table, where you can visualize your dream unfolding and growing. This can allow you to look at different aspects of your dream and what it represents for you.

It may be helpful to let your dream speak in each of the different dimensions that we are recurrently looking at in this book. Examine, dimension by dimension, the physical, emotional, mental, heart, self-expressive, intuitive, spiritual, contextual and temporal aspects of your dream. Looking at each of these different levels and how they interact or conflict is a good way to get to know your dream and to understand it in a multidimensional way.

Transforming Intuition

Intuition can be defined as inner knowing that bypasses the rational mind. The rational mind pieces things together slowly, bit by bit, through reason and analysis. It is largely based on understanding through breaking something down into component parts and laws of nature that can be studied and reproduced. Intuition is a kind of knowing that happens instantly, more like grasping a gestalt, or big-picture understanding of a problem that contains many component parts.

Many discussions about the source of intuition get into metaphysics, including the nature of consciousness and reality. Without getting into metaphysics, it is possible to look at intuition as the ability of consciousness to grasp connections between people and objects. This contrasts with the mental dimension, which is based on breaking things into parts and putting them back together again, one or two pieces at a time. In other words, intuition is more of a synthesis (bringing together) than an analysis (breaking apart). It is the ability of the mind to perceive things in relationship to larger contexts.

Some physicians may shy away from a concept like 'intuition,' believing it to be unscientific. However, intuition is a natural human attribute. It is also part of daily clinical work and even scientific discovery.

Scientists owe the discovery of the benzene ring and the discovery of how to measure the mass of an irregularly shaped object to intuition. For example, Friedrich August Kekule von Stradonitz (generally referred to as Kekule in the literature) had a dream that led to the discovery of the structure of the benzene ring. He described dreaming after being frustrated with a chemistry experiment. He saw atoms dancing before his eyes. These then transformed into snakes and one of the snakes bit its own tail. Later, in describing the dream to the German Chemical Society, Kekule stated that, 'As if by a flash of lightning I awoke; and ... I spent the rest of the night in working out the consequences of the hypothesis.'[38] It was thus that he solved the problem of the structural form of benzene. His dream revealed that these would fit into a ring, which he had not previously considered. Kekule encouraged his scientific colleagues, 'Let us learn to dream!'[39]

Another famous scientific discovery through intuition is Archimedes' discovery that he could measure the mass of an object via the amount of water it displaces. The story goes that he was pondering this problem when he took a bath and noticed the water level rise in the bathtub. He reportedly shouted '*Eureka!*' ('I've found it!') and ran through the streets naked, so excited was he by this 'aha' moment.[40]

You can apply this same process of intuitive synthesis and intellectual analysis to clinical work. Many clinicians describe having a sudden sense of a correct diagnosis when working with a client. A good clinician will still do the intellectual analysis of checking labs and doing a diagnostic work-up to either confirm or deny the intuition. Also, many clinicians have had the frustrating occurrence of not being able to figure out 'what is wrong' with a client. No matter how many diagnostic tests or algorithms are used, the diagnosis continues to be elusive. When intense intellectual analysis does not yield results, it can be helpful to set aside the intellectual approach to problem solving. Taking a nap, having a dream, relaxing the mind, taking a walk, taking a vacation – all these things may suddenly clear the way for an intuitive understanding to arise. By no means am I arguing that scientific reasoning and intellectual analysis be discarded; rather I am advocating that physicians include these approaches along with other methods of information-gathering and problem-solving.

Everyone has the ability to both analyze using the mental dimension and synthesize using the intuitive dimension. Everyone has intuitive abilities. Intuition is a skill that can be practiced and developed, just as logical thought and analysis can be practiced and developed. The real challenge is to bring this dimension of your Self into your day-to-day clinical and administrative work, so that you can grasp the bigger picture as well as the details. There are a number of books on developing intuition. Some of these are written by physicians, such as *Second Sight*, by Judith Orloff,[41] Norman Shealy's *Medical Intuition: A Science of the Soul*,[42] and Larry Dossey's *The Science of Premonitions*.[43] Intuition is a natural process of consciousness that will happen of its own accord if you create the space to allow it to arise.

Intuition Exercise

A simple intuitive exercise is to choose a question or problem on which to focus. This may be a question or problem pertaining to your own life or to a clinical dilemma. Sit in a comfortable position in a quiet place. Close your eyes and bring your awareness to your breathing for a few minutes. Observe the easy in-and-out flow of breath through your lungs. You can imagine the oxygen-rich blood coursing throughout your whole body. Then bring that problem or question to your mind again. See if you can remain in a relaxed state without getting into a frantic mental frenzy trying to solve the problem. Instead, be curious to see what kind of answers may arise on their own, not from your mind, but from your whole Self, from your consciousness and your unconscious. Feel free to allow visual or other sensory input to emerge in addition to thoughts. It takes patience and time to create this open state. In this state, intuition will happen of its own accord. You are not 'trying' to be intuitive; you are allowing yourself to create an open and relaxed state of consciousness within which your intuition will naturally function. Note any images, words, feelings, sounds, sights, sensations and memories that arise; this is how your intuition expresses itself.

Another way of doing this exercise is to write your question or problem on a piece of paper and put it under your pillow. As you go to sleep, ask your intuition for any suggestions or guidance about your question. The next morning, take a little time to see if any of your dreams during the night shed any light on your question. Remember that the response may be in dream symbolism, or may emerge as a concrete, direct answer from your unconscious mind. Remember the role dreaming played in Kekule's discoveries, and his injunction: Let us learn to dream!

It may feel odd to trust yourself in this way as the ways of intuition not only seem illogical; they are illogical. Kekule could have very easily dismissed dancing atoms and a snake biting its tail, but he was open to the possibility that there was a deeper meaning in these brief visual images. Intuition can be developed, but you need to allow yourself to 'think' in its language and be open to the synthesis that occurs in this dimension.

Transforming Spirit

Spirit is both internal and external. It is a force or energy that flows through all beings and things and also is in the matter that creates all beings and things. I think of it like light, sometimes a physical object or particle and other times an energy wave. It can be a source of guidance, as many people will report from their own explorations of spirit. Many people have stated that they have had the experience of receiving information or advice suddenly appearing in their consciousness. This can be called intuition, but where does it come from? Connection with the spiritual dimension is healing. Disconnection from spirit brings about feelings of lack, hopelessness, cynicism, self-hatred, hatred of others, hatred of existence and nihilism.

The function of spirit is to animate, create and to provide meaning, to *inspire*. The spiritual dimension is an intrinsic part of every being. While the dimensions of the physical, emotional, mental (all three comprising the ego), as well as heart, creative self-expression and intuition create a multilayered individual being, the dimension of spirit suddenly becomes somewhat confusing as to what is a separate, individual being and what is a living, interconnected patchwork of manifested spirit.

Psychiatrist Carl Jung has written that,

> Life has always seemed to me like a plant that lives on its rhizome. Its true life is invisible, hidden in the rhizome. The part that appears above ground lasts only a single summer. Then it withers away – an ephemeral apparition. When we think of the unending growth and decay of life and civilizations, we cannot escape the impression of absolute nullity. Yet I have never lost a sense of something that lives and endures underneath the eternal flux. What we see is the blossom, which passes. The rhizome remains.[44]

From this perspective, the individual plant is connected through a subterranean and unseen pathway of roots to the entire living universe of spirit. Sometimes I picture this as a form of shifting perspectives. The tighter in you focus, the more individual and material (physical) a person seems. The more you soften your focus, the more you see that what previously looked like an isolated individual becomes a part of a larger, living environment.

Developing awareness of your spiritual dimension can be done in many different ways. Spirit is similar to the function of the heart dimension in that it allows you to expand your awareness beyond the boundaries of the ego in order to feel compassionate connection to others and the world. However, the spiritual dimension goes beyond connection to others to include connection to the structure and events of the universe and the energy that creates you, and the universe and the flow of that energy between you and the universe. The simplest way to say this is that the spiritual dimension is an internal connection to God.

I by no means imply a God of any particular religion, but 'God' is easier to say than: the animating force of all life and existence, which is creative and drives birth, death and evolution, which is in all things and all things are of, and is the essence of love, giving and receiving in a purposeful way, and in being in harmony with this creative energy, you can understand that all things in life are purposeful, and that even painful experiences can be seen to be part of a larger whole in which you have the opportunity to grow in depth of understanding and wisdom as you come to accept the reality of who you are and how you fit into the world, and that love, acceptance, change and growth create all things and flow through all things, and that you are composed of atoms that were created through the birth and death of stars, going all the way back to the big bang in which scientists think that the universe began, initiating a series of stages of star life-cycles that at first consisted of low molecular weight atoms like hydrogen and helium, and through the collapse of these stars, heavier and heavier weight atoms were created, and that every living thing consists of matter that can trace its birth back to the point of the big bang and before that, who knows?

I mean something like that when I say, God, which is a nice shorthand. A creative force is a part of all spiritual and religious traditions, although the details and explanations vary. For those who are atheists, a spiritual dimension is still functioning as a larger sense of connection and purpose in the world.

In this book, I try to stay away from debates about belief and metaphysics. Personally, I have gone through many different phases in my own understanding of Spirit and God, and I have been influenced by various ideas, writings and teachings, as well as by good and bad life experiences. In the end, I am comfortable with the fact that my understanding of God and Spirit will continually change over the course of my life.

Sometimes I am uncomfortable with the idea of God as a being, and prefer to think of God as a force, or a law of nature. There have been times where I have been angry and have not wanted to use the word 'God.' That is my personal journey. I would say the same for everyone, that God is a personal challenge. Other people may influence your ideas and experiences of God, but ultimately, what really matters is your own, personal experience.

An important principle of the spiritual dimension is that life has a purpose, that life events are meaningful and that one of the purposes of life is to learn and grow and evolve. I think that this is a matter of internal, personal experience as well as a matter of personal choice, or perhaps what is called 'faith.' Looking at this from an intellectual, analytical standpoint, you could come up with three basic positions: 1) nothing in life has a 'deeper or higher' purpose; 2) some things are meaningful and some are not; 3) everything is meaningful and purposeful. In this exercise you are invited to explore these questions for yourself.

Looking for Meaning in Life Exercise

Sit in a comfortable place; bring your focus to your heart and your breathing. Ask yourself, 'Does anything in my life have meaning?' After pondering this for a while, ask yourself, 'Are some things in my life meaningful and others not meaningful?' Then ask yourself, 'Is every little thing in my life meaningful?' Notice how you feel through your whole Self as you experience these questions and observe the answers that arise from your whole Self.

Personally, I believe that meaning comes from a sense of connection. This is why we suffer so much from meaninglessness and despair in Western culture and why the pursuit of happiness through material objects is doomed to failure. This is the risk of only having a biomedical philosophy of life that relies on reductionism, objectification and separation – it may create knowledge, but it destroys meaning.

If meaning is a function of connection, a meaningful and fulfilled life can only be achieved through seeking connection. This is the foundation of holistic medicine and it is also the foundation of this book which has the goal of encouraging greater connection within Self, between doctor and patient, and within the culture of medicine. The following exercise focuses on developing the ability to connect with different levels of reality in order to enhance a sense of spirituality.

Zoom In/Zoom Out Exercise

A visualization to work on this sense of connection of the inner and outer can be done in which you focus on one individual atom in your body (things get a bit weird if you focus tighter in on this bit of 'matter,' whether you do it in a visualization, or if you just start reading what physicists think makes up an atom), and then you can gradually pan out: the atom is in a molecule – the molecule is in a fluid or material substance – which is in a sub-portion of an organ – which is in an organ – which is in a part of your body – which is part of your entire body – your body is in a physical location – this location is in a sub-region of a country – which is in a country – which is part of a continent – which is in a hemisphere of the Earth – which is the Earth – expanding out is the moon, orbiting the Earth – neighboring the Earth is Mars and Venus – expanding out through the planets of the solar system, reaching the sun and the debated far objects, like poor old Pluto, no longer considered a planet by the astronomers – and, man, look at all the 'empty' space around our solar system (you can delve into 'dark energy' and 'dark matter' in space between 'things' in another visualization) – and then another solar system – and another – and another – until the solar systems make up points of light in the Milky Way Galaxy – and then vast, 'empty' space – and then another galaxy – and another – and another – until the galaxies, consisting of hundreds of thousands, probably millions, maybe more, I am just estimating, are like single stars or points of light, and yet each contains within it multiple suns and their spheres of influence – and then the edge of the expanding universe – if you are adventurous, maybe you go past that edge, or maybe that is enough for today and you begin to come back down to your Self, step, by step, by step, by step, by step.

You can visit all of this space through this internal exercise. Did your consciousness actually extend to the reaches of the universe, or was this just an 'exercise of the imagination'? Did you actually bring your consciousness down to the reality of one of the atoms in your body, or was this just a fanciful 'exercise of the imagination'? I will leave those questions for you to address. The purpose of this exercise is to develop the ability to shift dimensions within yourself and the universe and to develop a sense of connection between your ego, your Self and the surround of your Self.

Transforming Context

Context shapes what you experience and how you interpret your experiences and even how you experience your sense of Self. It does this by supporting some things and restricting others. Some aspects of your context you may have actively chosen, others you may have chosen unconsciously and still others you may have been born into. In transforming your Self, you can make a conscious decision to understand your context and then to some extent you can also shape your context.

Context begins with very individual aspects of you and extends out into larger social systems. Context consists of your physical attributes, such as your gender and physical characteristics and temperament. Your family of origin is a context, as well as family attributes, such as culture, ethnic heritage, religious affiliations and socioeconomic variables. There are also contextual considerations such as the country in which you were born, the country in which you are living, the region of the country in which you live and its environmental characteristics. Another aspect of context is the historical time in which you live, as that can shape opportunities and expectations. All of these contextual elements are very important in understanding a human being, whether that human being is yourself or your client.

Working to transform your context is a very challenging undertaking. First, how can you know who you are, independent of your context? In other words, how can you have the perspective to see there is something you want to change about your environment when your environment is shaping your perception? Second, there is a very strong conditioning effect that your environment has on you, which we explored in the previous chapter. Third, you have to understand yourself and your environment on a deep enough level to see that you are creating and perpetuating certain aspects of your context through your unconscious motivations.

To transform context is kind of like working with the 'Serenity Prayer' (attributed to Reinhold Niebuhr): 'God, give us Grace to accept with serenity the things that cannot be changed, Courage to change the things which should be changed, and the Wisdom to distinguish the one from the other.'[45] People both create their lives and are created by their lives. Looking at your context allows you to be an active creator as well as a grateful recipient of your life.

Many people lead unfulfilling and frustrating lives because they view their context as unyielding and they do not see that they are in an active relationship with their context, both creating it and being created by it. To transform context you need to first be aware of it, then you need to be aware of yourself. Next you need to look at the goodness of fit between your context and your inner desires.

You can change your job, the size of your house, your car, even the country in which you live. All of these are relatively easy to change, although they may involve a lot of details and you may have different emotional attachments to these physical contexts. Different contexts may be supportive at one point in your life and restrictive at another point. The purpose of looking at your context is to determine the goodness of fit between your context and what you want to do in your life. As this book focuses on re-humanizing your medical practice, we will look at context in light of this goal.

To use a holistic framework to re-humanize your practice, you need to have a certain amount of time with your clients and a supportive space in which to work. If you have a lot of financial debts and physical responsibilities, these can get in the way of your ability to create the kind of practice that you desire because you may feel obligated to prioritize money over time with clients. Having a lot of expenses is one way of avoiding being able to create the kind of practice that you want and it also makes you feel helpless and powerless to consider other job options. Looking at your financial situation and simplifying it can help you to create your practice. Another way of saying all this is that in order to have a holistic practice, you need to be holistically living a fully human life, and that means that you are creating a life space that is sustainable, supportive, regenerative and inspirational. A fully human life requires a balance of action and reflection. It also requires adequate space and time for awareness and development of your physical body, emotions, mind, heart, self-expression, intuition and spirit.

To transform your context, you have to be aware of your Self and the mutually interactive way that you are constantly creating your context and how your context is shaping you. You may find that it is difficult to change something within your Self or to create a holistic medical practice without changing some factors in your context and environment. Conditioning can work in a positive or a negative way and you can restructure your context so that it is supportive of what you want to do rather than feeling like you are always being forced to do something you do not want to do. The concept of the Serenity Prayer can be quite useful in transforming your context as you work to develop patience to accept what you cannot change, courage to change what you can change, and the wisdom to know the difference.

Serenity Prayer Exercise

The first step in transforming your context is in applying the concept of the Serenity Prayer to every aspect of your life situation and your Self. What do you accept, what can you change, and how can you know the difference between the two? In taking the time for reflection and self-awareness, you can become aware of what things in your life are becoming intolerable and that you feel you must change. The more you connect to your inner awareness, the more strength you will have to carry on with the difficult task of transforming your context and environment. Life consists of action and reflection, and developing both of these faculties will assist you in transforming your context.

Transforming Time

You may find yourself living in a shotgun shack
You may find yourself in another part of the world
You may find yourself behind the wheel of a large automobile
You may find yourself in a beautiful house with a beautiful
   wife
You may ask yourself, well, how did I get here?
Talking Heads[46]

The goal of a fully human life is to make sure that you are consciously investing your time in a way that grows and supports your entire Self. Just like in the Talking Heads song, 'Once in a Lifetime,' you may ask yourself how your life has become what it is. Generally, this happens through making a lot of small choices without a lot of awareness until you find out you have created a big choice that you feel you never actually made.

In his book, *The Three Marriages: Reimagining Work, Self and Relationship*, poet David Whyte writes that you cannot 'balance' work, self, and relationship – that each dimension requires absolute commitment. He speaks of this commitment as being married to each of these dimensions in a 'marriage of marriages.'[47] Whyte writes that, 'each marriage represents a core conversation with life that seems necessary for almost all human beings and none of the marriages can be weakened or given up without a severe sense of internal damage.'[48] He raises interesting points about the dangers of trying to logically draw out a pie chart of your life and to strictly allocate your time and energy according to some abstraction of balance. How committed to your work are you if you never give extra? How committed to your relationship are you if you never give extra? How committed to your Self are you if you never give extra to your Self?

Another author, philosopher John Ralston Saul, in his book *On Equilibrium*, asks,

What is the expression of our humanness, if not to live our lives, struggling with the dynamic of an impossible balance? This is something which lies within each of us and therefore within our societies. To know, imagine, sense, think, to some extent even to understand, this constant dynamic is to express civilization's essential nature.[49]

Like Whyte, Saul indicates that balance is not found through a static, imposed grid, but rather by a continually shifting and living competing tension. Saul writes that to 'seek equilibrium is to engage in a dynamic of constant movement, constant tension … (t)o expect or demand resolution is to slip into ideology – a form of death.'[50] What Whyte and Saul argue for is a continually shifting focus between different competing (yet complementary) dimensions of human being. The balance or equilibrium is not found in a static moment (which might actually be, appropriately, quite unbalanced), but through the relationship and connection of tension over the dimension of time. In searching for balance or equilibrium, you should factor in change over time. As both Saul and Whyte point out, it is *normal* to be unbalanced and to feel pulled in different directions. Feeling the pull of tension is perhaps even what creates life. When looking at the temporal dimension, the question becomes: how do you work with shifting tensions across the span of your life?

Just as being 'unbalanced' may paradoxically be part of the 'balance' of life, so too may losing touch with ourselves be a necessary part of finding and truly becoming ourselves. Whyte writes, '(There) is no way of being fully human without at times being fully stuck or even completely absent; we are simply not made that way.'[51] This statement would seem to imply that there are times that we are necessarily less than fully human, that somehow we have lost touch with ourselves. Rebecca Solnit wanders through this theme in her book, *A Field Guide to Getting Lost.*

> The things we want are transformative, and we don't know or only think we know what is on the other side of that transformation. Love, wisdom, grace, inspiration – how do you go about finding these things that are in some ways about extending the boundaries of the self into unknown territory, about becoming someone else?[52]

This reminds us of the Talking Heads song at the start of this section where David Byrne says, 'well, how did I get here?' That question is integral to the dimension of time and the concept of personal growth. Solnit seems to say that we do not know how to look for those very things that we most want to find. If we cannot find them through analytical thought and linear pursuit, how then can we grow into *unknown territory* in order *to become someone else?* She suggests that it is through getting lost that we are able to find ourselves. She quotes Thoreau: not 'till we are lost, in other words, not until we have lost the world, do we begin to find ourselves.'[53] Finding one's Self and being fully human thus seem to require a considerable amount of time because these are not linear functions but require periodically losing touch with our humanity and also getting lost.

Losing Your Self Exercise

Imagine a time that you were very lost in your life. Remember the feelings of that time. Let yourself really sink into your memory of the time. See if you can add other contextual details to make the memory more vivid. Where were you living? What was a local restaurant? How did you get to school or work? What did you think about as you were going to sleep at night? See if you can really recreate that time of your life.

Looking back, what did you learn from that time of being lost? How important was that experience to who you are now? Can you imagine your life without that experience of being lost? Is it possible to shift your attitude to being lost in the future? Do you always need to be moving in a linear way through life?

Finding Your Self Across Time Exercise

Get five blank sheets of paper. Divide your life into 4 equal segments. If you are 40 years old these can be 10-year increments; if you are 32 it would be 8-year increments, for example. On the top of the first three sheets of paper, write 'Who I was at age (increment).' On the fourth sheet of paper, write, 'Who I am now.' On each of these four sheets of paper, write out some of these details about yourself at that age, such as:

Where were you living?
Who was your family?
With whom were you living?
Who were your friends?
Did you have pets; if so, who were they?
How did you like to spend your time?
What did you spend most of your time doing?
What did you love doing?

What did you hate doing?

What were your hobbies?

What did you do for fun?

What was your favorite place to be?

What did you want to do in the future?

Who did you love?

Start with the first page and look it over. Once you feel you have a sense of that time, turn the paper over and write out your response to each of these questions:

How would you have defined yourself at that time?

What was important to you?

What stressed you out?

What did you love?

Do this exercise for each of the four increments of your life. Pay attention to any themes that arise between the different ages and also to things that you felt strongly about, but that you no longer have in your life in the same way.

Next, take that blank fifth sheet of paper and write on the top: 'Who I want to be in the future.' As you write out your hopes for the future, take into consideration the themes from the past that perhaps you did not actively choose, but that seem to be themes of your life nonetheless.

Integrating the Self

After looking at these nine different dimensions of Self, it might seem a bit overwhelming to imagine how you could ever go through daily life aware of all these elements. The truth of the matter is that you already are all of these things and all these levels of awareness are happening at the same time. It is just that you have 'learned' to listen to certain dimensions of your experience and not others.

You can imagine your Self as nine different rooms in which nine different musicians are playing nine different instruments. Each room has its unique musician and instrument which represents a unique dimension of Self. That is, the physical, emotional, mental, heart, self-expressive, intuitive, spiritual, contextual and temporal dimensions are each represented by a room. You can run from room to room trying to hum the melody from the previous room, or you can sit down, expand your awareness, and experience all the rooms at once. This would require awareness of the whole house at once, instead of running around with a smaller, one-at-a-time room awareness. Then, you can hear the symphony of your Self.

Symphony of the Self Exercise

You can use the metaphor of different rooms of a house having different musicians with different instruments as a way of integrating a sense of Self. Visualize nine different rooms, one each for the physical, emotional, mental, heart, self-expressive, intuitive, spiritual, contextual and temporal dimensions. Now visualize a musical instrument that represents each dimension and visualize a representation of yourself in each room with that instrument. There are many different instruments that you can choose, for example: drums, bass guitar, guitar, piano, trumpet, saxophone, flute, bassoon, triangle, violin, cello, glockenspiel, maracas, trombone, moog, theremin and harp, to name just a few.

Now that you have chosen your orchestra, start with the physical dimension room and visualize yourself playing that instrument. Stay with it until you have a good sense of the sound, feel and mood of the room. Then add in the emotional dimension room and really sink into that experience. Continue to add additional rooms/instruments while holding the rhythm and melody of the previous rooms until you can get a sense of the Symphony of the Self playing all together.

Part IV

RE-HUMANIZING YOUR PRACTICE

Overview

It is difficult to outline general rules when creating a holistic practice as it is such an individual expression. I will recount the story of my own journey in holistic medicine to help show that the process utilizes all the different avenues of experience that you have available, including your body, emotions, mind, heart, creativity, intuition, spirit, context and time. Each dimension provides unique information which can be integrated for holistic decision-making.

If you do not understand the structure of the health care delivery system in which you are working, you will be frustrated when you bump up against its limitations. However, it is possible to create a holistic practice in any setting because it is defined through your experience and relationship with your Self. Just as people are constantly growing throughout their lives, your practice will continue to evolve over time.

We will review some pros and cons to using a holistic approach in a typical, contemporary medical setting, and examine options for working outside the contemporary medical system. One attractive option is to start your own practice. The growing trend in the US toward establishing so-called *micropractices* reflects the desire of physicians to promote *connectivity* over *productivity* and *quality care* over *quantity care*.

By its very nature, there is no 'one-size-fits-all' approach for creating a holistic practice. Any practice of medicine can be re-humanized. It is just more challenging to do this in some practice settings than in others.

Chapter 8

My Journey in Creating a Holistic Practice

The serious problems in life ... are never fully solved. If ever they should appear to be so it is a sure sign that something has been lost. The meaning and purpose of a problem seems to lie not in its solution but in our working at it incessantly.
Carl Jung[1]

I have worked in a number of different practice settings. Each setting had strengths and weaknesses in regard to working holistically with clients. Each setting also had different levels of dehumanization inherent in the way it was structured and which model of medicine was predominant. Some practices were a good fit for a while, and then they no longer supported the type of work I wanted to do. I really could say that creating a holistic practice started back when I was doing my undergraduate degree at University of Illinois, Urbana-Champaign, where I read widely through formal and informal study. I used the sciences as a base, getting a bachelor's degree in psychology and taking the pre-med curriculum. Then I added classes in anthropology, Zen Buddhism, world religions, philosophy and an independent study course on Carl Jung's work. All the while, I was reading literature and anything that interested me on the side. I have always maintained my own 'curriculum' that ran parallel to whatever I was formally studying.

Medical School

I went up to University of Illinois at Chicago Medical School, and it really challenged me to stay balanced. Quite literally, I tried to balance all the medical science reading and training with books from the humanities. I constantly had a few books of poetry, meditation or literature handy, and I also would paint, draw and journal. I did not keep up my physical fitness as well as, in retrospect, I could have.

An image stands out for me from medical school. At the end of the first year of study, my friend, Darin Dougherty, and I each stacked our books and notes for the year. We each posed for a picture next to our pile of knowledge, holding a cup of coffee, as that was a constant study companion. The stack of books came up close to my waist. That image stays with me because it was a time of great excitement. I was living in the 'big city' of Chicago (I grew up in a small farming community about 60 miles west of the city) and I was in medical school – studying to be a doctor! I loved the challenge. Part of the challenge was working at the edge of my limitations in regard to how much I could memorize and how much sleep I needed to function. Sometimes, I had to learn how to push beyond my comfort zone to work a 36-hour workday. I think working with one's limitations is a crucial part of becoming a professional in medicine. It is also an aspect of growing in self-knowledge. It can also be a source of stress and burnout.

While I take a critical stance toward the overuse of the biomedical model and the dehumanization of contemporary medicine, I would still become a doctor again. I have had a very interesting and fulfilling career that has allowed me to move to different parts of the US and even to New Zealand. To return to that photo, in addition to the excitement, I feel other emotions looking at it now. I have a sense of loss for that young, energetic and idealistic person. In my imagination the stack of books becomes larger and larger, until I am surrounded by a tower of books, notes and information. I do not mean to be overly dramatic, but I do think there is a loss that occurs with medical education. Some of that is a necessary part of growing up and becoming a professional, but I think we could make a more humane system and formally remind physicians in training that, in life and in medicine, they will need both information and their humanity.

Looking back, I constantly gravitated toward mentors who embodied this mixture of humanity and professionalism. Bob Molokie, for instance, was interesting, well-read, passionate about medicine and education, idealistic and compassionate. Bob was as comfortable discussing the poetry of Stephen Crane or the writing of Jerzy Kosinski as he was teaching about hematology and oncology. Learning from Bob was like having four different topics of discussion going at the same time. His style of teaching was that I was never wrong in answering a question. If I gave the incorrect answer, he would formulate the question that was appropriate to the answer I had given – then we would go back to the original question(s).

Also, early in medical school, I was lucky enough to get a summer research elective with Deb Klamen, a psychiatrist I continued to work with throughout my psychiatric residency training. Deb's project focused on symptoms of Posttraumatic Stress Disorder in residents in relationship to their internship year of training.[2] This project kick-started my own interest in looking at not just the treatment that is delivered to the patient, but the whole health care delivery system and the effect it has on the people who work in it. I really enjoyed working with Deb. She did not fit the 'typical' mold of a physician and she was a good role model for how a person can be themselves and be an excellent clinician, teacher and researcher. I ended up working with Deb and Linda Grossman on a series of papers about medical student attitudes toward different controversial topics, such as AIDS, homosexuality and abortion.[3,4,5] I loved doing literature reviews that looked at different aspects of medical education and at how to foster and preserve humanism and idealism.

Psychiatric Residency

I decided on psychiatric residency because it seemed to offer the broadest range of potential ways of working with patients. These included not only prescribing medication and understanding the brain, but also learning psychotherapy and understanding people's social worlds. I continued my education at the University of Illinois at Chicago because it valued of its multi-faceted approach to psychiatry. As a true geek, I loved learning about neuroscience, but my heart was really in other approaches such as psychotherapy and humanistic, creative ways of working with people.

About halfway through residency, I met Steve Weine. He spoke up a lot in grand rounds and would challenge people when they became stuck in one explanatory paradigm. He was a true critical thinker and was comfortable using many different conceptual paradigms to understand human beings. I gravitated to Steve as he had a larger perspective of not just psychiatry, but humanity. He had started the Project on Genocide, Psychiatry, and Witnessing and was doing a lot of work with people from the former Yugoslavia. Steve had a solid training in psychodynamic psychotherapy. He also had a strong humanist and humanitarian element. He thought within systems, but then would turn around and challenge the system of thought itself. As my psychotherapy supervisor, he challenged me to have an 'authentic' relationship with my clients, not just a relationship mediated by a particular theoretical model.

Steve also developed a Trauma Psychotherapy and Research elective in which I participated during my last year of residency. As Steve believed that biological reductionism, numbers and statistics were not the only way to achieve understanding, he encouraged me to undertake research that was actually a lot closer to literary criticism and biography than to a double-blind, placebo-controlled trial.

My topic was trauma and creativity in people who had lived through adversity and then became writers. More specifically I looked at the complexity of witnessing. *Witnessing* is a concept that incorporates the psychological effects of living through a trauma with a social and perhaps even political element of 'bearing witness' to inhumanity. In this way, it illuminates dehumanization and is a voice for re-humanization. I focused on two writers: Jerzy Kosinski and Louis-Ferdinand Celine.

During Kosinski's career, he was idolized as a Jewish child survivor of the Holocaust who wrote about his experiences in semi-autobiographical novels, particularly *The Painted Bird*. His book, *Being There*, was another popular work which was adapted for a film starring Peter Sellers. Near the end of his life, however, an article published in the *Village Voice* in 1991 revealed that Kosinski's books were more fiction than fact. He committed suicide around the time this information came to light.

Celine was a French cavalryman in World War I. He later became a physician and cared for the poor, children and animals. However, he also wrote a hateful anti-Semitic tract in the lead-up to World War II. He was convicted *in absentia* of collaboration with the Nazis, declared a national disgrace, and served a year in a Danish prison after the war. The explosive and open-ended style of Celine's books, *Journey to the End of Night* and *Death on the Installment Plan*, influenced many writers, including Beat Generation writers like Ginsberg, Burroughs and Kerouac.

Both Kosinski and Celine bore witness to personal and collective suffering, which won them respect and literary acclaim. However, both simultaneously played out tragic roles. Kosinski was tainted as a 'liar.' Celine was branded a 'collaborator' and 'anti-Semite.' Through studying these two writers' works and lives, I learned about the complexity of human beings' reactions to trauma. There is also a sense in the work of both men that writing is a double-edged sword that can be used for healing or hurting. And sometimes it seems that the healing and hurting are hopelessly intertwined.

Looking back on these three mentors, Bob, Deb and Steve, I see some common threads. All were passionately committed to working with clients, and all of them saw that part of the role of professionals is to question power, tradition and prevailing beliefs. All three helped to shape who I am today and I can see that this current book owes a great deal to these three humanitarians.

First Work

After psychiatric residency, I started off in a joint academic and Veterans Affairs position, at the University of Nebraska and Omaha Veterans Administration (VA). At the VA, I worked in the Posttraumatic Stress Disorder (PTSD) Clinic. Here, the interplay between the clinical work and my conceptual learning was very rich. PTSD is inherently a mind–body condition, and my clinical work and reading deepened my understanding of the interplay between different human dimensions. Seeing the disruptive effects of trauma on veterans' relationships made the social aspect of trauma very apparent. At the VA, I treated veterans who often had childhood trauma as well as war trauma and subsequent challenges in adapting back into society. It was also shortly after the first Gulf War and a number of clients were presenting with perplexing mind–body symptoms such as 'Gulf War syndrome' and fibromyalgia. I learned a great deal about mind and body interactions working with these traumatized populations. I came to appreciate both the benefits and limitations of a biomedical approach to working with human suffering, as I realized that 'managing' symptoms was really just the beginning of working with traumatized individuals.

The academic environment encouraged me to pursue scientific and humanistic interests, and I presented various papers at conferences. I am still particularly fond of a presentation called, 'Learning to Save the Self.' This presentation looked at Samuel Shem's (aka Stephen Bergman) views on trauma, identity and medical education as portrayed in his book, *The House of God*. Around the same time, I met Robert Coleman, who was my mentor in Omaha, and I learned a lot about poetry and even a little about pinot noir in our discussions. Robert started a book club with a group of psychiatric residents interested in medical humanities. This led to a group presentation on 'Poetry and Medicine' at the American Psychiatric Association annual conference.

This was an intellectually stimulating time in my life. I pursued my interest in writing about trauma and creativity, and did some writing on the post-punk band Joy Division. This led to a series of short articles on punk rock, trauma and transformation. I owe a lot to Steve Weine for taking my interest in music seriously and for showing me a way to do scholarly work on subjects that are often not taken seriously in medicine.

Back to the Source

After two years in Omaha, my wife Mary Pat and I decided to move back to the town where we went to university, Champaign-Urbana, Illinois. My own clinical work was going well in Nebraska, but I was unable to get anything I was working on published, either poetry or scholarly work. I tried to get a piece on Celine published, but it seemed it was not 'literary' enough for academic literature publications and was not 'medical' enough for medical publications. In retrospect, this was to be a lifelong challenge. As I have endeavored to develop literary and scholarly medical writing as well as holistic and integrative clinical work, I have often found that I do not seem to 'fit' squarely into the concept of what a psychiatrist should be. I suppose this is part of the 'road less travelled,' that there is no clear, ready-made path. While I would not give up my interests that have made my life so rich, I have often wished I could just find a job in which all of my professional interests 'fit.'

Our university days in Champaign-Urbana had been very full and rich, filled with music, friends, cafés and learning. Mary Pat and I thought that maybe if we went back to the 'source' we could reconnect with what was important to us and get a new start.

I took a job at a multi-specialty group practice, primarily to move back to Champaign-Urbana, rather than for the specific job. I worked there for three years. It was intensive clinical work without much time set aside for meetings, grand rounds or educational activities. I continued to pursue my own intellectual interests in trauma, spirituality, creativity and transformation. I also returned to study Jung and Nietzsche at a deeper level. (I had a series of notebooks which I entitled, *Die Untergang* – 'the going under,' as I was studying the depths of myself as well as Jungian and Nietzschean concepts.) During this time, I also enjoyed owning our first home, working in the gardens, painting and writing. We even 'got the band back together again,' and played some music with old friends from university.

Holistic Medicine

I started to study holistic medicine in greater depth. Through Jung and also studies on meditation, I had become familiar with conceptual models of how thoughts, emotions and the body interrelate and co-create human experience. But it was around this time that some personal experiences shifted my intellectual understanding into a more personal understanding. It was as if I had been studying intellectual concepts all those years, and had formed a complete intellectual system that was separate from my daily life and my physical reality. This shifted over a period of a couple months and it was a time of great excitement for me as I integrated intellectual and spiritual concepts into my daily life.

My studies in holistic medicine, up to that point, had been largely self-directed. I was particularly interested in consciousness, personal growth, creativity, meditation and spirituality. These pursuits were a good foundation for when I undertook more formal study of a systematic review of holistic medicine in preparation for the board certification exam through the American Board of Holistic Medicine (now the American Board of Integrative and Holistic Medicine). I also started intensive personal growth work in different healing modalities through the A'Claire School for Healing in the Chicago suburbs. Here I continued to focus on the interactions between mind–body–spirit through experiential learning. I developed a daily meditation practice and explored different forms of healing practices.

Eventually, I left the job at the multi-specialty clinic, largely due to a philosophical and financial shift in the larger organization. The clinic moved away from a *foundational* model of medicine (valuing compassion, professionalism and serving all income levels) to more of an *economic rationalist* model (tying physician incomes to billing rather than to work productivity and a philosophy of 'cherry-picking' the more lucrative insurance contracts). All the psychiatrists ended up leaving the department over the course of about a year. Allan Crandell was the head of the department, and I found in him another idealistic psychiatrist. Allan walked away from the clinic rather than compromising his values. For a long time, I did not know what I was going to do, but then one night I paused in the middle of a bite of blueberry pie. At that moment I made the decision to leave the clinic. I still did not know what I was going to do next, but I knew I had to leave. This decision was complicated by the fact of a two-year, 30-mile, non-compete clause, which meant that I could not work within 30 miles of this town of 100,000 people in the middle of cornfields. I did not want to move away from the area, so it meant buying a second car and commuting.

I took two jobs at two different community mental health centers in Mattoon and Paris, Illinois. It helped that Allan ended up working in Mattoon. He and I spent long hours driving the 1.5-hour round trip to work. It was very supportive to work with Allan, and it changed the burden of the non-compete clause into a fun, shared adventure. These were also purely clinical jobs without time off for lectures or many meetings. In my spare time, I continued my studies at the A'Claire School for Healing, and eventually became a teaching assistant there. Mary Pat and I regularly commuted 2.5 hours up to Chicago for weekend workshops and longer four-day intensives.

Healing School

Susan Matz, the founder of the school, had a PhD in nursing, so she understood the biomedical model very well, but she also studied holistic approaches to healing and personal growth. The focus of A'Claire was on healing through self-knowledge and self-awareness. Healing, in this paradigm, comes from connection – connection within Self, between people and to society. While we learned a number of different techniques for self-connection or for teaching others self-connection, Susan always reminded us that these were just tools and not to mistake the effect of the tool with the tool itself. We learned various techniques, such as focused awareness, visualization, expressive art projects, meditation and mind–body exercises. We studied personal defense patterns as well as group dynamics. There was a strong leadership component to our learning, particularly once I took on the role as a teaching assistant.

It was a really exciting time for me and I imagined that the early days of psychoanalysis and depth psychology must have been similar – the feeling of being on the cutting edge of a new movement of therapeutics and self-knowledge. I developed an experiential understanding of holism and mind–body–spirit connections, not just an intellectual knowledge, but an inner experience of how different dimensions of human experience influence one another. Another thing I really liked about the school was that it did not focus on personal growth in isolation. Rather, the more one grew in internal connection, the more one was encouraged to connect to the world. There was a strong social consciousness that connected the individual to the group and that fostered professional responsibility.

It was at A'Claire that I learned about the model of human experience based on the chakra system of physical, emotional, mental, heart, self-expression, intuition and spiritual dimensions. As I moved back into more mainstream psychiatric work, I realized that this model was very individualistic and that it needed to include both a dimension of social and environmental context and a temporal dimension of how a person grows and changes over time.

Private Practice: A Holistic Micropractice

During my time at A'Claire, I became more and more focused on the concept and practice of healing and moved away from more academic and literary pursuits. I experienced an increasing dissonance between my daily psychiatric practice of medication management and my studies of different healing modalities. While it scared me to jump off into private practice, I felt there was no other choice if I wanted to work clinically in a way that was consistent with my shifting views. I wanted a chance to put my healing philosophy into practice!

So, in January 2005, I opened the doors of a part-time private practice. A local psychiatrist retired and Allan left the area (he went up to Alaska to work with the Native Alaskan population). I was flooded with patients from both of their practices as well as my own practices over the years. Many previous patients from Champaign heard I was back in town and sought me out. I was over-booked before I even opened the doors. I remember staying at the office until 1 a.m. that first week as I tried to figure out how to see all the patients I had booked, write the notes, figure out my practice management software, figure out how to bill insurance, return calls to pharmacies and insurance companies, pursue refused payments, take patient calls and reschedule appointments. I had decided to do all the work myself and to take all forms of insurance right from the start, including Medicaid and Medicare. This was in accord with my philosophy of *learning the whole system of medicine*, from service delivery to payment. It took me months to sort out a rough balance between how many clients to see and how much time I needed for administrative work. Actually, this was probably one of the central learning processes of my practice and I really worked on this balance over and over during the 5 years of my practice. In the first year, I often welcomed the days that I could go to the community mental health center or the Developmental Services Center, where I worked with adults with intellectual disabilities and psychiatric symptoms. At those sites I could 'just see patients' and did not have to worry about all the administrative work associated with running a practice.

After one year, I went to full-time practice. I kept the 2-days-a-month job at the Developmental Services Center, as I really enjoyed that work and it gave me a welcome break from running my practice. Working with these clients continually challenged me to reassess the role of psychopharmacology for psychiatric symptoms in the context of impulsive and sometimes aggressive behavior. It was always a challenge to sort out the efficacy of the various biochemical, psychological, social, environmental and occupational interventions we employed. We were always working to discern what was an outburst related to psychosocial variables and what was a behavior related to a more enduring mental illness or syndrome that required longer-term pharmaceutical intervention. This was one of the best teams I have been in. We were able to employ some very good, consistent interventions as many of the clients lived in group homes run by the agency and also worked on site at the center during the day.

I had a lot of fulfillment in my private practice. I remember realizing one day, on a trip to the bank, that I was a 'small business owner.' For some reason, I felt pride and accomplishment in that. In my practice, I offered a wide range of services. I had a few clients who just wanted a routine 15 minute medication check for maintaining medicine they had been on for years. Most appointments were 30–45 minutes, though I usually tried to have some buffer so that I could lengthen appointments if needed. These were 90805 or 90807 (medication management and psychotherapy) insurance codes for either 30 or 45 minutes. I also did up to 1.5-hour appointments that focused on more holistic techniques with a lot of mind–body–consciousness work. One of the things I found rewarding was supporting clients to learn mind–body techniques that allowed them to work with their symptoms and experiences. This often led to significant reductions in medication, sometimes 'physical' medications as well as 'psychiatric.'

During this phase, I was continually reworking a philo-sophical approach that incorporated biomedical, pharmaco-logical interventions with creatively addressing symptoms through other dimensions. I was able to witness how changing something in an emotional, mental, compassionate, creative/self-expressive, intuitive, spiritual, contextual or temporal dimension could actually change the expression of biological, emotional and mental symptoms. I came to see the majority of depressive, anxiety, psychosomatic, posttraumatic and dissociative disorders as being partially or even completely responsive to non-medical interventions. I still prescribed a lot of medication, but that gradually decreased over time. Near the end of my private practice, I was growing increasingly uncomfortable with the maintenance use of sedatives and hypnotics and made addressing chronic use a priority in my practice. I came to view the chronic use of these medications was often unnecessary and interfered with personal growth, which was increasingly becoming a focus of my practice. Another way of saying this is that as I began to see the possibility for treatment and sometimes even cure through a holistic approach; the chronic use of these particular medications seemed more like symptom suppression rather than active treatment. I sent out a letter to all my clients saying that I was re-evaluating the routine use of these medica-tions, and that it would be my general policy (although I would evaluate on a case-by-case basis) to no longer prescribe these medications on a chronic basis.

Throughout the years of my private practice, I never had a shortage of clients. I became more and more discriminating about taking on new people, and I would make sure their goals were consistent with my philosophy. As my practice matured and I became more competent in the administrative side of things, I started to give workshops in the community on meditation, holistic approaches to working with depression or pain, and different holistic techniques. Eventually, this grew to a fortuitous opportunity to teach a Personal Growth class at Parkland College to health professional students (thank you, Sara Holmes!) and also to do some teaching at the University of Illinois Urbana-Champaign medical school. It seemed like I had come full-circle when I gave an invited lecture at the faculty and staff development day for the university; and I realized I was delivering the lecture in the same room where I had performed as a college sophomore in a rock band (opening for the band, Die Kreuzen, where we earned $5 each and it seemed like the 'big time!').

After years of balancing a focus between my clinical work in psychiatry and my work at the A'Claire School for Healing, the school suddenly closed. This was quite a shock to me as it had been such a large part of my life from 2001 to 2008, and indeed a large part of my identity. It was a chaotic and messy ending and I was at a loss as to how to move forward. Looking back, I am really glad the school ended when it did. There is always a balance between studying a particular modality in depth (and working with a small group of idealistic people who would like to transform the world) and having a breadth of experience and many different influences. I remember reading a meditation teacher's advice (I cannot remember who it was, but it is a common topic) that at some point in a spiritual search a student needs to settle with one teacher. There is also a tradition that a student needs to let go of a teacher in order to be true to themselves and their own path. As Shunryu Suzuki has written,

The purpose of studying Buddhism is not to study Buddhism, but to study ourselves. It is impossible to study ourselves without some teaching ... We need some teaching, but just by studying the teaching alone, it is impossible to know what 'I' in myself am. Through the teaching we may understand our human nature. But the teaching is not we ourselves; it is some explanation of ourselves. So if you are attached to the teaching, or to the teacher, that is a big mistake. The moment you meet a teacher, you should leave the teacher, and you should be independent. You need a teacher so that you can become independent. If you are not attached to him (or her) the teacher will show you the way to yourself ... You should not take what you have learned with a teacher for you yourself.[6]

The ending of the A'Claire School for Healing led to a major re-evaluation in my life. I continued to practice and to teach, and I felt like I had set a number of things in motion that needed to be brought to completion, but I continued to question how to move forward. My teaching at the community college had been rewarding and the class I ran for three semesters was always at full capacity. At the request of many of the students, I developed a follow-up class and was preparing to teach that. Around that time, though, I experienced growing tension with some of the science faculty at the college as well as with one of the deans. I had a television appearance cancelled last minute the evening before by the dean. A local TV station wanted to promote a series of workshops we had created to bring together faculty, students and holistic practitioners in the community. The class I had prepared was cancelled by the dean, even though it had full enrollment. Much of the tension focused on fears and worries by the faculty about holistic medicine being 'unscientific.' There was also a lack of understanding about the benefit of personal growth and self-knowledge for clinicians. When I was offered the spot to teach the class, I asked to what extent I should teach what I thought was important and to what extent I needed to censor or limit what I taught to make it more acceptable to an academic mentality. I was told to teach whatever I felt was important for the students to learn, so I developed a class that was focused on learning different topics of self-care and well-being through an experiential, personal growth framework.

The whole issue became very politically charged at the college. I remember one meeting with the science department, where one faculty member was challenging me on the therapeutic use of magnets. I could not understand why he was bringing this up, as it was not something I was advocating or teaching. He was upset by the apparent inability to do a placebo-blinded study with magnets because the patient could always put a piece of metal by the magnet to see if it was a 'real' magnet or a 'placebo' magnet. I could see how much the arguments against holistic medicine were fuelled by emotion and how uninformed these scientists were about the objections they raised. There are uses of magnets, like magnetic shoe inserts, that do not have a strong evidence base. However, there is a strong evidence base for the therapeutic use of electromagnetic fields for treating bone fractures, and several devices are approved through the FDA for this use. In the end, my class was cancelled, but I decided to offer it to the students who had signed up, as a seminar in the community. I called it, 'Being Fully Human.' I built on the idea of extending personal growth from the individual into community and global awareness. This encouraged students to put their self-knowledge into action in the world. The class also forced me to really think about what I was focusing on with this idea of *being fully human*. It seemed to me that human nature included the capacity both for great goodness and for great evil. We studied genocide and cults as well as positive movements for social change and social justice. I would like to do further work on this topic, and maybe someday this will come together in a book.

Around this same time, a number of friends and family

started to talk about moving away from the area. It seemed like a point of general transition in our social group. This external synchronicity led my wife and me to start thinking about moving away, too. Champaign-Urbana is a very comfortable place to live and I could easily imagine comfortably passing another 40 years there. From a professional standpoint, looking back, I had become somewhat isolated in my practice and I needed to reinvigorate my life and work. The intensive learning through A'Claire had been life-changing, but somehow I felt I had reached a dead end. I could not figure out how to move forward.

New Zealand, New Beginnings

My 42nd birthday was a low point in my life that served as a creative space which eventually opened up a new chapter. It was a time of intense questioning. The future I had imagined seemed to have collapsed in on itself. The externals of my life were the same; probably very few people knew what I was going through. I have a picture of myself opening a CD that Mary Pat had given me as a gift. It was *Safari* by Jovanotti (aka Lorenzo Cherubini). I could not even understand my birthday present (Jovanotti sings in Italian)! But Mary Pat had given me a translation of the lyrics for the song 'Fango.' In the picture, our cat Neo sits next to me. In another picture, our bird Cinnamon looks over my shoulder from outside of her cage. Neo had terminal cancer that year, and this, coupled with so many friends talking about moving away, led us to rethink our lives.

We talked about various places in the US that we could relocate to. We had been contemplating moving up to the Chicago area to be closer to the A'Claire School, but now that idea held no appeal. At some point, we thought about moving to New Zealand. This had long been a kind of running joke of sorts as well as a back-up plan of mine. Whenever I felt things were not going well in my life, I would think, 'Well, I can always move to New Zealand!' I knew that New Zealand needed doctors and psychiatrists and that they were continually advertising these jobs in medical journals. The idea of New Zealand appealed to me as it is a beautiful country with a unique ecosystem. I knew they had a public health system, a progressive reputation and that they were a nuclear-free zone.

I started reading a couple of books on New Zealand and looking online at various websites. I told Mary Pat that, due to my practice and teaching, I did not want to leave Champaign for a couple of years, but that we could start looking into New Zealand in the meantime. I noticed something strange though: I felt deflated and a sense of loss as I returned to my daily life. I realized I had been flooded with feelings of excitement, adventure and hope just reading about New Zealand. On reflection, hope and a sense of possibility were what I desperately needed. We made the decision to move, and eight months later we had a one-way ticket to New Zealand, with no clear plans for the future.

It was the best of times. It was the worst of times. I loved learning about the cultures, learning different words and phrases, learning to drive on the opposite side of the road, learning to pronounce 'garage' and 'tomato' differently and the challenge of all those Maori words. However, my first job was not the best fit for me. In the States, I was doing full-speed 'accidental networking' (as I called the process of following leads and seizing opportunities) – building, putting things together, meeting with different people and continuously creating and re-creating my practice. I was constantly forming networks between clinical work, the community and teaching at the local college and university. A frequent saying in New Zealand (I think it comes from Winston Churchill in World War II Britain) is 'Keep calm and carry on.' There are many humorous variations on this saying, but it reveals a very different cultural orientation from that of the US. I thought the best fit for a US mentality was 'Get excited and make things!' These two statements sum up a great deal of the culture clash for me in New Zealand. It was not so much the job, at a community mental health center in the New Zealand public health system, that was the issue as much as it was my adjustment to a different practice setting and a different culture. However, it was not a good fit for me at that time. It did not help that I was probably making cultural blunders along the way.

I did learn a lot. I worked in an Assertive Community Outreach Service team which specialized in working with clients who were difficult to engage and had high levels of risk to themselves or others. With standard treatment, these clients might have fallen through the cracks, had frequent hospitalizations, or harmed themselves or others. The treatment philosophy of this model was for the team to work intensively, even on a daily basis if needed, with these clients in order to keep them safe and healthy in the least restrictive and least expensive setting. Rather than expecting clients to conform to the health care delivery system, the system conformed itself to the client.

One of my favorite memories of that work was driving up in a van with the team to drop off weekly medications to one of our older, Maori clients. He was losing a lot of weight and we had scheduled a chest CT as he was a heavy smoker. He did not want to go, absolutely not, no way. I tried reasoning with him, explaining why the test was so important and how long we would have to wait for another one to be scheduled if he did not attend the appointment. We even offered to pick him up and take him to the clinic. Finally he said, 'I'll only go if you tell me that, as my doctor, you are ordering me to go for the test.' OK, I thought, we'll try that. So I said: 'You *have* to go for this test. As your doctor I am *ordering* you to have this test done tomorrow.' 'OK, I'll go,' he said, smiling as if it was no big deal and we had not spent five minutes disagreeing.

I also worked in the general community team. One of the most surprising issues of culture shock was realizing that I expect the job to provide a structured approach to work. In all my previous jobs, I had had a good orientation about what was expected of me and had been provided with all of the things that I needed to do the job. Then someone would tell me how many patients to see each day and that would structure my day.

Coming to work in another culture, I had an increased need for orientation and definition in my job. You were supposed to 'get on with it,' 'keep calm, carry on' and figure it out. All of my attempts at clarification seemed to be somehow culturally inappropriate. I had a period of time where I knew I should stop asking about policy and procedure manuals, but I just could not help myself, as I felt increasingly desperate to find someone to tell me how my job was supposed to work. I could not believe that I should be seeing fewer clients in this job, backed by a whole clinic, than I had seen in a solo private practice in which I did all the administrative work myself.

I had so many meetings to go to that it seemed like I barely had any time to see patients and do my own work. Also, there was a very collective, group sense of taking care of clients, whereas in the US and particularly in my private practice, I was used to being personally responsible for my clinical decisions and work. At the community mental health center I was constantly being asked to provide prescriptions and fill out forms for clients I had never met. This went against my sense of individual responsibility and liability. I was the newest doctor at the clinic, but I was the only one who was there five days a week. In New Zealand, doctors have six weeks of vacation and two weeks of educational leave, so it was hard to adjust to someone always being gone; I was constantly scrambling to cover other doctors' clients as well as my own. To me, it felt like the entire system was about to crash. That must have been my own cultural perception, as the system seems to keep ticking along here ('She'll be right,' as they say in New Zealand, meaning it will all work out in the end). It was helpful for me to read Mark Thorpe and Miranda Thorpe's work on acculturation in mental health professionals who are immigrants to New Zealand.[7] Mila Goldner-Vukov also describes cultural adjustments in working as a psychiatrist in New Zealand.[8]

In the stress of the tension between ingrained practice approaches and the reality of the work in this new system and culture, I began to feel my personality changing. I became more suspicious and cynical. My usual ways of coping were not working and there was a painful period of time when I knew they were not working, but had not yet abandoned these coping mechanisms and acculturated. I started saying that it had taken me only two months to 'burn out' in New Zealand. Again, part of this is a cultural adjustment coming from the US where psychiatrists are often viewed as high-cost prescribers. This view leads to a system designed to have maximal administrative and nursing support to enable the doctor to see as many patients as possible (in my experience, this was usually about 24 patients scheduled per day). In New Zealand, I gradually learned that the psychiatrist functions as much or more as a team leader as a direct-care clinician. I was surprised at myself that I just wanted someone to tell me what to do. It was a challenge adapting to a different model of care at the same time as a new culture (and really not even just one culture, but a multitude of cultures that the staff and patients came from).

Generally, I would put in at least a year before changing jobs, but I heard that a job had opened up at Buchanan Rehabilitation Centre. The more I learned about it, the better the fit seemed to be. Psychiatric rehabilitation has quite an overlap with holistic medicine, as it is based on working with the whole person, not just someone's biochemistry. It entails a focus on instilling hope and motivating and encouraging people to grow. At Buchanan, there were art groups, literacy training, job training, horticultural therapy, sports groups, cultural groups and a number of other physical exercise and socialization groups. I started two groups that staff and clients both seemed to enjoy: a yoga group and a philosophy and spirituality discussion group. It felt like I, myself, was going through rehabilitation, as I found that all of my previous skills were needed. These included not just medication management, but also individual and group psychotherapy and the ability to create flexible rehabilitation programs that worked for the whole person.

After about a year, the opportunity arose to take on the clinical director role at Buchanan. This was a whole different level of challenge! I have been increasingly interested in working with staff and professionals in order to create a practice that works holistically with individual clients. (Let me tell you, though, this is easier said than done!) As I have mentioned previously, the same principles apply to professionals as well as patients. It is impossible to create a health care delivery system that treats clients in a holistic way unless staff are also treated in a holistic way. In my private practice, I was very focused on the personal connection between myself and the clients with whom I worked. In New Zealand I was faced with the task of creating a health care delivery system in which all the individuals within it, clients and staff alike, were encouraged to grow in their full humanity. The idea of creating a structure or system that does not become beholden to its own functioning and demands, but rather fosters and supports human connection, growth, healing, recovery and rehabilitation, is an incredible challenge.

In New Zealand, I developed a renewed interest in many threads of my life that had been quite important in the past. I had somehow set these aside over the years. Living in a bicultural country and a multicultural city piqued my old interests in cross-cultural psychology, anthropology and comparative religions. Auckland has the largest population of Polynesian people of any city in the world. The mental health workplaces are like working in the United Nations; my colleagues and clients came from all over the world. My interest in psychotherapy was also renewed, as I was providing psychotherapy supervision. I read the literature about psychotherapy with clients with psychosis to develop ways of working the client population. I met a number of very inspirational colleagues, including Debbie Antcliff, who worked to set up and shape Buchanan into the compassionate place that it is today. Also, Patte Randal challenged me to extend my holistic approach to understanding psychosis. Even though in my own holistic practice I had developed a deep understanding for how many psychiatric symptoms and syndromes can respond to holistic interventions in human dimensions beyond the biological, I still had felt that psychoses were a different kettle of fish. I made a distinction between dissociative 'psychotic-like' experiences and other psychoses, which I viewed as more 'brain-related,' and 'biological.' Working with Patte and the Re-covery Model[9] she has developed has made me really push the boundaries of my understanding of psychosis. I began re-reading Jung, who is starting to seem like an old friend who shows up in my life every few years. Jung's work provides another way of understanding psychosis, in which symptoms are meaningful experiences, and not just malfunctioning brain chemistry. In Jung's approach, symptoms are an attempt at growth, rather than a malfunctioning and broken mechanism.

I hope that this digression into my own work at creating holistic practices in different settings can serve as an example and maybe even an inspiration for your own work. I had originally tried writing a chapter that developed generalized concepts about creating a holistic practice and re-humanizing medicine, but it seemed to lack life and to have too many details. It seemed that the book called for a personal example.

Every true holistic practice is an individual creation which is alive and evolving. Corporate and institutional practices rarely have this same aliveness and flexibility. This is why so many clients and professionals find them dehumanizing. No matter what setting you are working in, you can 'make a practice your own,' although this may be more or less difficult depending on the setting.

I thought it might be of interest if I listed some of the various classes I have taken and skills I have learned. I offer these not as a recommendation of what a holistic clinician must do so much as an example of what one holistic clinician has done. As I have often said in this book, to be a whole person requires personal growth work. Some people explore a few techniques or modalities in great depth; others sample many different modalities. There is no 'right' way for everyone to follow. So, for what it is worth, here is a list of the personal growth modalities and techniques that I have sampled over the years (which definitely does not imply 'expert' level of mastery): painting, drawing, playing music, weight lifting, jogging, karate, meditation, dream analysis, journaling, writing (poetry, fiction, non-fiction), psychotherapy, various types of yoga, tai chi, Aiki awareness (blending of Aikido and meditation techniques), energy healing, visualization, gardening, backpacking, walking, life coaching, fencing, group fitness classes, massage and working with a personal trainer at a gym. I have also read widely as well as studied certain topics and authors in depth. Both depth and breadth are important in developing the different dimensions of your Self.

I have become lost in the materialism of medicine and I have become lost in the spiritualism of personal growth. Both of these are valid aspects of humanity, but what I return to is the *human*, which includes within it the ideal of the spiritual and the practicalities of the physical. There are so many different things to learn and to do in this world. Open your eyes, your mind and your body to all the many different possibilities that exist.

Earlier I mentioned that I had been contemplating the words to the song 'Fango' by Jovanotti on my 42nd birthday, a low point for me. I will end this chapter with a few excerpts from that song:

'Fango' (Mud)

...

The TV says that the streets are dangerous
But the only danger I really see
Is not being able to feel anything

...

A sign tells you that everything is around you
But you look around and there is nothing
The old world that stays together
Thanks to those who
Are still brave enough to fall in love

...

A heartbeat inside the chest
The passion that makes projects grow
Hunger and thirst, evolution in action
The energy created with contact.
I know I am not alone
Even when I am alone
I know I am not alone
So I laugh, and I cry
And I mix with mud and the sky[10]

Chapter 9

Transforming Your Practice

We had been brought up to notice, to take 'life as it is' and turn
it on the spindle of compassionate action to make it more like
'life as it should be.' This is resistance.
Shem[1]

When physicians become disillusioned with contemporary
medicine, they often look to different techniques to add to their
practice. As we have explored in this book, a different technique
does not necessarily mean that a clinician is actually practicing in
a different way. Just because you substitute an herb for a pill does
not mean you are really meeting the whole person of the client. A
physician might also look at getting a different job or working
with a different population as a way of dealing with burnout and
disillusionment. In most cases, a frustrated physician will be
looking for a way of practicing that is less dehumanizing.

While it is true that *where* you work is important, it is even
more important *how* you work in order to re-humanize your Self,
the client and your practice. A holistic practice can be created in
any setting as it is really the physician or clinician who ultimately
makes the choices that determine whether the practice is
dehumanizing or re-humanizing. If a physician embarks on the
ongoing process of transformation of Self, the practice will
naturally evolve into one that promotes the whole human being.

Decision, Decisions

Once you have done some initial work on self-transformation,
you will naturally have a lot of questions about creating a
practice that grows out of your own full humanity and
encourages the full humanity of the client. For instance:

Do I work alone or with other clinicians?

Do I hire staff or do things myself?

Do I start a practice from scratch or join an existing practice?

Do I try to expand my current practice in a holistic way or do I quit my job and jump off into the unknown?

Creating a holistic practice means that you will ask and answer these questions in different ways than in a contemporary practice. You will ask, ponder and respond to them using your whole Self. A holistic practice asks that you take responsibility for the way a system runs, even if you did not create that system yourself. In many contemporary practices these days, physicians are employees with a limited ability to determine how the overall practice will run. A holistic approach means that you will evaluate and re-evaluate many aspects of your practice with which most doctors do not bother.

I have discussed some of the issues I faced in medical practice, and also described my own growth process in creating a holistic practice and my ongoing work on the counter-curriculum of re-humanization. Yet there are many paths that clinicians follow in creating a holistic practice. For many people, it is a gradual process of becoming aware of the limitations of contemporary medicine, searching for something different, learning new techniques, doing personal growth work and finally, making a paradigm shift (and then this sequence is repeated). As has been discussed earlier, there is the risk that the search process will only focus on replacing contemporary techniques with Complementary and Alternative Integrative Medicine (CAIM) techniques. In this manner, the physician may remain a technician, albeit a 'natural' one, but without a deeper paradigm shift beyond technique to relationship. This could be called 'changing one's shoes without walking into another room.'

Personal growth work (learning, evolving, reassessing, getting perspective, allowing one's own interests to develop and change over time) is where the formation of a new relationship to Self can take place. This work is crucial in developing an identity as a whole human being and healer, not just a technician. It can help you to be more aware of the many dimensions of your Self so that you can begin to work in a multidimensional, holistic way with clients. Changing how you invest your time and energy will lead to a change in your practice. Change is like a pebble cast into a pond as your action leads to ripples that lead to further questions.

Part of the shift to a holistic practice is that you trust yourself in the evolving process. There is no blueprint or plan or protocol you can follow to be holistic, as that comes from a sense of Self, although it may be helpful to learn about the business side of medicine. You have to go through a search for a solution that feels comfortable to you because a holistic practice is one that takes your unique individuality into account. You will go through many transitions and phases as you grow; I hope the example of my own life showed that.

You have within yourself tremendous resources beyond your rational mind and ego. Let your dreams, mind, intuition, emotions, spirit, drive for creative self-expression, and your heart all work together to guide you in asking questions and making decisions. As you work on personal transformation, this will lead to external transformation of your practice, and vice versa. Remember the old alchemical saying, 'As above, so below.'[2] This statement encapsulates the holistic philosophy that everything is interconnected and change in one dimension brings about change in other dimension.

Many people start out making small changes in their current practice until they hit the limitations within it. The options at that point are: to stop growing and allow the setting to determine your practice; to challenge the setting to grow; or, to leave that practice setting. Growth is a scary thing. In the short run, it is always easier to keep working where you are, in your comfort zone. It is particularly challenging to walk away and step out into the unknown. Every change brings up anxiety and fears. When I started my own practice, I worried about financial security and about other doctors judging me negatively. But I faced my fears, felt them, lived them, and eventually I grew through them, stronger and wiser. I got outside advice, I consulted with other business people in health care and I did my own personal work through various therapies and life coaching. I went to conferences and listened and learned. I read and read and read.

There is a lot to consider in starting a holistic practice. There are the big generalities, like time, space, energy, money and practice setting. Certain contextual realities in your life may influence your decisions. If you have a family or a lot of debt, you may not be able to just quit your job and hang out a private-practice shingle. Certain kinds of holistic practices may be easier to integrate into a contemporary medical practice. Certain clinics or medical groups will be more or less accepting of you changing the way you work. Regardless of where you practice, there are certain principles to consider. A holistic practice is one that minimizes the fragmentation of patient care. It also requires face-to-face time for doctor and patient to work together to create a space for healing.

Where to Work?

You can create a holistic practice in any practice setting, but every setting will have different supports and barriers to practicing holistically. A truly human interaction requires time and energy in order to create a space that encourages the physician to act from a state of wholeness and encourages the wholeness of the patient to emerge. When defined this way, you can see that any setting can be a holistic setting, as long as you have a modicum of leeway as to how you will use your time and energy. Ideally, you would have unlimited time, energy and space to interact with each individual in your practice. But that ideal will never be a reality. Neither you nor any health care delivery system on the planet has such unlimited resources.

In a private practice, you decide how much time to spend with a client. You have control over what kind of space you create. You also choose how much energy to put into different aspects of your practice. The drawbacks are that you are responsible for everything. Even if you hire other people, you are still responsible for what they are doing. To quote one of the Spider-Man movies: 'With great power comes great responsibility.'[3] As a physician, you do have a lot of power – if you are willing to accept responsibility for that power. Starting a private practice gives you a lot of power to create the practice that you want, but this responsibility may be more than you wish to take on or more than you can take on due to other considerations with your specialty, or personal considerations.

You can work for someone else, and that gives you more guaranteed income, more infrastructure support for your practice, and more colleagues with whom to share the work. The downside is that you lose some power over decisions about how to invest time and energy. You also have less control over creating the therapeutic space. You have to see how good of a fit it is if you want to use certain CAIM techniques in that practice.

When considering where to work, ask yourself if you feel inclined to work within an existing health care delivery system to expand its holistic capabilities, or outside of existing delivery systems to create your own practice. Personally, I have pursued both paths – they are both very rewarding ways to create a holistic practice, but they have different challenges and rewards. In my own life, I have trusted when fate seemed to pull or push me in one direction or another. The risk of staying within the mainstream is of having a narrower perspective. The risks of staying outside the mainstream are mainly to do with isolation and radicalization. There are also risks of moving back and forth, including never feeling fully at home in either setting, finding it difficult to build something lasting, and not being fully recognized for your abilities in either realm. Every life choice is one that you will revisit from time to time. Depending upon your path, you may move in and out of systems, at times feeling you belong within a larger organization and at other times feeling just the opposite.

Working inside the System

By 'system' I mean standard, contemporary medical practice in a clinic or hospital setting. If part of the basis for a holistic practice is face-to-face time spent with the patient, then there are tremendous pressures working against you here. These stem primarily from the *economic rationalist model* of medicine, in which financial considerations strongly influence the structure of the system. The *biomedical model* does not inherently push doctors to see patients for shorter visits, but it does indirectly encourage this through the belief that a technical intervention for a problem that has been reduced to the level of scientific materialism does not require getting to know the person being processed.

There are different ways to change your practice within a larger organization. You can work at an individual level and focus on your own practice, providing the best care possible within the given framework. Another option is to work within the organization to make policy changes. This is generally not an 'either/or' decision, although you do need to decide how much you want to make waves in the larger system, and how much you want to just try to focus on your individual patients. You choose how your energy is most effectively invested. Just like choosing investment in a 401(k) or superannuation retirement scheme, you can decide how much energy to put into policy change and how much to put into direct care with patients. If you decide to change the system, you will need to get involved at an administrative level and help make policy. Barring this, you can still advocate for a holistic perspective. For example, you can affect the professional culture by speaking out about clinical and systems issues that interfere with meeting the needs of the client as a whole human being.

Stealth Care

If you decide not to get involved at an administrative level, but to provide 'stealth' holistic care in a contemporary medical system, you may choose to keep a low profile. If you have a degree of professional autonomy, or if you are more senior in the organization, you can try this approach: ignore the administration and just focus on creating a sense of openness in yourself and thus an environment of openness for your client. This way, you will always be, to some extent, an island within the larger system. You may need to refer clients out for some techniques or modalities that your organization will not support. At some level, you will run into constraints from the administration, and have to decide if these are acceptable. People change over time. Decisions are never made finally and indefinitely. If you truly want to re-humanize medicine, you cannot make decisions based on fear of change and avoidance of discomfort.

Spending more time with patients is a revolutionary act, and you may be treated as a revolutionary (or as a 'problem provider'). If you spend more time with patients, you will either see fewer people per day, or you will work longer hours to see the same number of clients as your colleagues. If you are paid on a productivity basis your income will be lower if you see fewer patients. Even if your pay is not lower, seeing fewer patients will create conflict within the organization between you and the people scheduling appointments, other professional colleagues, and ultimately the administration. Spending time with patients can be viewed as a subversive act in the medical-industrial complex, because it lowers profits and productivity, so expect periodic pressure from all quarters. There is a balance here; I am not advocating seeing one patient a day.

Changing the System

Personally, I think 'stealth holistic care' will result in a very limited holistic practice because sooner or later you will most likely become engaged in a policy debate with the administration. This is because you are going against the short-term financial priorities of most organizations who want you to see more patients. While you might feel this is unfair, it is not really reasonable to expect a system to change to suit your needs without you putting some time and energy into administrative issues.

Some systems are more open to change than others. For instance, some organizations believe in holistic care from either a philosophical or financial perspective. Many mainstream health care delivery systems have incorporated stress reduction clinics, multidisciplinary pain clinics, or integrative/holistic options for working with cancer and other specific, complex conditions. People are willing to spend money out of pocket to have more holistic, humane and personalized care. Also, certain disease states, syndromes and situations are more conducive to a holistic approach, such as hospice care, cancer treatment or posttraumatic stress disorder. The bottom line in health care, supported by numerous studies, is that preventative spending saves money in the long run. Most holistic practices will have a strong preventative and rehabilitative emphasis. If an organization is structured in such a way as to recognize and realize cost-savings over time from preventative care, it may be more open to a holistic treatment philosophy. Some organizations are beginning to recognize that if they want quality care, they need to support their clinicians and allow them to have smaller caseloads so as to have more time with clients.

Even if you are lucky enough to be working in a setting that is open to growth, you may still run into a lot of judgment and ridicule from other physicians within the organization. You may also be pigeon-holed into working with only one client type.

There may be leeway for working holistically with hospice patients, cancer patients, children, or pregnant women, but not throughout the organization. In a way, this is another case of compartmentalization. Rather than having a holistic philosophy distributed throughout the larger system, you may have a holistic clinic for a certain patient population.

In the current era, there are a range of options for expanding contemporary medicine. In the US, there are federally funded research grants from the National Center for Complementary and Alternative Medicine (NCCAM), a branch of the National Institutes of Health. There are also various clinics and hospitals that vary along the progressive–opportunistic spectrum of providing holistic care. By this I mean that *progressive* organizations will provide holistic medicine because it is viewed as *good medicine*; whereas *opportunistic* organizations will provide holistic options because it is viewed as *profitable medicine*. It is possible in some hospitals and clinics in the US to get acupuncture, massage, energy work, yoga, tai chi, meditation and many other modalities of treatment that even 10 years ago would have been ridiculed. There is a growing literature on the benefits of stress reduction training, mindfulness, meditation, various exercise modalities and even prayer in improving treatment outcomes. Public opinion is very much in favor of holistic models that include scientific contemporary medicine as well as attention to human dimensions beyond the biochemical.

In other countries, like New Zealand, government initiatives may favor different kinds of holistically oriented care, such as collaborative models between general practitioners and mental health services. Also, certain teams within the public health care system may value a multidisciplinary team approach, for example, rehabilitation, brain injury, hospice, oncology and pain clinics. In psychiatry, services such as assertive community outreach, early psychosis intervention, maternal mental health, and rehabilitation specialize in working with clients with complex needs. These services tend to have smaller patient loads in order to do more intensive work. Other services that require a broader approach include cultural teams that work with Maori or Pacific Island clients, whose cultural beliefs are holistically oriented. The inclusion of family networks is crucial to successful health care interventions with individuals from these cultures.

To work for change within a system requires a lot of patience and the realization that you might not even be around when the change finally occurs. Humanitarian work is based on doing what you feel is right, not what you think will profit you or make your life easier. Parker Palmer's concept of the 'new professional,' discussed elsewhere in this book, provides a model in which the professional serves as the conscience of the organization. Thus, the 'new professional' has a duty and responsibility to challenge the organization to ensure that its policies are humane and supportive to all.

Working Outside the System

When it is not possible to carve out a holistic niche as described above, or when system limitations seem too great, physicians may choose instead to create a practice outside of existing systems. (Both approaches are necessary for reclaiming the art, heart and soul of medicine.) Some of the considerations you may face if you choose to work outside of the system include whether to work in a holistic group or start your own practice, and whether or not to hire office staff.

Working in a Holistic Group

If you decide to leave the system in which you are working, it is probably an easier option to plug in to a holistic practice that is already set up, but the cost is that you may be limited by that system. There may also be a contradiction in creating *systematized* holistic care, as the very definition of holistic practice is the connection of the multidimensionality of the physician and the patient. Having a holistic organization is a little bit like trying to organize an anarchist club. Even so, there are a growing number of small practices, group practices, clinics and even large medical centers that are using more holistic perspectives. Patients definitely are interested in this and are willing to pay money out of pocket for someone willing to spend more time with them and to relate to them as a whole person.

There are many different philosophies about holistic medicine, and many different motivations for a practice to call itself 'holistic.' A practice may just want the window dressings in order to market itself as holistic, much like the phenomenon of 'green washing' when a company puts on a façade of being eco-friendly without changing company practices. A practice may also focus on one specific technique or on an assembly-line model of quick techniques. While a practice like this might call itself 'holistic,' the way it is structured is more akin to a contemporary medical practice where the physician processes a large number of patients via techniques. A truly holistic practice will give you the space to spend more time with your patients. It will also encourage you to spend time on personal growth, and give you the space for both you and your clients to grow in all dimensions.

There are many benefits to working in a group setting. For one thing, there is a very real factor of isolation and loneliness if you have an individual practice. Working with others provides social support and also intellectual stimulation. People who have trained in other specialties or traditions bring depth and variety to a practice. It can be tempting, particularly for physicians, to be a 'super-' man or woman who does everything for everyone. However, the truth of modern medicine is that you will provide care within a referral network. This may be an internal network within an organization or an informal network between individual providers.

In the community mental health system in New Zealand, I

have seen a multidisciplinary approach to mental health implemented very well at times. Some clients really do need a lot of support. For these clients, having an occupational therapist, psychotherapist, social worker, employment specialist, nurse, social worker and psychiatrist working together can be exactly what is needed. The benefit of a multidisciplinary team is that it brings together multiple experts, with different perspectives, to care for the whole person. The risk is that care and responsibility can become fragmented and the *person* can be lost within the team *system*. For a team to work well together, I believe there has to be one person who is responsible for the overall coordination and functioning of the team. This cannot just be nominal responsibility. It has to be real responsibility and with authority to guide and direct treatment. Also, each individual within the team must establish an authentic relationship with the whole person of the client, even if they are only intervening at one specific technical dimension. This means that each member of the team has to know what important clinical and human information to feed back to the team. It also means that that team has to have functional multidisciplinary team meetings on a regular basis to discuss the technical interventions that are being done within the context of the larger, holistic perspective of the person.

I think it is easier for a single person to have a holistic perspective in working with another individual. It becomes much more difficult in multidisciplinary teams, when you combine competing paradigms, personalities and politics. It reminds me of the common 'telephone' exercise in which a message is whispered through a group of people, and it comes out the other end often bearing little resemblance to the original message. It is difficult enough for one person to manage his or her own perceptual distortions. In a group, distortions can grow exponentially.

Any practice setting has strengths and weaknesses. Every

clinician will have a unique combination of strengths and weaknesses according to his or her personality, specialty, client population and treatment philosophy. Knowing your Self will help you to make the decision about whether or not working in a holistic group is right for you.

Starting Your Own Practice

Starting a private practice in the US in this day and age is a challenge and goes against the mainstream. A *New York Times* article stated that in 2005, more than two-thirds of medical practices were physician-owned. Three years later, that number had decreased to less than 50%.[4] While private practice is diminishing, it is not yet extinct. In some ways, it continues to evolve; there is a growing trend toward doctors leaving the system and starting what have been called 'micropractices.'

In a *Wall Street Journal* article, primary care physician L. Gordon Moore voiced his frustration with being pressured to see 30 patients a day, for 15 minutes each. He described feeling so rushed that he found himself making prescription errors and no longer providing 'the best medical care.' Instead of passively complying with an untenable system, he quit his job and started a practice without a nurse, receptionist or waiting room. Micropractices always rely heavily on technology and keep overhead low. As the article says: '(By) keeping a tight lid on overhead costs, (Moore) hoped to see fewer patients – no more than about a dozen a day – and provide them better care, and still earn a decent wage for a doctor.'[5]

Moore went on to found Ideal Medical Practice, a non-profit organization that assists doctors in the US with remodeling primary health care delivery systems. The Ideal Medical Practice model has significant overlap with the philosophy of holistic medicine and is similar to the Patient-Centered Medical Home model.

The Ideal Medical Practice model has the following elements:

Care is driven by the patient's needs, goals and values.

Access is 24/7.

The care team uses technology to its fullest.

Patients can see their own physician whenever they choose.

The majority of the office visit is spent with the physician.

Overhead is low.

Patients are seen the same day they call the office.

Physicians are able to see fewer patients per day.

Practices measure themselves regularly.

Practices are proactive in their care of patients with chronic illness.

Physicians are satisfied and feel in control.[6,7]

I was surprised to learn that the type of private practice I had created actually had a name: a *micropractice*! It met all of the above elements of an 'Ideal Medical Practice,' except for being able to see patients the same day. I could always do that in urgent situations, but routine appointments were often booked out a couple months, unless I had a cancellation. In the beginning, I did everything myself, including answering phones, doing billing, phoning in prescriptions and even shoveling snow. In my last year of practice, when I did hire some part-time help, a receptionist, I had to rent another room and pay wages and taxes. My overhead went up, but nevertheless I did not want to see more patients to increase my income. Having an employee was another learning process and the monthly payroll taxes were an added time commitment. In the end, every change to your practice has implications. My quality of life went up, but my income went down.

Even though I did not know I had started a 'micropractice,' it served me very well at the time, and I can recommend it as an incredibly flexible model for holistic work. There are downsides, however. I sometimes felt that I was always working (most weekends I went in at least one day). On Saturdays, figuring that

I would already be in the office doing paperwork, I would fit in an appointment or two. However, then I would not get my administrative work done and would have to come in on Sunday to catch up. I rarely felt that I was completely caught up with everything in the practice.

Another downside of the micropractice model is that it can be very isolating working by yourself every day. It really helped when I started teaching, although that was a pay cut from clinical work. It also helped to have a couple of days a month of contract work outside of the office.

Another option is to start a more standard private practice, with a waiting room, receptionist, nurse and maybe even other staff. You do have to consider what your priorities are, though, because you could easily set up your own system that then *runs you*, as you have to see more patients to make enough money to pay for increased overhead.

In New Zealand, there are options for starting a private practice. For example, you can join an existing practice that provides support staff and services such as booking appointments and taking phone calls. At least in psychiatry, most doctors who work in private practice also work part-time in the public system.[8] The perks of the public system are great, in terms of continuing education leave and funds, and these complement work in the private sector. Incidentally, the New Zealand public sector is largely comprised of specialists; general practitioners (GPs) are usually either in private practice or belong to groups. Also, compared to the US, where there are more specialists than GPs, New Zealand and the UK have larger percentages of GPs, compared to the US.[9]

There are a myriad of decisions that go into starting your own practice and it is impossible to anticipate them all. There are many books about starting a medical practice. These are designed to maximize your profits by teaching you how to create a business plan, arrange financing, branding, marketing and advertising. Learning the business of medicine is always valuable, but it is crucial when starting your own practice. The difference between a holistic practice and another business is that you want your business model to support work with the whole person of the client, not only to maximize profits. Running your own practice clearly shows you how business model decisions affect your practice and vice versa. What is important in a holistic practice is following what is in your heart and balancing this with all the analytical business issues. Many decisions will logically follow from what kind of holistic practice you want to have.

Do It Yourself, or Hire Staff?

Running an office yourself is a challenge, but it can be done, and one tremendous benefit is that there is no barrier between you and the client. You answer the phone, you return the calls, you do the scheduling, you do the billing, you call the insurance company and haggle over authorization of sessions and medication. This may sound like a lot of work unrelated to the practice of medicine, but the infrastructure of a practice is what shapes what you are able to do within the practice.

There are two primary barriers to taking on a solo micro-practice: first, the business side of medicine is daunting because most doctors are not taught even basic business in medical school; second, many doctors feel that business and administrative work is beneath them and that it is a job for 'support staff.' A lack of knowledge can be remedied. One of the most helpful things for me was that I was still working part-time at a community mental health center when I opened my part-time private practice. I had some really helpful staff at the clinic who walked me through the basics of filling out billing paperwork and gave me advice about troubleshooting problems with insurance companies. An exaggerated feeling of self-importance is a little more challenging to change. Even though I did not think I had such a bad attitude in this regard, it was still quietly there. I grossly underestimated how much time all of these 'support' functions really took. This created a situation in which I often felt beleaguered and stressed because I was constantly scheduling more clinical time than I had administrative time to support.

If you run your entire practice yourself, there are a lot of benefits. Being involved in every aspect of a health care delivery system means you learn how the entire system works. You become aware of changes in policy and payment from insurance companies as soon as they occur. You are also a more informed boss if you ever do hire someone to take on aspects of the work. Finally, you have a lot more compassion for patients as they navigate through the system.

In contemporary medical practice, you, as the physician, make a lot of decisions without fully understanding the situation or having all the details. A nurse or secretary takes a call from a patient who is a frequent caller and tells you, 'It's the same old thing again.' You trust that the staff person is using good clinical judgment, but what if they are having a bad day or are angry with this particular patient? Secretaries have never been trained clinically. They may be naturally good with gauging clients, but even so, if they make mistakes *you* are personally liable for the clinical consequences.

Even relying on clinically trained people is not foolproof. You have to make independent, professional decisions whenever there is an issue that is within your scope of practice. Many doctors' offices run without the doctor being fully present for all the decision-making and sign-offs throughout the day. If you think you can hire office staff so that you do not have to think or do your job, you are increasing your liability risk. In fact, this is one reason why many doctors leave group practices. Like L. Gordon Moore in the *Wall Street Journal* article above, they feel that the pressures for high productivity interfere with the quality of patient care and promote mistakes. In order to avoid leaving a practice and just recreating the same thing, you have to carefully consider your staffing structure.

The point is not to be fearful of liability, but to see that liability follows responsibility and you are the person who is ultimately responsible for the people you hire and for their decisions. You generally have the most education and training as well as the professional and legal liability. You may make hundreds of decisions every day in a busy clinic setting. It is easier to say 'yes' to something and sign off than to slow down, say 'no,' and have to explain why. Hiring good staff could help simplify your decision-making process, but you are still the one responsible for those simplifications.

Take care not to recreate a fragmented contemporary medical model in your practice. Each person you hire puts a distance between you and your patient. Poor communication is the norm in medicine today, so do not just recreate what is 'normal,' because that is very dysfunctional.

Some of your decisions about hiring office staff will depend on your life circumstances. If you have small children or other serious personal responsibilities, it may not be practical to do everything yourself in your practice. It is all about priorities. Fully consider every decision you make, because any structural decision will shape your practice in ways you may not anticipate. Having a holistic practice means that you approach everything as interconnected systems. This means balancing awareness of how multiple dimensions affect one another, including your life context, clinical, business and administrative considerations.

Your decisions about staff will also depend on what type of practice you have. If a typical session with a patient is an hour or more, you may only see five or six patients a day. In this case, you may not need a secretary, or maybe just a part-time secretary to help with returning phone calls, taking messages and doing some of the initial footwork with insurance companies. If your practice is one in which you are seeing a patient every 15 minutes or less, you would be hard-pressed to run an office yourself, unless you blocked out a substantial amount of time for documentation, phone calls, and insurance issues. I do not think you can have a holistic practice if you are seeing your patients for 15 minutes. I have found that 30 minutes, at least in psychiatry, is the minimum time for most patients, assuming there is flexibility for longer visits when required.

The Evolution of a Holistic Practice

As I went through my education and my practice, I would sometimes remember an incident that M. Scott Peck wrote about in *The Road Less Travelled*. When he was in training he became frustrated that, to provide the level of care he felt was required, he was spending more time at work than his colleagues, who were leaving hours earlier than he was. He went to his supervisor, presented the problem, and waited to be given a solution. Much to Peck's annoyance, his supervisor just kept agreeing with him and repeating, 'I have heard you, and I am agreeing with you. You do have a problem.' Peck became more and more angry, wanting his supervisor to somehow solve the problem, so that he could continue giving the best care to his patients while also leaving work at the same time as his colleagues. Eventually, Peck realized the wisdom of what his supervisor was telling him. He wrote, 'My time was my responsibility ... My working hard was not a burden cast upon me by hardhearted fate or a hardhearted clinical director; it was the way I had chosen to live my life and order my priorities.'[10]

Managing time is a central challenge in any practice. It is up to you to decide how much time to spend with clients. This decision cannot be made based on what others are doing, or on what the minimum needed to get by is. It is based on moral and ethical principles of what level of care you feel is best for patients.

Every person grows and changes over time and every medical

practice evolves with time. Some things you learned in residency work well in the real world and some do not. Fad diagnoses and treatments come and go. Even within evidence-based medicine, treatments once thought to be safe and efficacious turn out to not work very well, or to have serious side effects. Some medications that seemed to have an evidence-base have been pulled from the market due to serious side effects. Many treatments work for some clients and not others.

A holistic practice also grows and evolves with time. Exciting new developments with a lot of hype turn out to not be that effective. Other innovations in medicine really change the field. Techniques once dismissed as quackery are found to be effective treatments. For instance, electricity was widely used as a thera-peutic modality in the early 20th century, but was gradually forced out of practice following the Flexner report of 1910 in the US. Electrical treatments in the form of trans-epidermal nerve stimulation (TENS) units are now used for pain management. Electromagnetic fields have been recognized to promote bone healing after a fracture.[11] Electrical stimulation, in the form of electro-convulsive therapy (ECT), is also used in psychiatry for treatment-resistant depression. Growth in any discipline occurs through periods of small, incremental change interspersed with occasional leaps forward. When growth occurs too quickly, it may be unsustainable. When growth occurs too slowly there is the risk of stagnation.

For most doctors, learning holistic medicine is something you do on your own, outside of a formal training program. This is why I refer to re-humanization as a counter-curriculum. As noted in chapter three, there are a few residency programs in the US that focus on holistic or integrative medicine. Even if you attend such a program, you will develop your own style and focus.

Since most physicians go step-wise toward a holistic practice, most holistic practices grow slowly and organically. At first, you may have a straightforward contemporary medical practice. You might start spending a little more time with patients, listening to all the things going on in their lives before writing a prescription. After taking some courses or doing some reading, you may be comfortable discussing holistic treatment options with patients, perhaps directly asking them, 'What about fish oil, or herbs, or exercise, or meditation?' This stage of your practice may feel a little clandestine. You are advertising yourself as a contemporary medical doctor and your colleagues think of you this way, so it may feel like you are leading a double life. In fact, you are. Your inner philosophy is changing, but your outer actions have not yet caught up with the change. Slowly, though, you may start to 'come out' to a few patients. In other words, you become more comfortable with who you are and how you want to practice, even though it may be a change from the lockstep of contemporary practice. It is wise to start things slowly, get your feet wet, see what works for you and your patients and what does not. It is also wise to gradually build your own self-confidence because your colleagues and your administration may not be supportive of what you are doing.

In the last 20 years, contemporary medicine in the United States has come to tolerate and sometimes even embrace CAIM and holistic medicine, but that is definitely not the case in every practice setting. The head of an in-patient unit where I had admitting privileges once criticized me for not studying enough 'real medicine.' He had just reviewed my yearly continuing medical education activities, noticing that I had attended an American Holistic Medicine Association conference, even though the program was accredited through the University of Minnesota.

An excellent reference for the legal aspects of including CAIM techniques in your practice is Michael Cohen, Mary Ruggie and Marc Micozzi's *The Practice of Integrative Medicine: A Legal and Operational Guide*. This book provides a clinical risk grid that breaks down techniques into one of four categories depending on the research base: a) research supports safety and efficacy, b) safety supported, but evidence regarding efficacy is inconclusive, c) efficacy supported, but evidence regarding safety is inconclusive and d) research indicates either serious risk or inefficacy.[12] As a lawyer interested in integrative medicine, Cohen's 'CAMLAW blog' is a great resource.[13]

Making the Change to a Holistic Practice

There is no 'one way' of building a holistic practice. At some point, you may start to feel constrained in your current job. Even if your colleagues and administration are supportive of your interests, you may find that it is time for a change within your institution and decide to openly practice holistically. If your current job is not supportive, it is time to move on. The decision largely depends on personal variables, such as your life situation, your finances, the type of holistic techniques you want to practice and the kind of job opportunities available in your area.

Some doctors reach a point where they stop taking on any new contemporary medical clients. In other practices, your clients may grow with you. Even if you leave a clinic job and start your own practice, many of your clients may want to follow you. Many clinics have restrictive covenants or non-compete clauses to try and prevent this, but if you are practicing more holistically your patients may not want to switch to another doctor. These clients may either follow you to wherever you have gone outside of the non-compete radius, or they may come back to your practice if you return at a later date. This was the case in my practices. Patients really value a doctor who spends time with them. You may be surprised how many people will travel or pay out of pocket to continue seeing you.

If, at some point, you are considering making a leap into a more outwardly holistic practice, you do want to make sure you have all your ducks in a row financially. You may need to plan for a few years before making the leap. Perhaps take on some extra work, or go on a budget to try and pay off some bills, like credit cards, car loans, student loans. (My wife and I went on a strict budget to pay off our student loans before I started my private practice, we even down-sized our house. At one point, I had to keep track of my change in order to afford a cup of coffee, even though I was on a physician's salary. It was worth it, though, to have financial freedom once we paid off our loans.) Or, you may just get to the point that something has to change – and quickly. This cannot always be planned; you may just wake up one day and say, 'I have to make a change.'

The reality of a truly holistic practice is that you will spend more time with patients, you will see fewer patients and this may mean you will earn less money. If you control your expenses, this may not lead to a major decrease in your income. It is safe to say, though, that in most holistic practices you will make less money than if you put the same amount of time and energy into a contemporary medical practice. This is OK, though, because you know from a holistic practice that money is not the primary value; it is just one dimension and variable in life – an important dimension, but still, just one dimension. You choose the model of medicine that provides the right balance for you.

You can work out the balancing of 'contemporary practice' and 'holistic practice' over time. It may be that contemporary medicine pays more than your holistic work. You may have to take on contract work or do more contemporary work to supplement the income from your holistic practice. In this way, the contemporary work can support the holistic work. Of course, it seems anti-holistic to compartmentalize your holistic work. Even if you were to take on contract work in a clinic doing 10-minute medication checks, you would still bring your holistic perspective with you, but you would have to refer for the more time-intensive work. The clinic may not want anything from you other than straightforward prescription of medication. This still may be part of your work, though, particularly if you are just starting a more holistic practice and need to supplement your income. To think in 'all or none' concepts is not an aspect of holistic medicine. Remember that your practice is evolving; do not fret too much if you have to make some compromises along the way.

Every doctor practicing holistically will have his or her own blend of CAIM approaches and contemporary practice. Within the life of your own practice, sometimes you may practice more within a contemporary framework and other times within a holistic framework. Similarly, there will be times when you focus more on one dimension of your holistic practice than others.

One aspect of holistic practice is knowing when you need to devote time and energy to one specific dimension, such as financial, conceptual, practical treatment, personal growth, professional education, business education, learning CAIM techniques, or keeping up with contemporary medical education. At different times, you may be learning to do business or admin-istrative things yourself, or else hiring people to work for you so you can focus on certain aspects of your business. To have a holistic focus is to be aware of the whole and yet still be able to put a lot of energy into one part of the whole as it is required.

As you go through this process, there will be periods when you are excited – everything is new and fresh! Other times, you will despair, feeling that you know 'nothing.' Sometimes you may feel pretty confident in your treatment approach, and other times you may feel compelled to get supervision or to learn about a new facet of your practice. Over years, you may go through this process of leaving one type of practice and growing into another.

There are two distortions regarding change in your practice: changing too quickly, and not changing at all. As the *I Ching* states: 'When change is necessary, there are two mistakes to be avoided. One lies in excessive haste and ruthlessness, which bring disaster. The other lies in excessive hesitation and conservatism which are also dangerous.'[14] People's fears and defenses can pull them into never changing and doing the same thing in repetition, or in constantly changing and chasing the 'newest' CAIM technique. Changing too little or too much can both be distractions from creating what, in your heart, you truly wish to create. Everyone is constantly creating in their lives and their practices (even if you work in a structured clinic). The question is where are you creating from – your fears – your mind – your heart – maybe from your whole Self? Life is a balance of change and stability. However, life is not constant stability; that is stagnation. Nor is it constant change; that is chaos.

Your work in holistic medicine will change over time and it may lead you through many different practice settings. Each setting offers benefits and restrictions as to how you want to practice. Each also offers new learning opportunities. It is possible to focus on connection and holistic medicine in any practice setting. You never know how all the pieces will fit together while you are gathering them. Focus on what you can learn in a particular setting. When you begin to feel constricted, re-evaluate whether there is room to grow in a different direction within your current setting, or whether it is time to move on to a new setting. Maybe it is even time to create your own health care system. Working to bring your full humanity into your practice of medicine is a continual process.

Creating a Holistic Practice Exercise

When you face those aspects of your practice that do not support living from all human dimensions, you will likely encounter internal and external resistance as to why you cannot change those aspects. Some of these resistances you may have to accept, but others may be possible to change. Whenever you tell yourself that you cannot change something in your life, sit down and really ask yourself why you believe those things cannot change.

It can be helpful to write down, as a thought experiment, some of your thoughts about change, including: 1) what you want to change; 2) why you want to change it; 3) the reasons why you feel you cannot change the context of your life; and 4) any idea, no matter how crazy, about how you could change. Putting excuses down in words often exposes them for what they are, whereas putting truths down in words will tend to strengthen truth. Try asking each of these questions from each of the different dimensions of yourself: how do you feel in your body; emotions; mind; heart; self-expression; intuition; and spirit?

Chapter 10

Holistic Decision Making

The poet's noblest work ... his life; and his poetry would grow
out of his life
Carl Bode, on Henry David Thoreau[1]

We often think of decisions as something that we make with our
logical, rational mind. Those of us who have gone through
medical education have become decision-making machines, and
have memorized and internalized algorithms and flow charts.
However, most important decisions are made with more than just
the mind. It is important to consider your feelings, if your 'heart
is in' a particular decision and what you are aware of intuitively.
You may even use spiritual guidance through prayer or
meditation to have a broader perspective when making
decisions. I have come to believe that the proper role of intellect
is to help you enact a plan once you have deeply felt a need for
change. Too much intellectualization can actually prevent you
from being aware of your true feelings and desires.

An example from my own life is from a time when I was
working at a for-profit, multi-specialty clinic (I mentioned this
decision in chapter eight, but it illustrates a point about decision-
making). Allan, the head of the psychiatry department, had
gathered together a group of caring and committed mental health
clinicians who definitely were not 'cog in the machine' clinicians.
Allan's philosophy seemed to be a kind of 'stealth, under the
radar' approach, where we practiced according to the care a
patient needed, rather than maximizing profit. Eventually, we
showed up on the radar when a change in clinic administration
came about.

The new administration began to institute what they called an *eat what you kill* reimbursement model. (Yes, they actually used those words to describe how supposedly caring, health professionals should get paid.) This meant that the higher earning specialties would no longer 'subsidize' the operating costs of the primary care specialties and psychiatry, which require a lot of direct patient contact time and do not have any high-income earning procedures. As it became clear how the clinic was going to be run, Allan announced he was leaving. Then another psychiatrist announced she would be leaving. The clinic administration and my other colleagues asked me what I planned to do. The administration even approached me and said I could develop a 'boutique' practice: I would be in charge and get rid of the 'dead wood,' their term for some of the clinic's professionals who were allegedly not pulling their weight. I disagreed with this analysis of why the psychiatry department was not making more money.

I did not know what I was going to do. I considered negotiating with the clinic to create an upscale holistic practice, but that was just a brief thought as I could not view my colleagues as 'dead wood.' I did not necessarily want to stay in this new environment, but the idea of facing a two-year non-compete clause in which I would have to work outside of a 30-mile radius did not appeal to me either. I knew that a job that complied with the non-compete would be a 45–75 minute drive to the next nearest communities. Believe it or not, I had never had a job to which I could not walk or ride my bike. Even in medical school and residency, I only had a couple of rotations where I had to drive to work.

I felt stuck. I did not want to stay and I did not feel I could go. The decision came in a flash while my wife and I were sitting at a restaurant, getting a late-night dessert. As I held a forkful of blueberry pie, I suddenly realized, I *have* to leave the clinic. This was not a reasoned, intellectual decision. In fact my intellect was screaming, 'No! I cannot do it! I do not want all that uncertainty and hassle!'

The decision was an inner sense of certainty that hit me full force between one bite of pie and the next. Once I had that certainty, then I jumped into action and my intellect became very helpful. Within a few weeks I had three job offers. I ended up taking the job that was furthest away – one I had almost not considered due to the distance. This job ended up being only be part-time, but the employer contracted me out to work at a neighboring community mental health center, which happened to be where Allan had taken a job. He and I got to spend many pleasant hours commuting together back and forth from work, as well as regularly getting coffee over lunch. What had seemed like a losing proposition actually turned out to be a great experience.

Decision-making is something that you can do with either your limited mind and ego, or by letting the choices percolate through your body, emotions, mind, heart, creative self-expression, intuition, spirituality, as well as through the dimensions of context and time – until a decision becomes clear with input from *your total Self*. Decisions made this way may 'freak out' your ego, but they can be truly transformative. Recall my description of my decision to move to New Zealand that balanced dreams, desires, excitement and hope with the 'What ifs' and 'You cannots' of the ego and intellect. It is not always easy to listen to your whole Self, trusting those dimensions beyond the limited ego. But if you work on being open to your own multidimensional nature, you will be guided and supported in deciding how to create a more holistic practice.

In the rest of the chapter, we will examine decision-making from each of the different human dimensions. While I did not consciously think about it at the time of writing, Rick Jarow, in his book, *Creating the Work You Love*, uses a similar framework, recommending that people consider input from their physical, emotional, mental, heart, self-expression, intuition and spirit dimensions in order to create work that is fulfilling and meaningful. We will be looking more specifically at holistic decision-making for a medical practice. The discussions below can apply to whether you are creating a practice from scratch, reassessing your current practice, or looking to join an existing group practice.

The Physical Level of Decision Making

At the physical level, you will be aware of your physical body in the physical space of the practice. (You will notice there is some overlap with the contextual dimension in a later section. This is because your physical body is the interface between 'you' and your environmental context.)

Whether you are looking at your current practice or at a new practice, you can use your physical body to gather a lot of valuable information. What does the office space look like from the outside? Is it visible and accessible, while feeling safe and protected? What is the physical plan of the office space? What are the first things that you notice as you walk into the clinic and waiting room? How does it feel to sit in the waiting room? What are the bathroom facilities like? How private do the offices feel; are they sound-proof? Is there adequate lighting and air flow (e.g. do the windows open)? Is the temperature comfortable?

Ask yourself whether you can afford the space. It is always wise to keep a low overhead in a holistic practice, as you may see fewer clients and have a lower income than in a profit-oriented practice. The higher your fixed expenses, the more you will feel pressured to make more money. Also, be wary of recreating a contemporary medical practice by having a big space and a bunch of employees to do the work. While this might appeal to your ego, it creates a larger overhead and layers of disconnection between you and your client.

What about the availability of public transportation? And proximity to other businesses? I always prefer to work somewhere that I can walk to get lunch or a cup of coffee as I find physical exercise very helpful for getting perspective and reducing stress.

All of these aspects are relevant if you are choosing your own office space. They also apply in a practice where you will be employed. Even if you do not have control over the larger clinic space, you can always decorate your office so that it is both an expression of who you are and also creates a welcoming and comforting space.

The Emotional Level of Decision Making

Your emotions may actually be what get your attention, causing you to reassess your current practice or start looking for other opportunities. If you notice you feel stressed, tense, irritable, anxious, sad, or angry in your current setting, the *problem* may not be your clients or your colleagues or the administration; it may be that *you* have changed and it is time for you to grow or change something in your life. You may realize this at the emotional level before you notice it at the intellectual level.

What is your emotional reaction as you walk through the physical space? Does it feel safe, secure, private, yet open, welcoming, and encouraging? How do you feel as you interact with the staff? How does the staff treat you and how do they interact with clients? What is the emotional tone of the place? Even if you have a great physical space, take a few minutes to feel what emotions the space evokes in you.

While medicine often tries to train us to ignore our emotional awareness, most people understand this level without too much difficulty. If you strongly rely on your thoughts, you might notice that when someone asks you what you feel, you answer, 'I think (such and such).' To develop the emotional level, ask yourself, 'What do I feel?' Keep asking yourself this until you can answer in terms of some feeling, such as angry, scared, happy, mad, shocked, peaceful, excited, petrified, curious, content, or indignant.

The Intellectual Level of Decision Making

Looking at the intellectual level of your thoughts can help to balance impulsive emotions. You do not want to quit your job if you have one bad day, but also, you do not want to use your intellect to convince you to stay in a job in which you are miserable. Your intellect can help you gain an objective sense of the variables involved in any decision. It excels at analysis and comparison.

In your current practice, your intellect may be helpful for analyzing the context of your feelings. For instance, there might be new management and it may not be clear how they will run the clinic. At the level of the intellect, you may decide to see how it works out over a set period of time, and to let your emotions simmer in the background until it becomes clear. Your intellect may also tell you that something is just not going to work, logically, with your current inner state and the external environment of the clinic.

If you are looking at moving, some of the things you will want to learn are the basics of any practice choice. The intellect loves to learn, to read, to get details, specifics, numbers and statistics. How much money will you make? Are you an employee, a partner, or an independent practitioner? If you are not a strict employee, how are expenses and profits divided up and paid? Are there hidden personal expenses, like having to pay support staff salaries, pay for your own phone line, advertising, or malpractice insurance? How is billing done? Who gets authorizations from insurance companies for visits? Are there call expectations? How are patients in crisis handled during office hours and after hours? Do you have to pay your own tail coverage for malpractice insurance if you leave the practice? Are there expectations that you will donate some of your services? (I actually spoke with a group who required that all clinicians do 10% of their work pro bono. I felt this was intrusive. I have also come to believe that free care undermines the sense of responsibility that is necessary for clients' healing. I would rather charge $5 for a visit than let it be free. It is not about the income for me, but rather clients' commitment to their own health and healing.)

There are other issues more specific to holistic medicine. Will the other clinicians accept the type of holistic work that you do? Due to prejudice, it may be rejected as 'unscientific,' or you just might be ridiculed. What kind of work are the other clinicians doing? Do you feel comfortable with it? Could you be held accountable if another clinician is sued? What kind of opportunities are available for your own personal and professional growth? Does the organization value change and growth, or expect you to perform 'X' number of techniques a day?

As a physician, you probably will not need to work on developing your intellectual ability. Medical education in the Western world already focuses heavily on that. The challenge is to balance your intellect with the other dimensions of your Self.

The Heart Level of Decision Making

When you are facing a decision, someone may ask you, 'Is your heart in it?' There is real meaning in this saying. Heart is different from emotion, as emotions are more fleeting and have a smaller scope than heart. Heart is what sustains you in the long run, what pumps you up, and what gives you a sense of strength to struggle against adversity for a cause or purpose.

Pay attention to how you feel in your heart. For some people this is quite easy, whereas others have to work at it. You can actually feel your heart open or close if you practice being aware of this dimension. As you focus on your heart, does your chest feel like it opens up or does it tighten up? You have to get to know yourself and what sorts of things make you afraid. Your heart could be trying to open to a possibility, but if your ego is afraid of change, you might close down or try to restrict this opening. Just as you need time and space in order to become aware of the flow of your emotions, you also need time and space to develop awareness of your heart. It takes practice and is like another language or layer to add to that of your physical body, emotions and mind.

To bring heart into your decision-making, you can ask yourself, *Is my heart in this decision?* Something may be great from an analytical level, but it might not be for you, even though it is great for someone else and a valuable service to the community. Many people go through life doing what they 'are supposed to do' or trying to make their parents or spouses happy. Some people even become doctors because it was someone else's idea, not their own. Opening your awareness to the wisdom of your heart is a scary thing because it can lead you in directions that your ego is afraid of going. As Howard Thurman said, 'Do not ask yourself what the world needs. Ask yourself what makes you come alive and then go do that. Because what the world needs is people who have come alive.'[2]

A challenging dilemma is when your emotions and intellect are saying, 'I have to get out of here,' and you feel like your heart is saying, 'But I have to take care of all these patients; I cannot abandon them.' This is a very complex situation in which you can feel pulled in different directions. (Using a multidimensional model of human experience actually provides a framework for understanding this sense of being pulled in different directions. This happens when different dimensions process your situation in different ways, with different values and priorities. Your challenge is to integrate or synthesize the different perspectives from within yourself to come to a decision). There may be times when you, for professional and ethical reasons, choose to stay in a situation for other people, even though you yourself are unhappy or suffering. It is true, after all, that the heart dimension is where you first transcend your ego in order to be compassionate toward others. However, this is a tricky situation; if your heart is gradually becoming depleted, you will soon have nothing left for yourself or to give to others.

Are you caught up in a situation in which you feel your clients are helpless without you? The two primary distortions of the heart dimension are to either give, give, give without receiving in turn, or avoid giving, leaving you 'cold-hearted,' analytical, clinical, aloof and unaffected. Healing the latter distortion is the focus of this book. The former distortion of the 'perpetual giver' can mislead you into believing self-sacrifice is the ultimate good. This could mean that you are creating dependency rather than empowerment for clients. Or that you have an exaggerated sense of importance and specialness, for instance that no other clinician understands your special clients the way you do. This view fosters dependency in clients, while growing your own narcissism.

Remember what the physical heart does. It receives the oxygen-depleted blood from the body and gives this to the lungs where it is re-oxygenated. Then the heart receives the richest blood in the body, replenishing the heart itself. This rich blood is then given away to the rest of the body.

The heart dimension works in a similar, metaphorical way. It can take in pain and suffering and transform and heal it, but it can only do this by balancing giving with receiving. A heart that gives without receiving and replenishing becomes weak, depressed and hopeless. A heart that receives without giving becomes engorged, stagnant and preoccupied with the ego. A heart that neither gives nor receives becomes like the caricature of the objective scientist, an island of intellect that stands aloof and disconnected. And as Philip K. Dick has written in his essay, 'Man, Android, and Machine,' that 'which is a mental and moral island *is not a man.*'[3]

If you recall, one of the ten principles of the AHMA is that *the physician teaches by example*. Sometimes the best thing you can do for patients with whom you are working is to quit. This 'quitting' may be metaphorical or literal. Metaphorically it may mean to quit *doing for them* and start *supporting* them to solve their own problems. This is similar to the concept behind the saying. 'If you give someone a fish they are full for a day, but if you teach them how to fish, they are full for a lifetime.' Having the courage to quit, when this is the most appropriate option, may also mean literally quitting your job, or an insurance plan. I remember having a contract with a particular insurance company that I felt was unethical in its treatment of doctors and clients. It was difficult to stop taking the insurance because I knew it would mean that some of my clients would no longer be able to see me, but I eventually chose to walk away from that contract. I can remember some patients telling me that they understood and supported my decision and that they were going to change insurance plans so they could continue working with me. Sometimes 'soldiering on' is not the best thing to do because it can be collusion with a malfunctioning system. Quitting a system sends it a clear message. It must then either respond or work harder to ignore the problem.

Developing the heart level of decision-making will ultimately support your own heart and others' hearts. But how can you develop your heart, particularly given all the statistics about burnout and physician dissatisfaction? In addition to this book, you may find it helpful to read books by other physician authors: Robin Youngson (*Time to Care*), Allan Peterkin (*Staying Human During Residency Training*) and Lee Lipsenthal (*Finding Balance in a Medical Life*). These all focus on how to bring more heart into medical practice. Gerald Arbuckle's *Humanizing Healthcare Reforms* has a similar focus, although it targets the system level, rather than the personal. Arbuckle appeals to strengthening the *foundational model* of health care, which has its basis in many of the assumptions and values of Christianity and Western human-itarianism. Eastern spirituality also has a strong tradition of focusing on compassion in action. For instance, Gandhi's book, *An Autobiography: The Story of My Experiments with Truth*, documents his own struggles on a personal level to live the concept of *Ahimsa*, 'not-hurting, non-violence.'[4] While Gandhi writes largely about operating in the political arena, many of the same concepts apply to professionals developing the heart dimension in medical practice.

The Creative Self-Expression Level and Decision Making

The creative self-expression dimension is like a structure or blueprint for your life. By developing awareness of this aspect of yourself, you sense areas in which you crave self-expression. Creativity and self-expression are linked; creativity means bringing your own perspective (expression) into what you are doing. It means you are engaged with what you are doing and not just following the guidelines someone else has assigned for what a practice is supposed to be. You are making it your own.

This dimension is quieter and steadier than your emotional dimension which may shout and scream and curse and cry. The dimension of self-expression is more like the current in water, a steady pressure encouraging you to move in a certain direction. If you ignore the current, you have to work harder just to stay in the same place. If you decide to do something challenging (that is true to an inner drive to create) and it is in alignment with the current, you will feel supported and will find you can rise to the challenge. This dimension is where you will discover your passion and what your dream job would be.

You do not need to be 'good' at something in order to long for self-expression in that area. In fact, it is often the areas in which you are least experienced that you have the greatest growth potential. An example of this from my own practice was the business end of things. While I was really excited about physically decorating my office and even making artwork specifically designed for the practice, I dreaded learning all of the business details. I had a good advisor at the time, Susan Matz, who encouraged me to learn every detail of the practice and to avoid hiring out any aspect of it, such as billing, until I understood it thoroughly. Luckily, my desire to create my own practice was strong enough that I faced my fear and jumped in with both feet. It was not always pretty; I made a lot of mistakes. For example, I did not collect all the money that I was entitled to with Medicare in the first year as I was learning the system. But in the end, I was running my own practice. I had created something that was new, unique and my own. And I found that I was continually growing and evolving with my practice.

Once my own holistic practice was established, I spent time trying to put together a holistic group practice. I had a vision of a big open space with a group of professionals from many mind–body disciplines, not just mental health. I pictured gardens, an art room and a cozy waiting room. I imagined how this center would differ from a psychiatric or medical clinic by interfacing with the community, because I believed that treating people in isolation is not the best care. I also wanted the center to be a place of learning and growth for people from the community; I imagined having yoga and exercise groups, as well as other kinds of creative and personal growth classes. I got to the point of looking at space with a few other people, but it just never quite came together. We found a beautiful house on the historic register that had room for everything I had envisaged. But the old building would have cost a lot of money to fix up. I eventually let go of this dream as we decided to move to New Zealand, and I closed my private practice.

As I mentioned earlier, my first job in New Zealand was a challenging transition for me. But when I walked into my second job, my eyes opened wide and I felt like I had found my dream job (as well as went through my own rehabilitation). The Buchanan Rehabilitation Centre had gardens and a horticultural therapist. There were groups that focused on exercise, physical health, culture, creativity and recovery. The setting was supportive for starting the Exploring Mental Health with Yoga group with Sneh Prasad, Bernie Howarth and Arishma Narayan all co-facilitating. We had a lot of fun in this group. We celebrated Holi (complete with colored powder, to the perpetual disappointment of the housekeepers, Vai, Karly and Karen) and Diwali (Deepawali) where we had great food and the opportunity to learn the cultural history of the festival. I also worked with staff on a philosophy and spirituality discussion group that was really interesting and rewarding. A number of staff helped out with this group, including Veronica Rodricks, Kiri Prentice, Mark Mercier and Peter Mutch. There were a number of great artists (Neil Dizon, Michael Cashmore, Peter M.) as well as musicians on staff (Pete Brown, Neil, Chris Koneferenisi) and these staff brought their intuition and creativity into our work. I should really list every staff member by name, as they all brought so much of themselves to work in a holistic way. We had around 70 staff members and 40 clients at the rehabilitation centre, so it was really intensive work. I came to appreciate each and every human being at Buchanan.

One of the things I really valued in the groups that I was involved with was the integration of staff, clients and students all participating in learning, teaching and doing different activities. It was kind of an 'All Do, All Learn, All Teach' model. You really have to use your intuition, though, in running these kind of groups, balancing the involvement of people at various levels in a way that is always focused on learning and fun while also being therapeutic.

I started doing, what I came to call, collaborative poetry writing with clients, sometimes one on one and other times with a few people. This was a great way to have human interactions that were not so 'clinical,' but brought up a lot of serious existential issues. I believe that the rhyming aspect and my interventions to shift emotional or thought blockages to refocus on the flow of words of poetry helped clients to structure and express strong emotions and disorganized thoughts. This provided a non-medical approach for working with emotions and traumas in a truly healing way. It also provided a source of self-esteem for clients to have their thoughts and words so closely attended to and valued. Some of these poems were then published in the BRC Magazine the staff and clients put together. The process of writing, for me, was very intuitive, I had to let go of trying to do psychotherapy, but at the same time I would challenge thoughts, actions and behaviors through introducing different themes to the narrative of the client. Oftentimes, this would be something paradoxical or would broaden the context of an absolute statement of the clients. I did not really think about it at the time, but I would say the guiding principles were to keep the emotions, thoughts and words flowing; to pay attention to both content as well as structure and form of the language, for instance rhyming, punning, repetitive structures within the poem; and that any experience can lead to learning and growth.

Prior to going to New Zealand, I had the desire to build a community center that included arts, physical exercise, nature, creative multidisciplinary staff all working together collaboratively. I was disappointed that it did not come together in the States, but then I came across a setting that had many of the components I had dreamed of. This goes to show that you should not give up on your dreams and you do not have to create everything from scratch. Sometimes what you see in your vision is already out there.

While this section is discussing the dimension of creativity and self-expression, this discussion of the work at Buchanan Rehabilitation Centre demonstrates how creativity can be used to integrate a number of dimensions in a holistic way, including aspects of care that are often lost in contemporary medical settings, such as the heart, creativity, intuition and spirituality. My daily work there really was a balance of all dimensions, ranging from physical concerns such as safety, risk, and psychiatric medication, all the way to the spiritual growth of clients and staff.

We will finish this section with a brief discussion of how self-expression can transform your practice. Stephen Bergman, aka Samuel Shem, the author of *The House of God*, has made a career of speaking up against dehumanization in medicine. In an article called 'Fiction as Resistance,' he explores the ways in which writing fiction can be used as a form of protest and resistance against dehumanizing systems. This brings together creativity, in the form of fiction writing, with self-expression of one's own experiences. Shem's writing always has the feel of a blend of autobiography and fiction as a way of reaching human truth. His advice is aimed not only at transforming the individual in isolation, but also transforming medicine into a more compassionate system. He lists four ways to 'resist the inhumanities in medicine:'

1. Learn our trade, in the world.
2. Beware of isolation. Isolation can be deadly; connection heals.
3. Speak up ... *speaking up is essential for our survival as human beings.*
4. Resist self-centeredness.[5]

Shem shows us that using our voice to speak up is healing for ourselves and also for medicine and society. Just as we have examined how the personal can become universal through poetry, so too can the personal become political, when we advocate for social change.

The Intuitive Dimension of Decision Making

Intuition is the realm of direct knowing that does not rely on the senses, the body, emotions, or the mind. Intuition is a sudden illumination, like when I suddenly knew, between two bites of pie, that I was leaving my job. The decision was just suddenly there. You can ignore intuition, but you can also develop greater awareness of the information available at this level to guide you and give you feedback on your decisions. Intuition is a sense just as much as vision, smell, hearing, touch and taste. In fact, sometimes it is called the 'sixth sense.' This dimension combines many facets of information over time and space into a felt sense. The language of intuition is the metaphorical language of dreams during sleep, for instance when a 'snake grasping its tail' represented the circular benzene ring in Kekule's dream.

There are many popular and professional books that discuss how to develop your intuition, but the important thing is to practice connecting to your own intuitive sense. Each morning, ask yourself, 'What do I sense about this day that is about to begin?' Or before seeing a patient: 'What do I sense this person will bring to this meeting?' This creates a feeling of openness as well as showing you any preconceived notions you might have. Similarly, when deciding about a change in your career, you can develop a sense of how you might grow in a particular practice. Intuition is more like daydreaming than analyzing something with your mind. Try to fantasize, dream and muse about what might unfold. Thinking is a form of doing. Intuition is more like allowing. Thinking can close down intuition; it wants an answer, an end, a goal. Intuition is a flowing stream; it encourages you to follow it and may suggest things you had never before imagined.

Intuition is known to be helpful in clinical work, in creative work and in scientific research. To use it to help create a holistic practice, you may need some time and space for intuition to arise to consciousness. Intuition bridges the line between consciousness and the unconscious. It is something that you know unconsciously, without intellectually assembling each piece of the puzzle. It can be an amazing thing when intuition pops fully formed into consciousness, but usually intuition takes some work. For example, you may exhaust yourself intellectually, thinking and re-thinking a problem until you give up – which is when intuition may suddenly 'pop out.' There are also techniques for allowing intuition to cross over into consciousness. These include: active imagination,[6] writing down your dreams, putting a question on a piece of paper before you go to sleep, sitting and watching the waves or the wind, or just shifting gears, taking a walk, working out, or even taking a bite of blueberry pie.

The Spiritual Dimension of Decision Making

What is a valid experience? For instance, if a dog bites me, is that a valid experience? It is an experience; and if I have a religious experience, well that is an experience too, and how shall I say that it is valid? You might say, 'Oh, you have an imagination, you have an illusion; you think that you had a religious experience.' Well, that does not concern me. Perhaps it is an illusion; how do I know?' There is no criterion. I can only say, 'I felt like this.' Of course, you can draw conclusions, and so you can ask, 'Are the conclusions you draw from it valid?' ... Is that interpretation valid? ... (T)here is a considerable difference in the interpretation of such experiences, but the experiences themselves are always valid because they exist. Carl Jung[7]

The spiritual dimension is the sense of how you fit into something larger than yourself. It is big-picture awareness, and it yields a sense of purpose and meaning in life. Jung's perspective on religious and spiritual experiences is that, while they may be intangible from a physical perspective and they are illogical from an intellectual perspective, these experiences are valid, belonging to a subjective domain of human existence. While Jung is speaking of more dramatic spiritual experiences, the spiritual dimension is part and parcel of everyday life. Even mundane decisions and experiences have a spiritual dimension.

Earlier, I mentioned an example of the spiritual dimension in action from my own life, when one day I had the sudden realization, 'I am a small business owner in this community.' I realized that I was a part of the community and that I offered a valuable and unique service. This did not happen until I had been practicing for a year or two and reflected on the connections I had made to the larger community. This sense of having created something and expressed a heretofore hidden aspect of myself gave me a tremendous sense of accomplishment and gratitude. The spiritual aspect of this experience was the sense of connection and pleasure I felt as I recognized how my individual work fit into the larger community. In starting my own practice, I had developed a systems-level awareness of how medicine works, and became aware of the interplay between the structure of health care delivery systems, and individual, social and economic variables. Through dealing with the everyday practicalities of running a practice, I had gradually developed a sense of the bigger picture, and a sense of connection that extended beyond the day-to-day.

I had another practical, spiritual experience when I sat down to write this book. I realized that, without trying to do so, I had worked in a number of different practice settings. Whereas I had always felt a little guilty about this, like I could not fit in or find the 'perfect' practice, I suddenly saw the experience of working in many different practice settings as an asset. Although I had not set out to move in and out of many different workplaces, in doing so, I had developed a working knowledge of many different practice models. This in turn gave me a greater understanding of the pros and cons of creating a holistic practice in varied settings. The spiritual level is often like this example; in retrospect, there is a meaning and purpose to what seems at first like a series of random events, or even failures. Where the mind and ego see failure, spirit may see opportunity for growth and learning.

Accessing the spiritual dimension in decision-making

requires that you give yourself time and space to sense the larger purpose of what you are doing. If you read autobiographical accounts of people who made big life changes, they often have the intuition that something is not right, followed by a sense of guidance or clarity that leads to a life-changing and meaningful experience. As the person trusts (or has faith in) this unseen and non-rational force, he or she eventually sees a deeper meaning in life. Trust and faith in the spiritual dimension can give you the support you need to follow your intuition. The spiritual is also what allows you to bring all the pieces of your life together into an integrated whole.

A sense of spiritual connection can transform what seems like a bad or terrible experience into the learning opportunity of a lifetime. Just as a person confronting death can learn how to truly live (even though he or she eventually dies), so too can the spiritual dimension give meaning and purpose to events that may seem purely negative at a personal, ego level. Some great examples of this can be found in Andrea Joy Cohen's book, *A Blessing in Disguise*. The book consists of 39 life stories told by people whom Cohen describes as 'modern-day spiritual alchemists (who) have digested and transformed events of their lives.'[8] The stories of these various doctors, artists and teachers range from topics like learning from 'failures,' to struggling with depression, even living through physical illness and cancer. Taken together, these accounts show that it is possible to learn from the 'bad' times in your life and to develop an appreciation of your life as a meaningful, ever-evolving whole. This ability is the purview and gift of the spiritual dimension.

To make decisions from the spiritual dimension means having trust in the validity of your experiences in the other dimensions. Many people look to prayer or guidance from their 'higher' Self, or from other metaphysical sources. Vaclav Havel, playwright, political dissident and the first president of Czechoslovakia after the fall of the Soviet Union, describes hope as an aspect of spirit.

In the extended quotation in chapter three, he also states that hope (and by implication spirituality) is not dependent upon religion or belief in God. As previously quoted, Havel describes hope as a 'state of mind,' 'a dimension of the soul' and 'an orientation of the spirit, an orientation of the heart. Further, he states that hope 'transcends the world that is immediately experienced, and it is anchored somewhere beyond its horizons ... its deepest roots are in the transcendental, just as the roots of human responsibility are ... I think that the deepest and most important form of hope ... is something we get, as it were, from "elsewhere."'[9]

The Contextual Dimension of Decision Making

Context is the external environment that surrounds your physical body. This consists of the actual physical environment as well as less material contexts such as family, culture and social influences. There is overlap between your physical dimension (your body) and the physical aspect of your contextual dimension. While the physical aspect of the contextual dimension is very obvious, people often overlook it because it is so obvious. For instance, there is the saying that a fish cannot describe what water is, because it has no perspective on life without water. Family, culture and social aspects of context are also often difficult to be aware of as they have shaped your perceptions, values and expectations. While it is easy for the individual to overlook his or her own particular context, the contextual dimension plays an important role in shaping peoples' lives.

Physician Esther Sternberg, who studies brain-immune system interactions, reviews concepts and research related to the healing effect of the external environment in her book, *Healing Spaces: The Science of Place and Well-Being*.[10] She examines the senses of vision, sound, smell and sensation, as well as larger healing environments, like the structure of buildings and nature.

Her book illuminates the growing body of evidence supporting what people innately have known for thousands of years: the environment can have a healing effect.

There is also a social aspect to the contextual dimension. For your practice, you can seek out social support. You can develop relationships with mentors and talk with friends and colleagues in the field. You can also hire consultants, life coaches or even psychotherapists to help you sort out what is important to you and how you would like your practice to evolve. As Samuel Shem reminds us, isolation 'can be deadly.'[11] A successful practice requires you to create a social environment that is supportive of your whole Self in your work.

Some aspects of your context are changeable, but others are not. You can actually examine your contextual situation using multidimensional awareness: look at it from the perspective of the physical, emotional, intellectual, heart, self-expressive, intuitive and spiritual dimensions. You will notice many contextual factors influencing your decisions around creating a practice.

The Temporal Dimension of Decision Making

The temporal dimension refers to where you are in terms of your own developmental phase of life. Your sense of this dimension will let you know whether or not the timing is good for you to make a change. For example, it may be difficult to start a private practice right out of residency, particularly if you move to a new town where you do not have an established network of contacts. Some choices you build up to over many years. But other opportunities may be time-limited events, like the marketing slogan, 'Hurry! This offer ends soon!'

In ancient times, people read 'signs' to see if the timing for a given undertaking was right. Astrology and divination developed partly for these purposes. While many people outright dismiss things like astrology signs, tarot cards, and reading palms or tea leaves, there are a couple of perspectives on how these techniques may be useful in decision-making. One explanation is that using any sort of divination technique temporarily puts the intellect on hold. This can allow one's own sense of self-expression, intuition and spirit to 'fill in the gaps.' This explanation is like using information and life events as 'Rorschach ink blots', which psychologists use to determine personality styles and unconscious patterns of association. In this way, you can learn about your Self through studying how events unfold in your life. This can be one way of understanding the practical use of divination techniques to tap into aspects of Self that are more unconscious in nature.

Another explanation draws on Carl Jung's concept of synchronicity, in which acausal (physically or logically unconnected) events can be meaningfully related. He gives an example of a patient telling him a dream about a beetle. During the telling of the dream, Jung heard a tapping at his window, went to the window, opened it and grabbed something, and then opened his hand and said to the patient, 'Do you mean a beetle like this one?' Oddly, the beetle was very similar to the one mentioned in the dream.[12]

Intuitive and emotional awareness of the non-logical meanings of events can often have a profound effect in guiding deeper understanding and life choices. This is a metaphysical explanation of the interconnected meaning of events that are not logically or causally connected (which sounds a lot like the workings of the spiritual dimension discussed above). Jung was interested in parapsychology and in looking for scientific evidence for the concept of synchronicity. He also was interested in tools like the *I Ching*, also called *The Book of Changes*, and he in fact wrote the introduction to the authoritative English translation of this book. One of the functions of the *I Ching* is to help determine how to make the right change at the right time. It balances inner, personal variables with external variables, in order to recommend a course of action that could be said to be 'in harmony with the Tao' (*Tao* is often translated as 'the Way'). As also referenced in a previous chapter, the *I Ching* states that '(w)hen change is necessary, there are two mistakes to be avoided. One lies in excessive haste and ruthlessness, which brings disaster. The other lies in excessive hesitation and conservatism which are also dangerous.'[13] I am not saying that you should make your decisions according to your astrological horoscope, but when you are stuck, looking for symbols, patterns and examining your dreams might help you to clarify how you feel about different possibilities.

As a human being, you develop over time and you may find that you are very passionate about a particular topic, treatment modality, patient population, or practice for a time. But then, gradually, it may become clear that it is time for you to move on to something new. An exaggerated and humorous representation of this can be found in the movie, *Adaptation*.[14] Chris Cooper plays character John Laroche, a kind of 'mad genius,' orchid thief and collector. In an interview with Meryl Streep's character, he gives an example of his motivation and passion, namely his deep love of learning about fish earlier in his life. He follows this passion with all his being, and it shapes his life, until one day he realizes he is completely finished with it. At that point he says, 'Fuck fish!' He is so over fish that he does not even set foot in the ocean again. 'And I love the ocean,' he adds.

A lot of people do not have the depth of passion of John Laroche. Also many life decisions occur without such a clear demarcation of being 'over and done' with something. Still, many people can gradually have the sense that they are 'done with' something, that it is an end of an era, that it was good while it lasted, but they are ready to move on. While it may be that a person is well and truly done with something in their life, in retrospect each of these different phases can be facets of a larger calling.

In the past few years, I have rediscovered and remembered

the relevance of things I had intensely studied in the past. Coming to New Zealand renewed my interest in culture that had been dormant for a while. Also, I have thought I was 'done with' Jung on a number of occasions, but find myself drawn back to revisit his writings every few years. I have come to believe that it is rare for me to ever be completely 'done with' something I have been deeply interested in. These interests can be used as a way of learning who you are. As Jung has written, there 'is no linear evolution; there is only a circumambulation of the self.'[15] The problems of the self are revisited in a spiral fashion. Patte Randal has a similar concept in her 'Re-covery Model.' She uses a spiral image to describe how people revisit certain patterns again and again in their lives. However, people have the choice as to whether these will be 'vicious' or 'victorious' cycles of re-covering the same ground.[16] Growth, development and recurring patterns are an aspect of time. Sometimes development can only be seen looking back or during times in life when you are in a period of re-evaluation.

Integrating Dimensional Information for Decision Making

I have mentioned that as you get in touch with different dimensions of your Self, you may notice contradictory information. This is normal and expected. This is what gives human beings a richness and complexity, that they can simultaneously hold contradictory truths at different levels. Decision-making then becomes about negotiating and compromising between different internal aspects of your Self. This is also why applying a Cognitive Behavioral Therapy approach of 'change your thoughts, change your mood,' or a New Age mantra of 'visualize what you desire,' can seem so simplistic and untrue at one level, while being true at other levels. It is impossible to fully know one's Self. An attitude of wonder and curiosity is probably more appropriate than a rationalistic or spiritualistic engineering approach.

So how do you compromise or negotiate between conflicting and contradictory information from different dimensions? Excellent question! I do not have an answer for that one, other than recommending that you are patient with your Self, tolerant of ambiguity and allow a decision to solidify over time. First, be aware of the conflicting information. Second, allow the conflicting positions to interact, like a large meeting in the United Nations. Third, see if a consensus arises. Finally, prioritize and negotiate. For instance, you might take on a very busy new job with many responsibilities. However, you might negotiate for a little extra time off, even unpaid, to take a dream vacation.

I am also a fan of 'trying on ideas' by doing some initial work beyond the purely conceptual. For instance, when my wife and I were considering moving to New Zealand, I bought a few books and looked at jobs online. When I mentally decided we might try it, but not for a few years, I began to notice that my life seemed dull and routine and that I no longer enjoyed the things I used to enjoy. When I started to think about moving to New Zealand, I noticed that it seemed like I had become more alive. This observation led me to implement the decision sooner rather than later, even though I did not think it made sense from a purely mental perspective.

Making Decisions with Your Whole Self Exercise
Focus on a question you have about a particular decision in your life. Write the question on a piece of paper, or simply hold the question in your awareness. You can now work through each dimension to explore it from different perspectives. Start with the spiritual dimension. Allow yourself to feel into the 'big picture' level of meaning and purpose regarding the decision. How do different aspects of the decision lead to different possibilities for who you are as a person in the world? How might the decision affect your personal mission, goal and values in life?

Next, move to the level of intuition. Do not work or push your brain to think. Let different aspects of the decision come together and separate. Decision-making at this level is almost like watching a kaleidoscope make different patterns before your eyes, as you daydream about what the patterns look like.

Now move to the level of creative self-expression. Do not worry about practicalities or limitations at this point; just focus on what you are drawn to create in your life and with your life. What are the projects you have always dreamed of? Does this decision move you closer to your dreams? At this level, you are more actively engaged, as if you are influencing the way that the kaleidoscope pieces are coming together.

The next level is your heart. Take a deep breath and feel into the center of your chest. Notice the changes in your heart as you examine different aspects of the decision. It may be a great decision, but if your heart is not fully in it, it will be a chore rather than a joy. See if you can notice a feeling of your heart opening or closing when you work with the decision.

Now you can move to your mind and intellect. Your intellect is great at focusing the information from the other dimensions into a concrete plan. Maybe you are dreaming about being an astronaut. That may be very unlikely to happen, but you can ask yourself if there are any alternatives that capture the essence of being an astronaut. Maybe you could learn scuba diving – a more realistic way to explore another realm. Once you have this attainable dream, you can use your mind to think, develop a plan, organize and reality-test your dreams.

After your intellect has shaped the input from the other dimensions, how do you feel, emotionally, about all of your options? Are you excited about the intellect's proposal, or has it taken all the fun and adventure out of it? Feel back and forth through different aspects of the decision.

Finally, you arrive at the dimension of physical reality. There are a few more steps before implementing your decision. You can use body awareness as another tool in making decisions. As you explore *different aspects of the decision, what do you notice in your body? Are there butterflies in your stomach from excitement or anxiety? Do you have a headache, or feel dizzy or tired? Are you having a feeling of panic? Do you feel more alive? Does your body feel more solid and connected? Take notice of how your body responds to your decisions. Using body sensations can be challenging. Your body might be panicking over a decision about which the rest of your Self is very excited, but which calls for a lot of change at the physical level. Not all anxiety is bad or to be avoided. Sometimes the best decision for you is the one you are most anxious about. If you are patient with your bodily feelings, you will notice that you will pass through different waves of sensation and it may take a while to get to how you really feel deep within your Self.*

From the physical dimension, expand your awareness to consider your context. How does the context of your physical environment and your social situation provide new information about your decision? If you are moving forward with a change, how can you mobilize resources and support?

Now, consider the temporal dimension. Can you implement the decision right now? Will it take years of planning because it is a long-term goal, like becoming a doctor? Are there many steps that you will have to negotiate and organize over a period of time? How does the decision fit into the timeline of your life?

Now that you have gathered information from these nine different dimensions, the work of integrating them begins. You could do this in different ways, maybe just by an overall gestalt feeling, or by a vote from each dimension. At one level, you may feel incredibly excited. In another dimension, you may be terrified. How do you work with both of these contradictory feelings? That is the work of integration.

The process of integrating information from different dimensions into a holistic decision is a skill you develop over time. It is the same process that goes on at all levels, whether you are engaged in personal growth and the pursuit of self-knowledge, working with an individual client, developing your practice, or working for social change to transform the culture of medicine. This holistic work of examining, valuing and balancing different kinds of information is the work of transformation.

Part V

RE-HUMANIZING
THE CULTURE OF MEDICINE

Overview

The last section of the book looks at transforming and re-humanizing the culture of medicine and re-establishing healing relationships at all levels of medicine. We will examine the role of leadership, and explore healing and connection. The concept of healing is all about connection and interconnection, and it provides a counterbalance for the disconnection and dehumanization in contemporary medicine.

Chapter 11

Leading the Transformation of Medicine

Q: 'What is the most important issue in health care today?'
A: 'The major challenge we face is how to spiritualize and humanize medicine, how to infuse it with a compassionate quality that answers our inner needs as well as to the needs of our physical bodies,'
Larry Dossey[1]

Re-humanizing medicine begins with an individual human being, the clinician. This is not just an isolated exercise, however. The way health care professionals treat themselves influences how they treat other people and this, in turn, influences larger health care delivery systems. From a holistic perspective, what happens at one level influences other levels. The personal growth of the clinician ultimately leads to system change. In this sense, 'the personal is political,' as stated by Carol Hanisch.[2]

Worldwide, we are in a time of dramatic change in health care systems. We are still working to find a way out of the global financial crisis, and health care costs are continuing to increase. While the US has particularly high health care costs relative to other developed economies, all countries are struggling to keep health care affordable. Change and health care reform are becoming the norm. Medicine is a unique field because, even if it were run very efficiently, it could still be dehumanizing and dissatisfying for staff and clients. Good medicine must include something more than efficiency and technical competence.

The Quality Revolution Meets the Compassion Revolution
We are in the midst of a worldwide Quality Revolution. The Quality Revolution champions cost containment, improved

safety and standardized treatment protocols. It largely grows out of the *biomedical* and *economic rationalist* models of medicine. However, it also proposes patient-centered care and a 'continuous healing relationship.'[3] When the Quality Revolution speaks of a continuous healing relationship, it is referring to quick access to the health care delivery system. However, the choice of the term 'healing' is interesting. On the one hand, this may be an attempt to co-opt the word 'healing' to denote access, but on the other hand, it creates the possibility of a change in the therapeutic relationship, a recognition that true healing is part of the debate on health care reform. Similarly, the focus on individualized, patient-centered treatment opens the door for meaningful collaborative care between professionals and patients.

The Compassion Revolution grows out of the values of the *foundational* and *traditional* models, in that it views a compassionate relationship between the full human being of the doctor and the patient as transformative and healing, above and beyond it being a vehicle for biomedical intervention. When the Compassion Revolution speaks of a 'continuous healing relationship,' this is closer to the American Holistic Medical Association's principle that *'love is life's most powerful healer.'*[4]

So the current climate of health care reform presents many possibilities. At the intersection between the Quality and Compassion Revolution lies both tension and opportunity. Even if the Quality and Compassion revolutions have different motivations for speaking of 'healing relationships' and 'patient-centered care', it is hopeful that the language is converging and this legitimizes a compassionate and holistic approach to medicine. At this point, we need leadership that can encompass both principles. I am calling this *holistic leadership*, as it takes into account many different dimensions and principles and creates a framework to support human growth and healing within complex systems.

Holistic leadership aims to transform the culture of medicine.

It aims at human growth and system growth. It highlights the connection between personal, clinical and organizational growth. And it recognizes the multidimensionality of individual human beings and of relationships between human beings.

Hand in hand with reducing costs and increasing quality and efficiency, we need *human* leadership in medicine. By this I mean human beings championing humane treatment. This is a different kind of leadership than the *economic rationalist model* of a CEO or CMO directing change from the top of a hierarchy. That kind of leadership is 'old school,' disconnected leadership. What we need is holistic leadership distributed throughout the system at all levels. Every person involved in health care delivery has responsibility and a leadership role to fill, even the patient.

Holistic Leadership

Holistic leadership includes all the standard aspects of leadership, such as the concerns about quality issues in medicine, safety, efficacy and cost-effectiveness. However, it does not stop at the level of an efficient system, but includes an awareness of human needs.

Holistic leadership is personal, growing out of an individual's awareness of his or her own physical, emotional, mental, heart, self-expressive, intuitive, spiritual, contextual and temporal dimensions. The ability to balance and choose between these, often conflicting, multiple dimensions of Self can be considered *internal leadership*. From a solid base of internal leadership, leadership is possible at professional and organizational levels. *Professional leadership* focuses on clinical issues between individuals and within small teams. *Organizational leadership* considers interactions at a systems level.

Any of these leadership levels – internal, professional, or organizational – can be approached in a simplistic or complex way. Each level has infinite complexity. An individual could dedicate a lifetime to developing internal leadership and not reach the end of possible growth. This is the path of mystics such as monks and nuns of different denominations. It is also possible to devote a lifetime to the study and practice of professional leadership or organizational leadership. What holistic leadership does is to show that it is necessary to connect these different dimensions of leadership development.

Holistic leadership is ultimately about people – not ideas, numbers, percentages or dollars. It is not only about the 'latest and the best,' but is also about the 'deepest, most true and authentic.' Transformation at a personal level is what fuels trans-formation at clinical and organizational levels.

Gandhi as an Example of Holistic Leadership

A brief study of Mohandas K. Gandhi's book, *An Autobiography: The Story of My Experiments with Truth*, shows how internal personal growth and the transformation of organizational systems are interconnected. You do not have to aspire to the accomplishments of Gandhi, but his life provides a good template for understanding the internal, professional and organi-zational aspects of holistic leadership.

Internal Leadership

Gandhi tirelessly worked on personal growth his whole life. In early adulthood he struggled with fears and anxiety that kept him from speaking in public forums. As a young lawyer, he had to excuse himself from his first case because he could not speak in front of the court. He struggled to understand and master his sexual passions and his relationship to his wife, to whom he was married as an adolescent. He constantly worked on his diet, examining the relationship between *ahimsa* (non-harming) and his daily nourishment. He briefly tried eating meat, but the decision to avoid killing animals for his food was relatively easy for him. The more difficult and lifelong struggle was whether he should take in animal products such as milk. Even when on a hunger strike or when ill, his doctors would plead with him to take some milk, but he would resist on the basis of his spiritual and moral convictions.

Particularly to a Westerner reading Gandhi's *Experiments with Truth*, it may seem that he was extreme, or even obsessed with certain topics, such as his diet. However, it was through his internal work that he was able to know himself and to develop internal leadership. This allowed him to choose spiritual and heart-based dimensions of himself over physical desires and the fears of the ego.

Professional Leadership

Despite his anxiety, Gandhi chose to become a lawyer, a profession that required public speaking. While he did do a great deal of internal work, he did not solve his personal issues prior to taking on professional issues. So often in life, it is by reaching beyond our capabilities that we grow. For Gandhi, we could hypothesize that encountering social injustice allowed him to bring his internal spiritual and compassionate strength into the world to help people. His sense of moral outrage turned out to be stronger than his fear of public speaking.

Gandhi went to South Africa at the age of 24, where he spent the next 21 years of his life. It was here that he gradually found his voice speaking out on human rights issues. The first major case he worked on taught him the 'true practice of law.' This case was between two Indian businessmen who were related to each other. While Gandhi understood how to win the case for his client, he saw that winning in this situation would damage the relationship between these relatives and within the larger Indian community. He was able to convince both sides to settle out of court in a way that preserved each person's dignity and did not bankrupt either party. Gandhi wrote, 'I had learnt to find out the better side of human nature and to enter men's hearts. I realized that the true function of a lawyer was to unite parties riven asunder.'[5] This is quite a holistic description of a lawyer, and it resonates with holistic medicine's focus on reconnecting that which has been separated.

Organizational Leadership

Through his internal and professional leadership, Gandhi eventually reached the place where he started working to challenge and change the system. In South Africa, he saw how people with darker skin were treated by the ruling white government. His unshakeable belief in morality, justice and fairness pushed him into the limelight, taking on a challenge to a bill that took away rights for Indians living in South Africa. Working with challenging internal issues led him to work with challenging external issues involving discrimination and human rights.

On his return to India, he continued to be pulled into larger leadership roles because of his inability to tolerate injustice and discrimination. This is the Gandhi of popular imagination, who led non-violent protests that eventually led to India gaining independence from Great Britain. It is not that he was done with his internal struggles or his professional, interpersonal work – that continued as before – but he also took on another level of leadership that was larger than individual or professional interests and was concerned with all people, the whole of society.

Gandhi continues to serve as an international role model for non-violent change. He has greatly influenced others' struggles around the world. For instance, Martin Luther King, Jr. studied Gandhi's leadership methods, particularly his belief in non-violent resistance. This influenced King's work as one of the leaders of the Civil Rights Movement in the United States which attained greater equality for African-Americans. One also has to wonder how much Gandhi may have influenced his one time opponent, South African leader Jan Smuts. While Smuts resisted reform of segregation in South Africa, he later went on to be one of the founding members of the League of Nations and also wrote the book *Holism and Evolution*, which is generally credited as having popularized the term 'holism' as a principle of the interconnection of things.[6]

Gandhi's Holistic Leadership

We can see from this outline of Gandhi's life and work that he tirelessly worked on leadership issues at the internal, professional and organizational levels. His work at each level supported work at other levels. He is a true example of the personal being political.

You may be thinking, 'That is all fine and good, but I am no Gandhi, and I do not have as lofty a goal as freedom of a people.' The beauty of Gandhi's life is that he started out so awkward and shy. It could be argued that working with his limitations and putting himself in challenging situations in which he had to reach beyond his personal comfort zone is what allowed him to accomplish such great things. He was also a lawyer, a profession which has some similarities with the profession of medicine, particularly in regard to the emphasis on professional ethics and ideals. Gandhi is a great inspiration for how you can change yourself, your practice and the larger culture, if you truly work at all three levels of leadership.

Medicine and the Three Levels of Leadership

In examining holistic leadership in Gandhi's life and work, we see three levels of leadership: an internal, personal level; a professional, interpersonal level; and an organizational, systems level. Holistic leadership does not separate the personal from the professional or the professional from the organizational. Instead, leadership is found in each of these different domains, and strengthening one level supports other levels as well. As Wilber stated about the growth of human consciousness, 'it transcends *and* includes'[7] the preceding dimensions. It is the same with the three levels of holistic leadership; each level transcends *and* includes the preceding dimension. We can examine these three levels of holistic leadership as they pertain to medicine.

The first level of medical leadership is within the physician's or clinician's Self. This is *internal leadership* and it involves knowing one's Self and developing strong values and ethics. Internal leadership is developed through personal growth work. Its aim is self-knowledge and personal understanding. If we view the physician's Self as the tool for working with patients and the systems that serve them, then it is reasonable to say that the more developed the tool, the more developed this work will be.

The nine-dimensional model of human beings described in this book recognizes that each individual is a multiplicity of different dimensions and experiences. If an individual is viewed as a simple unity, internal leadership does not make much sense. However, if individuals are viewed as a multiplicity, leadership is an issue for every individual. We have discussed the concept of the ego which consists of the first three dimensions of the physical, emotional and mental aspects. We could say that the ego is a level of leadership that integrates and regulates the individual's experience of these three dimensions. Ego leadership would thus maximize the individual's physical, emotional and mental potential.

We have also discussed the concept of the Self, which includes all nine of the human dimensions. From the perspective of the Self, the ego is one aspect of a larger whole. The Self adds dimensions of the heart, creative self-expression, intuition, spirituality, context and time. These dimensions are larger than the ego's preoccupation with the individual and show how the individual is connected to 'higher' aspects of Self as well as to other people and the environment. Internal leadership, informed by Self-awareness, leads to concerns that transcend the individual.

The second level of holistic medical leadership is *professional leadership* in the day-to-day clinical practice of medicine – seeing patients, interacting with a medical team and making medical decisions. Professional leadership is exercised at an interpersonal level. You do not need to have a formal leadership title; you are already in a leadership role by virtue of your profession. The most important thing is that you are providing leadership from the heart as well as the mind. Holistic professional leadership brings awareness of your own body, emotions, mind, heart, creativity, intuition, spirituality, context and temporal dimension. When you are aware of these dimensions within your Self, you can advocate for these human realities in any kind of clinical decision-making. For instance, you can prescribe the correct medication to a patient, but if they have lost hope in life, they may not take it. Through your own self-connection, you can connect with this patient and help address the hopelessness (which may stem from the heart and spiritual dimensions) to improve the person's capacity for self-care.

If you approach your job through your ego, you will not be aware of the reality that you are a leader in your daily work. You will also treat your job, your colleagues and your patients as 'things' that are there to gratify your ego. If you have already developed internal leadership within your Self, your day-to-day work and decisions will be informed by your heart and your spirit.

The third level of medical leadership is *organizational leadership* in the larger health care delivery system. This means looking beyond your specialty, your clinic, even your organization, to larger systems. At an organizational level, you will see where systems interact well and where they do not. Leadership at this level means that you do not just complain about a problem, you work to address it to whatever degree you have the capacity. If we take Gandhi as a model, we could say that where you find you lack capacity, you challenge yourself to grow.

Re-humanization of Self, practice and medical culture grows out of a holistic framework for understanding problems and decisions at the internal, professional and organizational levels. Dehumanization occurs through the fixed use of less than nine dimensions of human being. Rehumanization, then, would be the approach to problems and experience from the full nine dimensions of human being. Holistic leadership is, thus, leadership that includes all nine human dimensions.

The Compassion Revolution and Holistic Leadership

In short, the fundamental insight of twentieth-century physics has yet to penetrate the social world: *relationships are more fundamental than things.*
Senge, Scharmer, Jaworski and Flowers[8]

Across many different fields, including medicine, business, education, social services and the non-profit sector, there is an interlocking network of thinkers promoting new forms of leadership that are based on compassion, reflection, mindfulness and collaboration. There is a larger re-evaluation and re-valuation of society occurring. Writers like Peter Block,[9] Frances Westley,[10] Peter Drucker,[11] Margaret Wheatley,[12] Peter Senge[13] and Adam Kahane[14] have developed new models of leadership that promote collaboration while being comfortable with chaos and complexity. These leadership styles are holistic and systems-oriented and promote respect for human beings working at all levels within a system. These styles of embedded leadership are an evolution beyond the old models of strict hierarchy and leadership from above. This new leadership is concerned with the transformation and growth of human beings and organizations. For instance, I heard Peter Block speak at the Authentic Leadership In Action (ALIA) conference in Nova Scotia in 2012, where he said that the 'task of leadership is to sustain faith.'[15] These proponents for a new style for leadership have faith in the humanity of the people working in systems. They understand that humanity must be preserved and promoted in individuals if we want systems that act humanely.

Another example of this new leadership style can be found in the book *Presence: Human Purpose and the Field of the Future*, by Peter Senge, C. Otto Scharmer, Joseph Jaworski and Betty Sue Flowers. *Presence* has sections that discuss 'parts and wholes,' different kinds of thinking and knowing, 'seeing with the heart,' and even a chapter called, 'Leadership: Becoming a Human Being.'[16] The authors blend the wisdom of scientists, spiritual leaders, leaders of cultural change and business leaders into a new theory of change applied to business and social services. This book is just one example of a larger cultural shift toward a holistic way of being and working that views the individual, groups and systems as interconnected. This holistic perspective includes a focus on human dimensions that often are not considered in business, such as subjectivity, compassion, intuition and spirituality.

Another example of new leadership is the work of Tony Schwartz. His book, *The Way We're Working Isn't Working*, focuses on re-humanizing business. We have reviewed his idea that successful businesses must attend to the physical, emotional, mental and spiritual needs of their employees. Schwartz has started a consulting firm called The Energy Project which works to bring these ideas into corporate consciousness. He recognizes the need for compassion and caring in business and concludes that a 'workplace culture characterized by appreciation and high regard for employees undeniably drives higher engagement and loyalty.'[17] One study that Schwartz cites looked at 90,000 employees in 18 countries and found that the greatest predictor of employee engagement was 'whether senior management was perceived to be sincerely interested in employees' wellbeing.'[18] Thus, we can see that there is a growing awareness in business of the importance of caring relationships between employers and employees.

Returning to the field of medicine, Parker Palmer, Robin Youngson and many others[19] are working to bring compassion and human values back into health care. We can consider this a Compassion Revolution consistent with the goal of re-humanizing medicine. Parker Palmer calls for a *new professional* and Youngson writes about *compassionate leadership*. Regardless of the terminology, a similar goal and process is pursued by each of these visionaries. That goal is the transformation of the individual which, in turn, leads to the transformation of organizations and institutions. This is holistic leadership in medicine.

If we choose to exercise holistic leadership within ourselves, with our patients, and in our health care delivery systems and societies, we may feel that we are acting alone. However, judging by the examples above, there is a ground swell of support in creating new models for the 21st century. The work of Parker Palmer and Robin Youngson provides examples of this societal change applied to health care.

The New Professional

The new professional is 'a person who not only is competent in his or her discipline but also has the skill and the will to resist and help transform the institutional pathologies that threaten the profession's highest standards,' (Parker Palmer).[20]

Parker Palmer's life and work exemplifies what he has called an 'undivided life.'[21] He draws on his own personal struggles, such as his work with his own depression and what this taught him about his 'true self.'[22] He has also written about his spiritual journey and how it influenced his views on education.[23] Palmer champions an approach to education that values compassion, professionalism, subjectivity and spirituality.

Parker Palmer's concept of the 'new professional' is a very good example of holistic leadership. Palmer writes from the perspective of an educator, but he has also written specifically on medical education after his work attracted the attention of the American Council for Graduate Medical Education (ACGME) in the US. His organization, Courage and Renewal, has started an annual conference called 'Integrity in Health Care.'

Palmer addresses a number of concerns about dehuman-ization and re-humanization in medicine. He views the role of education to be personal transformation as well as the trans-mission of knowledge, and provides a critique of the current one-sided emphasis on objective facts. For instance he describes *objectivism* in education as 'obsessed with the purity of knowledge,' adding that objectivism 'wants to avoid the mess of subjectivity at all costs – even if the cost is the "decivilizing" kind of knowledge that renders us unfit for the messiness of life.'[24] According to Palmer, objectivism affects more than just the student; institutions that over-promote objectivism can dehumanize teachers and students. Palmer states that 'the very institutions in which we practice our crafts pose some of the gravest threats to professional standards and personal integrity. Yet higher education does little, if anything, to prepare students to confront, challenge, and help change the institutional condi-tions under which they will soon be working.'[25] This is what Palmer seeks to redress with his concept of the new professional – an ethical framework to counterbalance institutional forces.

Just as the present book promotes the development of all the dimensions of Self, so too does Palmer's concept of the new professional encourage the development of human dimensions beyond the intellectual. Rather than seeing subjectivity as a weakness to be eradicated, Palmer sees it as a resource for the individual facing difficult decisions. He writes that the 'education of the new professional would not teach emotional distancing as a strategy for survival. Instead it would teach students to stay close to emotions that might become sources of energy to challenge and change institutions.'[26]

Palmer sees the transformation of the whole individual as the key to the transformation of organizational structures, stating that 'the capacity to translate private feelings into public issues, when warranted, has been an engine of every movement for social change.'[27] It is, thus, the connection between the personal and the social which provides the foundation for holistic leadership that is transformative. Furthermore, to be effective in systems, individuals must be subjectified rather than objectified. This process of subjectification is similar to my 'counter-curriculum of re-humanization'. For Palmer, there is thus a tension between the objectification of knowledge in the institution which is counterbalanced by the role of the new professional, who uses subjectivity in the form of emotional and compassionate dimensions as well as through the development of a strong set of personal ethics and values which set up the new professional as the conscience of the institution.

In his chapter, 'The New Professional: Education for Transformation,' Palmer uses the example of physicians in training to elaborate his concept of the *new professional*. This provides a good working example of holistic leadership, in which the individual and the social are interconnected. Palmer traces the story of a junior resident (postgraduate medical trainee, or 'registrar' in UK-influenced systems) who was on call in the hospital, over-worked and under-supported, in a scenario that led to a possibly preventable death of a patient. While Palmer has a keen critique of the institution, he also holds the young professional responsible for her actions. The professional is not a member of a disenfranchised underclass who lacks any power (although professionals are subject to the use of power within the institution in which they work). In appealing to professionalism, subjectivity, the role of emotion in learning and the transformative power of education, Palmer asks professionals to step up and to challenge institutional policies that are dehumanizing and unhealthy. In a sense, each professional has the responsibility to use their own heart to be the moral compass for the institution, rather than letting institutions make ethical decisions, a situation in which the physician becomes a technician simply following orders.

Palmer's critique of institutions is that they do not empower the individuals in the system to take responsibility. He also critiques the overuse of certain kinds of knowledge and analysis in institutions.

> When systems analysis is our only approach to a catastrophe of this sort, it becomes one more way we allow the logic of institutions, which is about self-preservation, to overwhelm the logic of the human heart, which is about love and duty. In the process, systems analysis can contribute to the long-term decline of compassion, responsibility, and courage in our culture.[28]

He continues by asking how 'medical residents might be educated to confront institutional inhumanity of this sort instead of collaborating with it through action or inaction.'[29] While Palmer clearly finds fault with institutional policies that throw inexperienced students into overwhelming roles without sufficient support, he also challenges the student to step up into the responsibility of a new professional.

> Not just the system failed in this case. The heart of the healer failed as well, a heart that surely knew what was occurring but refused to recognize the fact. And it is the heart of the healer, not the system, that education has the best chance to touch and transform … What caused the 'heart failure' in this resident, apparently leaving her with the sense that she had no option but to play the stacked hand she had been dealt? Can we think of her not as a victim but as a moral agent uniquely positioned to challenge and help change the insti-

tution before, during, and after the moment of crisis? If so, what might happen in residency programs to support the healer's heart – and the courage to follow it – when conditions under which medicine is practiced threaten the heart's imperatives?[30]

Palmer sees the human heart, not as a place of 'soft' science and fuzzy logic, but rather as the location of courage, ethics and ultimately professionalism. He critiques contemporary medicine without becoming anti-science, advocating that we use other human aspects, in addition to the analytical mind, to support professional and ethical responsibility and action. This view transforms the one-dimensional medical technician into a multi-dimensional, complex, full human being, who uses science and the heart to best serve his or her patients.

It is this focus on the individual human heart that is at the foundation of holistic leadership in which personal transformation leads to professional and organizational transformation. A transformed individual is no longer an isolated object, but rather a connected subject who can act as a moral agent within the institution. Palmer writes that at the 'heart of every profession is an implicit affirmation that the mission of the profession must never be confused with the institutional structures in which it is pursued ... We need professionals who are 'in but not of' their institutions, whose allegiance to the core values of their fields calls them to resist the institutional diminishment of those values.'[31] This dual position of new professionals being 'in but not of' the institution allows them to draw on their own subjectivity of Self while working in the institution. It allows them to bring dimensions of compassion and spirituality into their work.

It may seem that one person is no match for the heartless bureaucracies – with their layers of guidelines and protocols – in which we practice. The power of the individual lies in the fact that they can be 'in but not of' the bureaucracy. As an individual human being, you have your own internal source of information and support through your emotions, heart and spirituality. Subjective connection to your Self supplies the inner strength to challenge institutions. Individual professionals can draw upon their own truths. It is this inner truth that is the source of ethical responsibility. So, in this sense, the individual is separate from the institution. However, Palmer also shows that it is just these separate individuals who create institutions.

> In fact, institutions are us! The shadows that institutions cast over our ethical lives are external manifestations of our own inner shadows, individual and collective. If institutions are rigid, it is because we fear change. If institutions are competitive, it is because we value winning over all else. If institutions are heedless of human need, it is because something in us is heedless as well. If we are even partly responsible for creating institutional dynamics, we possess some degree of power to alter them.[32]

Palmer thus sees individuals as having several kinds of power in institutions; first, institutions are made up of independent human beings who are trained professionals. Second, the acts of the institution are comprised of the acts of the individuals within those institutions. In order to educate new professionals to view their role as ethical agents within institutions, Palmer presents 'five immodest proposals:'

1. We must help our students debunk the myth that institutions possess autonomous, even ultimate, power over our lives.
2. We must validate the importance of our students' emotions as well as their intellect.
3. We must teach our students how 'to mine' their emotions

for knowledge.

4. We must teach them how to cultivate community for the sake of both knowing and doing.

5. We must teach – and model for – our students what it means to be on the journey toward 'an undivided life.'[33]

Palmer's concept of the 'new professional' supports the idea of holistic leadership that links personal growth with institutional change. His example of how medical trainees can become moral agents through trusting their own subjectivity provides a challenge to students to grow in professionalism. It also is a challenge to medical education and health care employers to support 'the healer's heart.' In the old model of leadership, the empowerment of 'followers' diminished the power of 'leaders.' In the model of holistic leadership, the stronger each individual, the stronger the system.

Compassionate Leadership

Robin Youngson, an anesthesiologist in New Zealand, serves as a great example of holistic leadership in medicine. He shares his own personal journey as part of his work to enhance compassion in medicine, relating his and his family's experience of the medical system when his daughter was seriously injured and had a prolonged hospitalization. Being on the 'other side' of the doctor–patient relationship was shocking to Youngson, and he saw that something seriously important had been lost from medicine: compassion. He used his own and his family's pain as motivation to take on the culture of medicine.[34]

Youngson started an organization called Hearts in Healthcare. Through this organization and his book, *Time to Care: How to Love Your Patients and Your Job*, he puts the call out to bring compassion back into medicine. Youngson sees individual change as the driver of institutional change. 'The only person who can make the change is you. And when enough people like you choose this different path, then the whole system will change.'[35] He calls for individual responsibility, leading to individual change, compassionate leadership and eventually system change. Youngson argues that individuals can always change the way that they practice in favor of re-humanization instead of dehumanization. 'As an individual you may not be able to redesign your workplace but you can change the way you relate to patients and work with colleagues. You do not need permission from your boss, or even approval from your peers.'[36] Change occurs when people mindfully pursue and practice different behaviors. As Youngson says, healing 'occurs when you open up a sacred space between practitioner and patient. You need to be deliberate in creating the conditions for this deep connection.'[37]

Youngson's work is another example of the Compassion Revolution. With a more holistic and re-humanized model of health care, the division between technician and patient breaks down and we have instead a 'sacred space' in which two human beings come together for the purpose of healing. Part of the Compassion Revolution includes attention to the health care provider as a human being as well as a renewed focus on the whole person of the patient. Palmer and Youngson both focus on the growth and development of the clinician as a human being and as a human leader. Another book on this subject is *Patients Come Second: Leading Change by Changing the Way You Lead*, by Britt Berrett and Paul Spiegelman.[38] This book states it plainly; you cannot achieve good health care outcomes unless employees are also cared for and nurtured in a compassionate way.

Compassion is a very important factor in holistic leadership and it is necessary for the expression of human love, caring and spirituality. Compassion supports the individual to bring out what is best in him- or herself and it also provides a supportive matrix for bringing out the best in clinical interactions and in the larger institution.

We are thus seeing a growing interest in the well-being and

personal growth of employees, and in particular 'new professionals.' While the Compassion Revolution seems to be spreading
in medicine, it is not unique to medicine, but is happening in
other areas of society as well.

Compassion as a Revolutionary Act

So if you stand up for caring, compassion and the humble
service of patients and communities, you are a threat to established and powerful interests.
Robin Youngson[39]

The role of the paramodern leader is to foster a subversion of
reality that persistently undermines the ordinary. The stark
fact is that many health care institutions never succeed in
reinventing themselves because people lack the courage and
imagination to challenge deeply held assumptions about
existing strategies and processes and, in response, to think
and act in fundamentally altered ways.
Gerald Arbuckle[40]

Arbuckle and Youngson refer to compassion and health care
reform as 'subversion' and a 'threat to established interests.'
Palmer writes that institutions are a threat to professionalism. I
speak of a Compassion Revolution and a counter-curriculum.
These concepts represent a form of creative resistance in order to
re-humanize medicine. I agree with these authors' appraisals that
re-humanization is in opposition to the objectifying agenda of the
biomedical and economic rationalist models. It may seem absurd
to say that promoting compassion and human potential in
medicine is revolutionary and may oppose the organizational
structure of contemporary medicine. Not to be overly dramatic or
to overstate the parallel with Gandhi as a holistic leader, but
Gandhi also stood for compassion in terms of the concept of

Ahimsa[41] as well as non-violence with the concept of *Satyagraha*.[42] He was definitely revolutionary as his values of compassion, non-violence and human rights were violently opposed by the power structures of his day, the South African and British colonial government in India. Historically, compassion seems to be revolutionary when we look at the lives of Gandhi, Martin Luther King, Jr. and Jesus. It is possible that the organizational structures of contemporary medicine may oppose holistic and compassionate perspectives, particularly if they are at odds with the profits of the economic rationalist model or the objectivity of the biomedical model.

Another perspective on why re-humanizing medicine might seem revolutionary can be found in the history of science and ideas. The study of the development of human thought, science, philosophy and psychology can be viewed as a dialectical progression. We embrace first one, than another explanatory model. These explanatory models are often contradictory. For a while, we vacillate back and forth between thesis and antithesis until we achieve synthesis.[43]

The history of psychology reveals this back-and-forth progression. One of the most fundamental debates is between nature and nurture, which is the debate between biology and genetics on the one hand and social learning and environment on the other hand. Even just looking at the history of the last hundred years of psychology, we can go from the exploration of the unconscious of Freudian and Jungian psychoanalysis, to the positivist and empirical work of the behaviorists, to the focus on human potential and subjective states of humanistic psychology, and finally to the current hegemony of the cognitive-behaviorists' focus on evidence-based treatments. Ideas are developed up to the point where their further development actually is a detriment to other forms of understanding.

Recognizing a similar dialectic in medicine and looking for a holistic synthesis has been the focus of this book. Ideally, my view is that a synthesis of holistic and contemporary medicine is needed. I do admit that at times my arguments may fall into the antithesis position in relation to the thesis of contemporary medicine. My goal, however, is not to just oppose contemporary medicine, but to move forward toward a synthesis of oppositions.

During the recent history of medicine, it has become more scientific, evidence-based and empirical, resulting in many benefits to health care professionals, patients and society. However, further objectification in medicine threatens other human aspects that are equally essential to progress and well-being. What is required is a synthesis of science and humanism, not a triumph of humanism over science or a triumph of science over humanism.

Further progress in the scientific, technologic and economic aspects of medicine will not truly be progress if we lose our humanity. Progress in medicine, at this point in history, will occur through counterbalancing the predominantly objective and reductionist approach to human beings in medicine, which stems from the biomedical and economic rationalist models.

If we choose to work to bring compassion back into medicine and if we work to re-humanize medicine, we can expect that it will be a difficult challenge. However, one person, in this case – *you* – can make a difference in the culture of medicine. You do this by connecting the dimensions within you (connecting to your Self), by connecting to the patients with whom you work and finally by promoting connection within systems. Holistic leadership starts with knowing your Self and then expands out from there.

Chapter 12

Reconnection and Re-humanization in Medicine

The rise of complementary medicine, and the holism that it embodies ... represents ... a healing force within the healing profession itself.
Vincent Di Stefano[1]

Disconnection and Dehumanization in Medicine

Physicians are taught to strive to be objective, and yet objectivity is detachment and disconnection from the people we are attempting to care for. Science fiction author Philip K. Dick illustrates this point in his essay, 'The Android and the Human.'

> A native of Africa is said to view his surroundings as pulsing with purpose, a life, that is actually within himself; once these childish projections are withdrawn, he sees that the world is dead and that life resides solely within himself. When he reaches this sophisticated point he is said to be either mature or sane. Or scientific. But one wonders: Has he not also, in this process, reified – that is made into a thing – other people? Stones and rocks and trees may now be inanimate for him, but what about his friends? Has he now made them into stones, too?[2]

We might very well ask whether the process that Philip K. Dick describes above also happens in medical education and in health care delivery systems. As we have earlier discussed, dehumanizing someone (making them into a stone) also *dehumanizes the dehumanizer*[3] (makes the self into a stone). From a scientific technician standpoint, it is OK to treat others as objects or stones, as long as one performs technical interventions appropriately. The practice of medicine, however, calls for more than two stones knocking together.

Palmer discusses this theme of what we have lost in moving from a 'primitive' perspective to an 'objective and scientific' perspective. He writes that, 'if the problem with primitive knowledge was the over-identification of the knower with the known, our problem now is the disconnection of knower and known. In our quest to free knowledge from the tangles of subjectivity, we have broken the knower loose from the web of life itself.'[4] Palmer traces the root of the word 'objective' to its Latin root, meaning 'to put against, to oppose.'[5] Thus, in all our striving to become objective, we are putting ourselves in opposition to the person who, ostensibly, we wish to heal.

In medicine, doctors acculturate by deadening aspects of their human *responsiveness*, thus feeling they are no longer *responsible* for certain dimensions of the human being in front of them. The medical acculturation process encourages disconnection as pseudo-professionalism. The internal struggle that faces every physician is whether or not they will choose to dehumanize themselves. This question is prior to the decision to dehumanize or objectify patients. Decisions not to feel or to deny internal or external reality may seem protective, but they come at a cost of fragmenting and compartmentalizing different human dimensions, in other words turning oneself to stone.

Re-humanizing Ourselves

If it is possible to dehumanize and disconnect, it is possible to re-humanize and reconnect. That which has been split apart and broken can once again be made whole. This is a universal spiritual principle: rebirth, rejuvenation and re-humanization is possible through reconnecting with something larger than the individual ego. It is possible to *re-member* and *re-collect* full human being. This requires bringing back together that which has been separated or disconnected.

The present book has suggested a way forward, proposing a nine-dimensional model of human being. This model acknowledges that along with the ego-based dimensions of body, emotions and mind, human beings also are comprised of heart, self-expressive, intuitive, spiritual, contextual and temporal dimensions. The utility of the nine-dimensional model is that it reminds us of who we are and who others are when we engage in clinical work. It does not mean that we cannot, temporarily and for some greater purpose, focus on one dimension and set the others aside. It does mean, however, that we must bring the pieces back together once we are done analyzing them in isolation.

What does this mean practically? It could be as simple as remembering to ask the patient in front of you about each of these different dimensions. This requires you to become internally fluent with each of these dimensions – not just the physical, but also the heart and the spiritual. I realize that in most contemporary practice settings, finding the time to do a nine-dimensional review of symptoms is probably unrealistic, given all of the other pressing clinical and administrative work that must be done. In this case, doctors must develop the ability to effectively and correctly triage between dimensions. For instance, an obvious case of 'strep throat' can be approached from a purely biomedical perspective, perhaps with a question or two about whether the person is overly stressed. However, for recurrent infections or more chronic conditions, repeated applications of a purely biomedical approach may have diminishing returns. Depression, anxiety, insomnia, chronic pain, diabetes, hypertension, hypercholesterolemia and fatigue (just to name a few) all benefit from biomedical intervention *plus* lifestyle modification, *plus* a holistic approach that examines the contributions of all nine dimensions. A skilled holistic clinician can develop the ability to hone in on a particularly pertinent dimension after biomedical consideration. For instance, some depressions are more related to the heart (lack of self-love or problems connecting with others), some are related to a lack of creative self-expression (as the person holds themselves back from life), while others are related to a spiritual loss of meaning and purpose.

A counter-curriculum of re-humanization for medical professionals is proposed as a counterpoint to biomedical, economic rationalist medicine. This involves reconnecting to the aspects of Self that are sometimes 'left behind' as medical professionals become socialized to the contemporary medical system. As clinicians reconnect to all dimensions of themselves, they undergo a transformative process of re-humanization, which informs not only their lives but also their practice of medicine. Humanitarian values that drew many clinicians to the profession in the first place – compassion, caring and love – are reawakened. This in turn affects the doctor–patient relationship. A deeper relationship to Self leads to a more complex and holistic relationship with clients. Embracing the whole Self and taking a more holistic approach to client care also influences the culture of medicine and health care delivery systems, resulting in a holistic approach to leadership that reinvigorates and ultimately transforms both medical professionals and the systems of which they are a part.

A holistic perspective continually draws attention to the connection between elements. This synthetic process applies equally to internal relationships within the Self; interpersonal relationships between people; and to the functioning of organizations. Michael Murphy discusses the ancient Greek term *antakolouthia* in his book, *The Future of the Body*. He writes that the Stoic philosophers used this term to express the view that 'every virtue requires others to complete it.'[6] He goes on to state that this concept of the interconnectedness and interdependency of traits was fundamental to Greek philosophy. *Antakolouthia* draws our attention to connection, relationship and community. It explains why it is difficult to have a discussion about the benefits of holistic medicine by isolating variables. The very nature of the holistic paradigm is not in breaking things apart, but in looking at the connection between things: whether this is the connection between mind and body, the connection between doctor and patient, or the connection between individual and society. Connection can be seen as the root concept in understanding holistic medicine. It can be simply stated that the shortcomings of contemporary medicine all stem from impaired connection: super-sub-specialization, compartmentalization of services, interchangeability of 'service providers,' excessive application of protocols to people, excessive technological orientation of clinicians/technicians, and the chronic time pressure that inhibits real human interconnection. All these things lead to the creation of a bureaucratic delivery system based on isolated elements and variables rather than a system that promotes a healing connection.

Any disconnection can be viewed as a source of suffering, whether this is disconnection within Self or between selves. Re-humanization can, thus, be seen as re-establishing connection between the dimensions of human being, not only within the person of the patient, but also within the physician, and between the physician and patient. Re-humanization promotes a new sense of relationship and community.

It is hard work being a good human being. I do not want to make it seem that it is easy to be both a technician and a healer. I often find myself slipping in and out of these modes. Is it possible to use a reductionist and a holistic paradigm simultaneously? I think it is debatable whether it is truly possible to be in both states at the same time. It may be that we have to develop the capacity for moving back and forth between these different modes of being and ways of perceiving the world. Cohen has spoken of the need for negotiating a 'medical pluralism'[7] to integrate different paradigms of health and illness. This is what I argue for in this book, a pluralism of different medical models in order to best address the full humanity of physician and clients. We, as physicians, must familiarize ourselves with different paradigms and frames of reference in order to become comfortable shifting between different models of medicine. As I have said, it is not that the biomedical model is false, but just that it is not the whole truth. To perceive the whole truth of a human being requires that we first develop the capacity to be a whole human being ourselves.

I hope that the holistic framework of human being provided in this book has led to some transformation of your Self, your practice, and maybe even the culture of medicine.

Thank you.

Epilogue

It has been over a year since I 'finished' this book and a lot has happened in the intervening time. I finished up my work in New Zealand and moved back to the United States. This is an ongoing transition with all the details of an international move. It is also a full circle for me in a number of ways. I am back in the US. I have started work at the VA, which was also my first job out of residency. Yet, this is also a new beginning as I have never lived in the Northwest of the US and things are always continually changing. I am reminded of the New Zealand *koru*, the spiral new growth of ferns, which symbolizes new beginnings. The *koru* looks kind of like a question mark with one end connected to the earth and the other end a spiral which is tightly curled in the center and gradually opens up as you move from center to periphery. Out of this spiral, you can imagine perpetually new experiences to unfurl, while at the same time these experiences are related to past and future events in the places where different points on the curled spiral touch each other. I have come full circle to a point of completion and new beginning.

I started this book while I was in the US running my private practice. The book started out as a place for me to share what I had learned in creating a private practice and specifically a holistic practice. The word holistic can mean a lot of things to different people and I sought to redefine it as a state of being or philosophy rather than any particular type of CAIM technique. By focusing on the state of being of the physician, in addition to technical knowledge, holistic medicine reintegrates the person of the physician back into the doctor-patient relationship. Transformation of health care, thus, begins with the transformation of the physician.

The editing, re-writes and revisions of the book occurred while I worked in the public system in New Zealand. This move to New Zealand expanded my understanding of culture and healthcare delivery systems. When I took the job at Buchanan Rehabilitation Centre, I was lucky enough to have one day off a week that I could dedicate to writing. This allowed me the time to finish the book. I realized that creating a holistic medical practice was really just part of a larger topic that was a recurrent theme in my life: re-humanization. I wondered if what I had learned for myself could be useful to others as well. This is where the idea of the *counter-curriculum* arose. (Actually, I owe the title of the book to Vincent Di Stefano who wrote an endorsement for the book. When he mentioned the idea of *re-humanizing medicine*, it clicked for me that what I was really passionate and enthusiastic about was re-humanization and holistic medicine is just one pathway for that. This led to a re-write of the book.)

The concept of re-humanization implies that some degree of dehumanization has occurred. In the writing of this book, I have often struggled with some of the concepts I have used, such as 'being fully human.' What does this mean exactly? What does it mean to be 'more' or 'less' human? Is it not somewhat circular reasoning to say that human beings should strive to be fully human beings? Even if we can adequately define what 'being fully human' means, we can still ask what supports the argument for *why* doctors should work to develop their full humanity in order to practice medicine beyond being good technicians. The primary dilemma that I faced in medical school was a struggle between materialism and my sense of idealism and spirituality. I felt that in embracing a strictly biological materialist perspective, I was losing important, but difficult to name, parts of myself and this led to a loss of the ability to connect to people in a human way. My own re-humanization has worked to counter the philosophical position of materialism and to rekindle my idealism and spirituality. (This is an ongoing process, just as one must periodically re-align the wheels of the car to make sure that small misalignments do not cause unnecessary wear and tear on the car, make driving more difficult. It only takes small adjustments if done regularly, but if you ignore these small deviations, you can end up far off course and not know how you came to be so lost.)

It can be argued that idealism and humanism are ends in and of themselves, but I had difficulty philosophically justifying these positions. When I read Amit Goswami's perspective from quantum physics that consciousness is primary and matter is secondary to consciousness, it dawned on me that we will treat ourselves and others differently depending on our ultimate definition of the reality of what it means to be human. If human reality is based on matter, then we will function from a position of materialist reductionism. If human reality is based on consciousness or spirit (or deep respect for the immaterial dimensions of human being) then matter is secondary and medicine becomes a spiritual practice in addition to a technical endeavor. It follows, then, that we need to treat people/patients as whole human beings because there is something sacred about people, relationships and our jobs. I in no way mean that this sacredness or spirituality is related to any particular religious creed, but rather that it is founded upon a view of human reality in which biological materialism is contextualized within a larger perspective.

Historically, Medicine grew out of a religious and spiritual context, but with the rise of science and technology, we have moved away from anything that cannot be reduced to a number and we have become skeptical and wary of the spiritual dimension. It can be argued that if, as physicians and clinicians, we have narrowed our focus from the whole human being to the biological and the objective, we have dehumanized both ourselves and our patients. If all that clinical work asks of us is to be an efficient technician, there is no need to attend to our own personal growth. The gift of the current discussions about whole person care is that it asks us to attend to the whole person of ourselves in order to meet the whole person of the client.

In trying to write a satisfactory conclusion to this book, I have started and scrapped numerous attempts at bringing together a holistic 'list' or breakdown of the ultimate reason why a holistic framework in medicine is needed. I kept coming to the same unsatisfactory feeling that in breaking down and listing holistic benefits and concepts, I was diluting the strengths of holistic medicine. Thus, I feel obliged to admit in this epilogue that the ultimate reason why people need to be treated as fully human beings is not to be found in science; rather it is to be found in poetry, spirituality and the heart. It is illogical (and actually dehumanizing) to insist that there is an evidence-based reason for why we need to treat the whole person of the patient and why we need to attend to our own full humanity. This statement creates a dilemma for physicians, clinicians and institutions working for medicine to be a completely evidence-based practice. Techniques can and should be evidence-based, but authentic human interaction cannot be based on what 'research shows' or on expert opinion. Authentic human interaction grows out of the struggle of being or the manifestation of individuality and connection between two people. Healing is everything that happens around the technique, procedure or protocol that is implemented.

When I think back to my career crisis during my university days, I realize that the two books that influenced me to study medicine, and particularly psychiatry, were books about bringing a spiritual approach to working with people. Carl Jung's *Modern Man in Search of a Soul* obviously has a spiritual focus. M. Scott Peck's *The Road Less Travelled* also looks at personal growth and spirituality. I realize that the counter-curriculum and compassion revolution are both based on a re-spiritualization of human beings as an antidote to the materialization of human beings that is so prevalent in society and medical culture.

I went into medicine to help people and I have found that a treatment model of purely evidence-based biological reductionism leaves important aspects of human suffering untouched. While connection and healing require us, as physicians, to give the gift of our ever more limited resources of time and attention, there are many small, quick human-based interventions that are possible throughout the clinical day. If we look at the practice of medicine as a sacred, spiritual practice and an ethical, professional practice, then we can see that we should always be reflecting and harmonizing our thoughts and actions with the timeless ideals of healing. A kind word, a pause in the hallway, a quick touch for one of our fellow human beings who is lost and hurting goes a long, long, long way. We have to remember that sickness is not something that just happens to 'patients.' The education process and practice of contemporary medicine can also make us, the physicians and clinicians, sick – in the sense that our humanity can slowly leak away if we lose our idealism. Re-humanizing medicine requires that we bring more to clinical encounters than our minds filled with numbers, dosages and protocols. We must also attend to our hearts and our spirits and first heal ourselves.

There is no certificate possible for 'being fully human.' In trying to conclude this book, I have not been able to find an airtight explanation, which does not resort to circular reasoning or appeal to spirituality as justification, for why we should be fully human. Perhaps the best conclusion mirrors the process I find myself in, continually asking the question, 'what does it mean to be fully human?' By engaging ourselves personally, ethically and philosophically and continuing to ask and answer this question we create the potential for transforming our Selves, our practices, and the culture of medicine.

David Kopacz
Seattle, Washington
United States
January 23, 2014

References and Notes

Introduction

1. E.M. Forster, *Howard's End* (London: Hodder & Stoughton, 2011), Kindle Edition.

2. Plato, cited in Shaun Holt and Iona MacDonald, *Natural Remedies That Really Work: A New Zealand Guide* (Nelson: Craig Potton Publishing, 2010), 17.

3. C.H. Griffith and J.F. Wilson, 'The Loss of Student Idealism in the 3rd Year Clinical Clerkships,' *Evaluation & the Health Professions*, 24 (2001).

4. C.H. Griffith and J.F. Wilson, 'The Loss of Idealism throughout Internship,' *Evaluation & the Health Professions*, 26 (2003).

5. Debra Klamen, Linda Grossman and David Kopacz, 'Posttraumatic Stress Disorder Symptoms in Resident Physicians Related to Their Internship,' *Academic Psychiatry*, Vol. 19, No. 3 (Fall 1995).

6. Debra Klamen, Linda Grossman and David Kopacz, 'Medical Student Homophobia,' *Journal of Homosexuality*, Vol. 37, No. 1 (1999).

7. Debra Klamen, Linda Grossman and David Kopacz, 'Attitudes about Abortion among Second-Year Medical Students,' *Medical Teacher*, Vol. 18, No. 4 (1996).

8. David Kopacz, Debra Klamen and Linda Grossman, 'Medical Students and AIDS: Knowledge, Attitudes and Implications for Education,' *Health, Education and Research*, Vol. 14, No. 1 (1999).

9. Since I am writing as a physician (discussion of differences in US/UK usage below), I will use the words 'physician,' 'doctor,' 'clinician,' and 'health professional,' interchangeably throughout the text. I admit that there are power issues of hierarchy and authoritarianism to consider in the choice of terminology, but there is also a long tradition of

medical ethics and humanitarianism associated with the medical profession. I choose to reinvigorate our terminology rather than attempt to use politically correct terminology that can actually lead to more dehumanization. The use of a term like 'service provider' is an attempt to find a generic word that can be used to describe anyone providing a 'service.' Although this is currently a 'politically correct' term, it translates the therapeutic relationship into dehumanized language in which 'service provider' and 'service user' come together in a generic business transaction. I will interchangeably use the terms 'patient, 'client,' 'human being,' and 'person,' rather than the more politically correct 'consumer' or 'service user,' which seems more appropriate to a discussion of fast food than for a book focusing on healing and human connection. While the motivation behind using service provider/service user language is to empower clients, I don't think the shorthand of 'SPs' and 'SUs' is anything but dehumanizing to all involved.

There is also a cultural difference in the way that the words 'doctor' and 'physician' are used in the United States and Commonwealth countries following UK usage. In the US, 'doctor' and 'physician' are used interchangeably and could be referring to a GP, a specialist, or a surgeon. In Commonwealth countries, there is a distinction between someone who is a 'physician' and someone who is a 'surgeon,' and these would not be used interchangeably. It seems to me that it might also be more common for a specialist, for instance a psychiatrist, such as myself, to be considered a 'doctor,' but not necessarily a 'physician,' which would be reserved more for an internist or GP. I apologize for any confusion for Commonwealth readers in using these terms interchangeably. I do think that there is merit in considering the group of all doctors, surgeons, GPs together as a group given the focus on medical profession-alism. I also do think that many of the discussions in this book are pertinent to other medical professionals and also professionals in other fields, such as education and business.

10. I use the terms 'humanitarian' and 'humanistic' inter-changeably in this book to reorient clinicians to human needs and realities, but not to refer to specific belief systems or worldviews, such as 'secular humanism.' I will attempt an operational definition of what it means to be 'fully human' at a later point in the book.

11. Stephen J. Swensen, Gregg S. Meyer, Eugene C. Nelson, Gordon C. Hunt, Jr., David B. Pryor, Jed I. Weissberg, Gary S. Kaplan, Jennifer Daley, Gary R. Yates, Mark R. Chassin, Brent C. James and Donald M. Berwick, 'Cottage Industry to Postindustrial Care – The Revolution in Health Care Delivery,' *New England Journal of Medicine* 2010; 362:e12, February 4, 2010, http://www.nejm.org/doi/full/10.1056/NEJMp0911199.

12. Swensen, 'Cottage Industry to Postindustrial Care.'

13. Kelli Harding and Harold Pincus, 'Improving the Quality of Psychiatric Care: Aligning Research, Policy, and Practice,' *Focus*, vol. 9, No. 2 (Spring 2011).

Part I: PERSPECTIVES ON CONTEMPORARY MEDICINE

1. The term 'contemporary' is used to show that the contem-porary paradigm is simply that, the way that most physi-cians practice of medicine at this point in time at the beginning of the 21st century. The word 'contemporary' also reminds us that medicine is an ever-evolving field that is shaped by individuals in a particular context and time. Individuals are, in turn, influenced by changes in the medical profession, science, politics, economics, organiza-tional systems and social context.

The word 'contemporary' is less biased than other terms that are often used (such as 'traditional,' 'scientific,' or 'orthodox') that imply that the one paradigm is more correct than other paradigms. During the contemporary time, doctors have gone from being highly autonomous decision makers (true professionals) to interchangeable technicians and 'providers' in a bureaucratic and corporate system. Also during this time, there has been a shift from primary care to specialty care and this has created layers of fragmentation as more doctors specialize in only one dimension or organ system of their clients.

2. Gerald Arbuckle was born in New Zealand, educated in the UK and currently lives in Australia. He has been a consultant for health care organizations in the US, Canada and Australia. His book is truly international in its review of health care organizations and health care reform in English-speaking countries. He brings a welcome perspective as an anthropologist who is able to observe the cultural assumptions of different aspects within contemporary medicine. His primary argument in his book is on making sure that we include the values of the foundational model in health care. He discusses these different models in: Gerald Arbuckle, *Humanizing Healthcare Reforms* (London: Jessica Kingsley Publishers, 2013), 67–104.

Chapter 1: Dehumanization in Contemporary Medicine

1. Tony Schwartz, Jean Gomes, and Catherine McCarthy. *The Way We're Working Isn't Working* (New York: Free Press, 2010), 3.
2. Samuel Shem, *The House of God* (New York: Dell, 1978), 14.
3. Shem, *House*, 364.
4. Shem, *House*, 420.
5. Michael Krasner, Ronald Epstein, Howard Beckman, Anthony Suchman, Benjamin Chapman, Christopher

Mooney and Timothy Quill, 'Association of an Educational Program in Mindful Communication with Burnout, Empathy, and Attitudes among Primary Care Physicians,' *Journal of the American Medical Association*, Vol. 302, No. 12 (2009).

6. Lee Lipsenthal, *Finding Balance in a Medical Life* (San Anselmo: Finding Balance, Inc., 2007).

7. Allan D. Peterkin, *Staying Human During Residency Training* (Buffalo: University of Toronto Press, 2008).

8. Lois Surgenor, Ruth Spearing, Jacqueline Horn, Annette Beautrais, Roger Mulder and Peggy Chan, 'Burnout in hospital-based medical consultants in the New Zealand Public Health System,' *The New Zealand Medical Journal*, Vol. 122, No. 1300 (2009).

9. Anthony Dowell, Travis Westcott, Deborah McLeod and Stephen Hamilton, 'A Survey of Job Satisfaction, Sources of Stress and Psychological Symptoms among New Zealand Health Professionals,' *The New Zealand Medical Journal*, Vol. 114 (2001).

10. Marcus Henning, Susan Hawken and Andrew Hill, 'The Quality of Life of New Zealand Doctors and Medical Students: What Can Be Done to Avoid Burnout?' *The New Zealand Medical Journal*, Vol. 122, No. 1307 (2009).

11. M. Kluger, K. Townend, and T. Laidlaw, 'Job Satisfaction, Stress and Burnout in Australian Specialist Anaesthetists,' *Anaesthesia*, Vol. 58 (2003).

12. Y. Shehabi, G. Dobb and I. Jenkins, 'Burnout Syndrome among Australian Intensivists: A Survey,' *Critical Care and Resuscitation*, Vol. 10 (2008).

13. *Improving the Health of the NHS Workforce*, Report of the Partnership on the Health of the NHS Workforce (London: The Nuffield Trust, 1998).

14. R. Burbeck, S. Coomber, S. Robinson and C. Todd, 'Occupational Stress in Consultants in Accident and

Emergency Medicine: A National Survey of Levels of Stress at Work,' *Emergency Medicine*, Vol. 19 (2002).

15. F. Joseph Lee, Moira Stewart and Judith Brown, 'Stress, Burnout, and Strategies for Reducing Them: What's the Situation among Canadian Family Physicians?' *Canadian Family Physician*, Vol. 54 (2008).

16. H. Thommasen, M. Lavanchy, I. Connelly, J. Berkowitz and S. Grzybowski, 'Mental Health, Job Satisfaction, and Intention to Relocate: Opinions of Physicians in Rural British Columbia,' *Canadian Family Physician*, Vol. 47 (2001).

17. Robin Youngson, *Time to Care: How to Love Your Patients and Your Job* (Raglan: RebelHeart Publishers, 2012).

18. Wendy Levinson, Debra Roter, John Mullooly, Valerie Dull and Richard Frankel. 'Physician-Patient Communication: The Relationship with Malpractice Claims among Primary Care Physicians and Surgeons,' *Journal of the American Medical Association* Vol. 277, No. 7 (Feb 19, 1997): 553–559.

19. Jonathon R.B. Halbesleben and Cheryl Rathert, 'Linking Physician Burnout and Patient Outcomes: Exploring the Dyadic Relationship between Physicians and Patients,' *Health Care Management Review*, Vol. 33, No. 1 (January/March 2008), doi: 10.1097/01.HMR.0000304493. 87898.72.

20. Britt Berrett and Paul Spiegelman, *Patients Come Second: Leading Change by Changing the Way You Lead* (Austin: Greenleaf Book Group Press, 2013).

21. 'Patients Come Second' website, Britt Berrett and Paul Spiegelman, accessed January 3, 2013, http://patientscomesecond.com/.

22. 'National Survey of Physicians, Part III: Doctors' Opinions about their Profession,' Kaiser Family Foundation website, pdf available at:
http://www.kff.org/kaiserpolls/20020426c-index.cfm.

23. Phillip Miller, Louis Goodman, and Tim Norbeck, *In Their Own Words: 12,000 Physicians Reveal Their Thoughts on*

Medical Practice in America (Garden City: Morgan James, 2010), 22.

24. Miller, Goodman, and Norbeck, *Words*, 21.

25. Michelle Mudge-Riley, foreword to Richard Fernandez, *Physicians in Transition: Doctors Who Successfully Reinvented Themselves* (Denver: Wise Media Group, 2010).

26. Arbuckle, *Humanizing*, 71.

27. Arbuckle, *Humanizing*, 83.

28. Arbuckle, *Humanizing*, 96.

29. Arbuckle, *Humanizing*, 92.

30. Vincent Di Stefano, *Holism and Complementary Medicine: Origins and Principles* (Crows Nest: Allen & Unwin, 2006), 41.

31. Robert Audi, ed., 'Logical Positivism,' *The Cambridge Dictionary of Philosophy* (New York: Cambridge University Press, 2009), 514–516.

32. Arbuckle, *Humanizing*, 95.

33. Mark Schwartz, Steven Durning, Mark Linzer and Karen Hauer, 'Changes in Medical Students' Views of Internal Medicine Careers From 1990 to 2007,' *Archives of Internal Medicine* 171(8), (2011): 744–749.

34. Jerome Groopman, *How Doctors Think* (Boston: Mariner Books, 2007), 5.

35. Groopman, *Doctors*, 6.

36. Steve Hickey and Hilary Roberts, 'Evidence-Based Medicine: Neither Good Evidence nor Good Medicine,' *Journal of Integrative Medicine, Official Journal of the Australasian Integrative Medicine Association*, Vol. 16, No. 3 (2011).

37. C. Antonioli and M. Reveley, 'Randomised controlled trial of animal facilitated therapy with dolphins in the treatment of depression,' *British Medical Journal*, 26; 331(7527) (2005): 1231.

38. William Barrett, *The Illusion of Technique: A Search for*

Meaning in a Technological Civilization (New York: Anchor Press, 1978), 19.

39. Philip K. Dick, 'The Android and the Human,' (1972) in *The Shifting Realities of Philip K. Dick: Selected Literary and Philosophical Writings*, ed. Lawrence Sutin (New York: Vintage Books, 1995), 183–210.

40. Barrett, *Technique*, 8.

41. US Department of Health and Human Services, 'Health, United States, 2007,' available at http://www.cdc.gov/nchs/data/hus/hus07.pdf.

42. Data from 2005/2006 for New Zealand, cited in Gareth Morgan and Geoff Simmons, with John McCrystal, *Health Cheque: The truth we should all know about New Zealand's public health system* (Auckland: Public Interest Publishing, 2009), 47.

43. Data from 2000, cited in 'Issues facing the NHS' (26 September 2008), British Medical Association website, accessed March 25, 2012.
http://www.bma.org/uk/healthcare_policy/nhsissuesfaqs.jsp

44. 'The Cost of Care,' Posted Dec 18, 2009, NGM Blog Central, *National Geographic*, cited in The Society Pages, http://thesocietypages.org/graphicsociology/2011/04/26/cost-of-health-care-by-country-national-geographic/.

45. Michael Kennedy, *A Brief History of Disease, Science, and Medicine* (Mission Viejo: Asklepiad Press, 2004), 445. Also see Paul Starr, *The Social Transformation of American Medicine* (New York: Basic Books, 1982), 393–405.

46. Christopher Chabris and Daniel Simons. *The Invisible Gorilla* (New York: Broadway Paperbacks, 2009).

47. Troyen Brennan, David Rothman, Linda Blank, David Blumenthal, Susan Chimonas, Jordan Cohen, Janlori Goldman, Jerome Kassirer, Harry Kimball, James Naughton and Neil Smelser, 'Health Industry Practices That Create

Conflicts of Interest: A policy proposal for academic medical centers,' *Journal of the American Medical Association*, Vol. 295, No. 4 (January 25, 2006): 429–433.

48. Ray Moynihan and Alan Cassels, *Selling Sickness: How drug companies are turning us all into patients* (New York: Nation Books, 2005), x.

49. Moynihan and Cassels, *Sickness*, xii.

50. Qiuping Gu, Charles Dillon, and Vicki Burt, 'Prescription Drug Use Continues to Increase: U.S. Prescription Drug Data for 2007–2008,' *NCHS Data Brief*, No. 42, September 2010, U.S. Department of Health & Human Services, accessed March 25, 2012, http://www.cdc.gov/nchs/data/databriefs/db42.pdf.

51. Ashley Wazana, 'Physician and the Pharmaceutical Industry: Is a Gift Ever Just a Gift?' *Journal of the American Medical Association*, Vol. 283, No. 3 (January 19, 2000): 373–380.

52. Brennan, 'Health Industry Practices,' 429–433.

53. Jason Dana and George Lowenstein, 'A Social Science Perspective on Gifts to Physicians from Industry,' *Journal of the American Medical Association*, Vol. 290, No. 2 (July 9, 2003): 252–255.

54. Dana and Lowenstein, 'Gifts,' 253.

55. Wazana, 'Gift,' 378.

56. Niteesh Choudhry, Henry Stelfox, Allan Detsky, 'Relationships between Authors of Clinical Practice Guidelines and the Pharmaceutical Industry,' *Journal of the American Medical Association*, Vol. 287, No. 5 (February 6, 2002): 612–617.

57. Marcia Angell, 'The Epidemic of Mental Illness: Why?' *The New York Review of Books*, June 23, 2011.

58. Marcia Angell, 'The Illusions of Psychiatry,' *The New York Review of Books*, July 14, 2011.

59. Brennan, 'Health Industry Practices,' 430.

60. Brennan, 'Health Industry Practices,' 429.

61. 'No Free Lunch' website: http://www.nofreelunch.org, accessed January 5, 2013.

62. Robert Stoller, *Observing the Erotic Imagination* (New Haven: Yale University Press, 1992), 32.

63. Stoller, *Observing*, 32.

64. Audi ed., 'Martin Buber,' *The Cambridge Dictionary of Philosophy*, 104.

65. A comment on the term 'detachment.' This term is sometimes used in spiritual and religious writing as the opposite of attachment, such as Buddhist and Hindu contexts. Attachment in this context is seen as a form of clinging or dependency of the ego to material reality. Detachment is thus a goal to be cultivated, in a sense that is somewhat congruous with the Christian concept of 'being in, but not of the world.' Personally, I prefer the term 'non-attachment' in this context, as it illustrates the opposition to attachment, but avoids the confusion of the negative associations of 'detachment' to a general Western audience. I think the terminology is complicated enough, but the concept is even more complicated when balancing a life-affirming, but non-attached approach to life without falling into the negative sense of detachment, dissociation, or the coldness that comes from the lack of engagement and human connectivity. Quite seriously, this topic could easily be a book length discussion, but for this book I will be using the term 'detachment' in its negative sense. My apologies to readers for whom 'detachment' is viewed in a positive sense of spiritual attainment.

66. Peter Salgo, 'The Doctor Will See You for Exactly Seven Minutes,' *The New York Times*, March 22, 2006.

67. Michel Foucault, *The Birth of the Clinic* (New York: Vintage Books, 1994), 38.

68. 'Patient-Centered Medical Home (PCMH),' American

Academy of Family Physicians website, accessed November 19, 2012,

http://www.aafp.org/online/en/home/membership/ initiatives/pcmh.html.

69. 'Patient-Centered Medical Home Checklist,' American Academy of Family Physicians website, accessed November 19, 2012,

http://www.aafp.org/online/etc/medialab/aafp_org/ documents/membership/pcmh/checklist.Par.00001.File.tmp/ PCMHCklist.pdf.

70. American Academy of Family Physicians, 'Patient-Centered Medical Home.'

71. Harding and Pincus, 'Improving.'

72. The Institute of Medicine, '10 Rules for Patient/Consumer Expectations of Their Health Care' cited in Harding and Pincus, 'Improving,' originally from the Institute of Medicine's, *To Err is Human: Building a Safer, Health System*, 2000.

Chapter 2: Health and Illness: Paradigms and Perspectives

1. Groopman, *Doctors*, 6.

2. John Beahrs, *Limits of Scientific Psychiatry* (New York: Brunner/Mazel 1986), xvii.

3. William Cameron, *Informal Sociology: A Casual Introduction to Sociological Thinking*, cited in the Quote Investigator website, accessed February 21, 2012,

http://quoteinvestigator.com.

Interestingly, and quite fitting to this current chapter, this quote is often attributed to Albert Einstein, because it fits Einstein's persona and seems like something he *might* have said. Einstein's cultural persona is of the absent-minded scientist, but also the wise sage who cuts through the obfuscation of science to speak simple human truths.

4. Rupert Sheldrake, *The Science Delusion: Freeing the Spirit of*

Enquiry (London: Coronet, 2012).

5. Beahrs, *Limits*, 135.

6. Beahrs, *Limits*, xiii.

7. Beahrs, *Limits*, 155.

8. Groopman, *Doctors*, 5.

9. Groopman, *Doctors*, 5.

10. Groopman, *Doctors*: attribution error (44); affective error (47); confirmation bias (65); commission bias (169); satisfaction of search error (169); vertical line failure (170); false positive/negative (180); availability errors (196); and cognitive errors (260).

11. Another interesting book that describes common cognitive errors is Chabris and Simons' *The Invisible Gorilla*. They state that we 'all believe that we are capable of seeing what's in front of us, of accurately remembering important events from our past, of understanding the limits of our knowledge, or properly determining cause and effect,' but these beliefs, 'mask critically important limitations in our cognitive abilities,' (xii). Their book examines common mistakes in human attention, memory and decision-making. They conducted the fascinating study which showed that people not seeing what was right in front of their face during a counting task with 50 percent of people engaged in a cognitive counting task failed to see a person in a gorilla suit walk on to a basketball court. This speaks to the mind's ability to filter out information when it is engaged in another cognitive task. If something as obvious as a gorilla goes unnoticed, just think how many cognitive errors physicians make while trying to fit a patient into the appropriate protocol!

12. Attributed to Max von Laue speaking about de Broglie's thesis that electrons have wave properties. Wikiquote website, accessed August 27, 2013, http://en.wikiquote.org/wiki/Talk:Quantum_mechanics.

13. For the story of Semmelweis, see Kennedy, *History*, 138–139. Also Robert Becker, *The Body Electric: Electromagnetism and the Foundation of Life* (New York: Harper, 1985), 331. Becker's chapter on the politics of science is also relevant to this discussion, pgs. 330–347.

14. Robert Becker and Gary Selden, *The Body Electric: Electromagnetism and the Foundation of Life* (New York: Harper, 1985).

15. Becker and Selden, *Body Electric*.

16. Becker and Selden, *Body Electric*, 20.

17. Elkins, *Humanistic Psychology: A Clinical Manifesto* (Colorado Springs: University of the Rockies Press, 2009), 46.

18. Elkins, *Humanistic*, 2–3.

19. Elkins, *Humanistic*, 2–3.

20. Ronald Levant, 2001, p. 219, cited in Elkins, *Humanistic*, 61–62.

21. Orlinsky (1994) reviewed more than 2,000 studies and identified therapist-related variables that influence therapeutic outcomes. These are summarized by Lambert and Barley (2002) and cited by Elkins, *Humanistic*, 79.

22. The following books are good references on social support and health from a number of different perspectives:
    Dean Ornish, *Love and Survival: 8 Pathways to Intimacy and Health* (New York: HarperCollins, 1998).
    Ranjan Roy, *Social Support, Health, and Illness: A Complicated Relationship* (Toronto: University of Toronto Press, 2011).
    Gail Bernice Holland, *A Call for Connection: Solutions for Creating a Whole New Culture* (Novato: New World Library, 1998).
    Martin E. P. Seligman, *Flourish: A Visionary New Understanding of Happiness and Well-being* (New York: Free Press, 2011).
    Allan D. Peterkin, *Staying Human During Residency Training* (Toronto: University of Toronto Press, 2008).
    Lee Lipsenthal, *Finding Balance in a Medical Life* (San Anselmo: Finding Balance, Inc., 2007).

23. Amit Goswami, *The Quantum Doctor* (Charlottesville: Hampton Roads, 2004), 35.

24. Goswami, *Doctor*, 4.

25. Goswami, *Doctor*, 5.

26. Goswami, *Doctor*, 4.

27. Goswami, *Doctor*, 10.

28. Goswami, *Doctor*, 64–65.

29. Goswami, *Doctor*, 33.

30. Goswami, *Doctor*, 20.

31. Niels Bohr, cited in Deepak Chopra, foreword to Goswami, *Doctor*, x.

32. Werner Heisenberg, cited in Chopra, foreword to Goswami, *Doctor*, xi.

33. Chopra, foreword to Goswami, *Doctor*, xi.

34. Michael H. Cohen, *Healing at the Borderland of Medicine and Religion* (Chapel Hill: University of North Carolina Press, 2006), 3.

35. Cohen, *Healing*, 16.

36. Cohen, *Healing*, 7.

37. Also see Bivens, *Alternative Medicine? A History*. She outlines how open or closed different medical systems have been when they encounter differing explanations for health and illness. Roberta Bivens, *Alternative Medicine? A History* (Oxford: Oxford University Press, 2007).

38. Cohen, *Healing*, 12.

39. Larry Dossey, *Reinventing Medicine: Beyond Mind-Body to a New Era of Healing* (San Francisco: HarperSanFrancisco, 1999), 12.

40. Dame Julian of Norwich from *Revelations of Divine Love*, cited in J.M. Cohen and J-F. Phipps, *The Common Experience* (Los Angeles: J.P. Tarcher, 1979), 111.

41. Lao Tzu, *Tao Te Ching*, trans. D.C. Lau (New York: Penguin Classics, 1963), 57.

42. Chuang Tzu, *Basic Writings*, trans. Burton Watson (New

York: Columbia University Press, 1964), 4344.

43. Chuang Tzu, *Writings*, 45.

44. Elkins, *Humanistic*, 111.

45. *D.H. Lawrence, The Complete Poems*, 1977, p. 620, cited in Elkins, *Humanistic*, 130–131.

46. Angela Belli and Jack Coulehan (eds.), *Blood and Bone* (Iowa City: University of Iowa Press, 1998), xiii–xiv.

47. Johanna Shapiro, *The Inner World of Medical Students: Listening to Their Voices in Poetry* (New York: Radcliffe Publishing, 2009), 12–33.

48. Shapiro, *Inner World*, 5.

49. Shapiro, *Inner World*, 6.

50. Shapiro, *Inner World*, 8.

51. Shapiro, *Inner World*, 8.

52. Louis Kavar, *The Integrated Self: A Holistic Approach to Spirituality and Mental Health Practice* (Washington: O-Books, 2012), 18.

53. Paul Starr, *The Social Transformation of American Medicine: The rise of a sovereign profession and the making of a vast industry* (New York: Basic Books, 1982), 3.

54. Michel Foucault, *The Birth of the Clinic* (New York: Vintage Books, 1994), 39.

55. Michel Foucault, *The Foucault Reader*, ed. Paul Rabinow (New York: Pantheon, 1984), 180.

56. Ivan Illich, *Limits to Medicine, Medical Nemesis: The Expropriation of Health* (New York: Marion Boyers, 1976), 8.

57. Illich, *Limits*, 34.

58. Illich, *Limits*, 41.

59. Illich, *Limits*, 41.

60. Illich, *Limits*, 9.

61. Illich, *Limits*, 35.

62. I will use the term 'Western,' following Watters' use, to refer to industrialized countries that embrace principles of science and economics. Since I have been living in New

Zealand, I realize that the East/West reference does not make much sense from the geographical perspective of the Southern Hemisphere. However, there is not another easy-to-use term, that I am aware of, that does not have some inherent baggage or imprecision. 'Industrialized' is one possible term, although I don't think it captures the cultural difference as well. Generally, 'Western' seems to refer to the culture and societies that are derived from European Caucasians and this may be more fundamental than how industrialized a country is. This is quite an interesting topic that requires discussion beyond the parameters of this book. For the purposes of this book, we can assume that the term 'Western' equates to societies that embrace the biomedical and economic rationalist models.

63. Ethan Watters, *Crazy Like Us: The Globalization of the American Psyche* (New York: Free Press, 2010), 1.
64. Ethan Watters, *Crazy*, 2.
65. Arthur Kleinman, cited in Watters, *Crazy*, 107.
66. For histories of policies toward indigenous people, see Dee Brown, *Bury My Heart at Wounded Knee* (New York: Holt, 2001), and Michael King, *The Penguin History of New Zealand* (Camberwell: Penguin, 2003). It can be argued that European colonists engaged in genocide in many instances, in the sense of systematically trying to eliminate and extinguish indigenous cultures.
67. Ethan Watters, *Crazy*, 106.
68. Ethan Watters, *Crazy*, 107.
69. Ethan Watters, *Crazy*, 91.
70. Patrick Bracken, cited in Watters, *Crazy*, 122–123.
71. Ethan Watters, *Crazy*, 123.
72. Rebecca Solnit, *A Paradise Built in Hell: The Extraordinary Communities That Arise in Disaster* (New York: Penguin, 2009), 8.
73. Solnit, *Paradise*, 118.

74. For ease of transfer to e-book format, I have left out special characters found in the Maori language, such as the macron over the 'a' in the word Maori.

   A brief pronunciation guide can be found on 'The New Zealand History Online' page. That source provides a rough guide to pronouncing Maori vowels as follows:

   'a' as in far

   'e' as in desk

   'i' as in fee, me, see

   'o' as in awe (not 'oh')

   'u' as in sue, boot

   The letters 'wh' are pronounced close to the 'f' sound in English. '100 Maori words every New Zealander should know,' from the 'The New Zealand History Online,' accessed January 2, 2013,

   http://www.nzhistory.net.nz/culture/maori-language-week/100-maori-words.

75. Mason Durie, *Whaiora: Maori Health Development*, second edition (South Melbourne: Oxford University Press, 1998), 73.

76. Durie, *Whaiora*, 68.

77. 1996 data cited in Mason Durie, *Mauri Ora: The Dynamics of Maori Health* (South Melbourne: Oxford University Press, 2001), 6.

78. Durie, *Whaiora*, 70–71.

79. Durie, *Whaiora*, 2.

80. All of the quotes in this paragraph are taken from table 12, Durie, *Whaiora*, 69.

81. Durie, *Whaiora*, 71.

Part II: HOLISTIC MEDICINE: A FRAMEWORK FOR THE WHOLE HUMAN BEING

1. Patricia Barnes, Barbara Bloom and Richard Nahin, 'Complementary and Alternative Medicine Use Among

Adults and Children: United States, 2007,' *National Health Statistics Report*, No. 12, December 2008, from the National Center for Complementary and Alternative Medicine website, pdf available at, http://nccam.nih.gov/news/camstats/2007.

2. Kris Wilson, Claire Dowson and Dee Mangin, 'Prevalence of complementary and alternative medicine use in Christchurch, New Zealand: children attending general practice versus paediatric outpatients,' *Journal of the New Zealand Medical Association*, Vol. 120, No. 1251 (March 23, 2007).

3. Raymond Khoury, foreword to Vincent Di Stefano, *Holism and Complementary Medicine: Origins and Principles* (Crows Nest: Allen & Unwin, 2006), vii.

4. Khoury, foreword to Di Stefano, *Holism*, vii.

5. Shaun Holt and Iona MacDonald, *Natural Remedies That Really Work: A New Zealand Guide* (Nelson: Craig Potton Publishing, 2010), 18.

6. Holt and MacDonald, *Natural Remedies*, 18.

Chapter 3: Redefining Medicine

1. Vincent Di Stefano, *Holism and Complementary Medicine: Origins and Principles* (Crows Nest: Allen & Unwin, 2006), xxii.

2. Michael H. Cohen, Mary Ruggie and Marc Micozzi, *The Practice of Integrative Medicine: A Legal and Operational Guide* (New York: Springer Publishing, 2007), 3.

3. Starr, *Socialization*, 47–54, 79–144.

4. Bivens, *Alternative*, 89–106.

5. Shaun Holt and Iona MacDonald, *Natural Remedies*, 21–22.

6. Guy Eslick, Peter Howe, Caroline Smith, Ros Priest and Alan Bensoussan, 'Benefits of Fish Oil Supplementation in Hyperlipidemia: A Systematic Review and Meta-analysis,' *International Journal of Cardiology*, Vol. 136, No. 1 (July 2009).

7. David Mischoulon, 'Ask the Expert: Depression and Dysthymia,' *Focus*, Vol. 10 (2012).

8. National Center for Complementary and Alternative Medicine (NCCAM), http://nccam.nih.gov/.

9. Nancy Pearson and Margaret Chesney, 'The CAM Education Program of the National Center for Complementary and Alternative Medicine: An Overview,' *Academic Medicine*, Vol. 82, No. 10 (October 2007).

10. Australasian Integrative Medicine Association (AIMA) website, http://www.aima.net.au/about_aima.html.

11. Arizona Center for Integrative Medicine website, http://integrativemedicine.arizona.edu/about/index.html.

12. The Consortium of Academic Health Centers for Integrative Medicine, http://www.imconsortium.org/.

13. The George Family Foundation was started by Penny and Bill George. It is a philanthropic organization devoted to fostering integrative health and healing, leadership, spirituality and community. http://www.georgefamilyfoundation.org/index.htm

14. Thomson Healthcare, *PDR for Herbal Medicines*, fourth edition (Montvale: Thomson Reuters, 2007).

15. For an excellent review of the philosophical concept of holism throughout medical history, see Australian osteopath Vincent Di Stefano's book, *Holism and Complementary Medicine: Origins and Principles*. Di Stefano's thinking is very similar to my own and in regard to the philosophy of holistic medicine, the distinction between alternative technique and philosophy, and also in the broader hope of moving beyond the technical treatment of the illness to healing and transforming medicine and society. The book includes quotes from his study of attitudes of many complementary and

holistic health professionals. The study which the interviews are drawn from, 'The Meaning of Natural Medicine: An Interpretative Study,' can be found at Di Stefano's website: http://thehealingproject.net.au/.

16. The American Board of Integrative and Holistic Medicine website, accessed January 17, 2014.
https://www.abihm.org

17. The American Board of Integrative Medicine on the American Board of Physician Specialties website, accessed January 17, 2014.
http://www.abpsus.org/integrative-medicine

Chapter 4: Principles of Holistic Medicine

1. '10 Principles of Holistic Medicine,' American Holistic Medical Association website, accessed April 1, 2012.
http://www.holisticmedicine.org/content.asp?pl=2&sl=22&contentid=22

2. Lewis Hyde, *The Gift: Creativity and the Artist in the Modern World* (New York: Vintage, 1979), 48–49.

3. Hyde, *Gift*, 49.

4. Hyde, *Gift*, 65.

5. M. Scott Peck, *The Road Less Travelled* (London: Arrow, 1978), 69.

6. Peck, *Road*, 111.

7. Dr. Francis Weld Peabody quoted in Jerome Groopman, *How Doctors Think* (Boston: Mariner Books, 2007), 54.

8. Dean Ornish, *Love and Survival: 8 Pathways to Intimacy and Health* (New York: HarperCollins, 1998).

9. Ranjan Roy, *Social Support, Health, and Illness: A Complicated Relationship* (Buffalo: University of Toronto Press, 2011).

10. Carl Gustav Jung, 'In memory of Sigmund Freud' (1932), *The Collected Works of C. G. Jung, vol. 15: The Spirit in Man, Art, and Literature* (Princeton: Princeton University Press, 1971), para. 68.

11. Vaclav Havel, *Disturbing the Peace*, trans. Paul Wilson (New York: Vintage, 1990), 180–181. I truly love this passage and hoped to quote it in extended form, however I wasn't able to obtain electronic and UK permission to reproduce an extended quote, so I will just give a few excerpts. I do encourage reading the full quote in context. All the quotations in this paragraph are from this same source.

12. Levinson, 'Physician-Patient Communication.'

13. Carl Gustav Jung, *Memories, Dreams, Reflections* (New York: Vintage, 1989), 396.

14. Peck, *Road*, 69.

15. American Board of Integrative Holistic Medicine website, http://www.abihm.org/.

16. The Police, 'Rehumanize Yourself,' from the album *Ghost in the Machine*, A&M Records, 1981.

17. Illich, *Limits*, 133.

18. Andrea Joy Cohen, *A Blessing in Disguise* (New York: Berkley Books, 2008).

19. Carl Gustav Jung, *Modern Man in Search of a Soul* (Orlando: Harcourt Harvest, 1955).

20. Richard Bach, *Illusions* (New York: Dell/Eleanor Friede, 1977).

21. Carl Gustav Jung, from 'On the Psychology of the Unconscious,' *Two Essays, Collected Works 7*, in Storr, *The Essential Jung*, 164.

Chapter 5: A Holistic Framework for Being Human

1. Murphy, *Future of the Body*, 552.

2. George Engel, 'The need for a new medical model: a challenge for biomedicine,' *Science*, 196 (4286), (1977).

3. Engel, 'New Medical Model' 129.

4. Nassir Ghaemi, *The Rise and Fall of the Biopsychosocial Model: Reconciling Art and Science in Psychiatry* (Baltimore: Johns Hopkins University Press, 2010).

5. D.P. Sulmasy, 'A biopsychosocial-spiritual model for the care

of patients at the end of life,' *Gerontologist*, Oct; 42 Spec. No. 3, (2002): 24–33.

6. Leila Kozak, Lorin Boynton, Jacob Bentley and Emma Bezy, 'Introducing spirituality, religion and culture curricula in the psychiatry residency programme,' *Medical Humanities*, 36 (2010): 48–51.

7. Parker Palmer, *To Know As We Are Known: Education as a Spiritual Journey* (New York: HarperOne, 1993), xxiii.

8. Palmer, *To Know*, 21.

9. Carl Gustav Jung, *The Psychology of Kundalini Yoga* (Princeton: Princeton University Press, 1999), 85.

10. Jung, *Kundalini*, 61.

11. Jung, *Kundalini*, 34.

12. Anodea Judith, *Eastern Body, Western Mind*,(Berkeley: Celestial Arts, 1996), vi.

13. Judith, *Eastern Body*, ix.

14. Barbara Brennan, *Hands of Light* (New York: Bantam, 1988).

15. Susan Matz, *The Art of Energy Healing, Volume 1: The Foundation* (Nevada City: Blue Dolphin, 2005). There are a total of six volumes in this series.

16. Richard Gerber, *Vibrational Medicine* (Rochester: Bear & Company, 2001).

17. Goswami, *Doctor*, 141–152.

18. Goswami, *Doctor*, 145.

19. Rick Jarow, *Creating the Work You Love* (Rochester: Destiny Books, 1995).

20. David Kopacz, *Finding Your Self* (unpublished, limited number of copies printed by Stipes Publishing, 2008, 2009 for a class at Parkland College, Champaign, Illinois).

21. Schwartz, *Working*.

22. David Matsumoto ed., 'hierarchy of needs,' *The Cambridge Dictionary of Philosophy*, 234.

23. Ken Wilber, *A Brief History of Everything*, second edition (Shambhala, Boston: 2011), Kindle Edition.

24. Ken Wilber, cited in Tony Schwartz, *What Really Matters: Searching for Wisdom in America* (New York: Bantam Books, 1995), 353.

25. Ken Wilber, Diagram 5, The Four Quadrants, from Ken Wilber Online, Shambhala Publications website, accessed April 21, 2012, http://wilber.shambhala.com/html/books/kosmos/excerpt6/part1.cfm/.

26. Candace Pert, *Molecules of Emotion: The Science Behind Mind-Body Medicine* (New York: Simon and Schuster; 1999).

27. Peter Salovey, Jerusha Detweiler, Wayne Steward and Alexander Rothman, 'Emotional States and Physical Health,' *American Psychologist*, Vol. 55, No. 1 (January 2000): 110–121.

28. Martin Seligman, *Flourish: A Visionary New Understanding of Happiness and Well-being* (New York: Free Press, 2011).

29. Dean Ornish, *Love and Survival: 8 Pathways to Intimacy and Health* (New York: HarperCollins, 1998).

30. Roy, *Social Support*.

31. Karen Baikie and Kay Wilhelm, 'Emotional and Physical Health Benefits of Expressive Writing,' *Advances in Psychiatric Treatment*, 11 (2005): 338–346.

32. David Tacey, *Gods and Diseases: Making Sense of our Physical and Mental Wellbeing* (Sydney: HarperCollins, 2011).

33. Cohen, *Healing*.

34. Barbara Mainguy, Michael Valenti Pickren and Lewis Mehl-Madrona, 'Relationships Between Level of Spiritual Transformation and Medical Outcome,' *Advances in Mind-Body Medicine*, 27(1) (2013): 4–11.

35. Judith, *Eastern Body*, 105–168.

36. Wilber in Schwartz, *Matters*, 353.

37. Betty Edwards, *Drawing on the Artist Within* (New York: Fireside, 1986), 39.

38. Tacey, *Gods*, 34.

39. Tacey, *Gods*, 209.

40. Levinson, 'Physician-Patient Communication.'

41. Tacey, *Gods*, 57.

Part III: RE-HUMANIZING YOUR SELF

Chapter 6: Physician, Know Thyself

1. Friedrich Nietzsche, *Thus Spake Zarathustra*, Part I, Chapter XXII, Section 2, in *The Portable Nietzsche*, ed. and trans. Walter Kaufmann (New York: Penguin Books, 1982), 189.

2. David Matsumoto ed., 'classical conditioning,' *The Cambridge Dictionary of Psychology*, 108.

3. M.B. Niemi, M. Harting, W. Kou, A. Del Rey, H.O. Besedovsky, M. Schedlowski and G. Pacheco-Lopez, 'Taste-immunosuppression Engram: Reinforcement and Extinction,' *Journal of Neuroimmunology*, 188(1–2) (2007): 74–9.

4. Terry Gray, Vice President for Technology Strategy, University of Washington, Seattle, website, accessed April 3, 2012,
http://staff.washington.edu/gray/misc/which-half.html.
Gray states, 'I first heard it attributed to a University of Chicago President addressing an incoming Freshman class: "Half of everything we teach you is wrong ... unfortunately, we don't know which half."'
Gray then lists a number of different people who have said or written similar things, including two from medicine: 'Richard Ruhling, MD: One of my professors, John Peterson, MD, was taught at Harvard that half of medical education was not true; the only problem was, they didn't know which half.' 'John L. Meade, MD, FACEP: When I started medical school, a professor told us that half of what we would be taught in the next 4 years was wrong; unfortunately, we didn't know which half was wrong just yet.'

5. Palmer, *Courage*, 100.

6. Palmer, *Courage*, 173.
7. J. Krishnamurti, *Total Freedom* (San Francisco: Harper SanFrancisco, 1996), 116.
8. Krishnamurti, *Freedom*, 44.
9. Krishnamurti, *Freedom*, 29.
10. David Kopacz, 'Learning to Save the Self: Samuel Shem's Portrayal of Trauma and Medical Education,' presented at the annual conference of the International Society for Traumatic Stress Studies, Washington D.C. (1998).
11. Shem, *House*, 6–7.
12. Laurence Gonzales, *Deep Survival: Who Lives, Who Dies, and Why* (New York: W.W. Norton, 2005), 142–143.
13. Gonzales, *Survival*, 122–123.
14. Betty Edwards, *Drawing on the Artist Within* (New York: Fireside, 1986), 11.
15. Edwards, *Drawing*, 12.
16. Edwards, *Drawing*, 11.
17. Edwards, *Drawing*, 13.
18. Edwards, cited in Schwartz, *Matters*, 191. *What Really Matters: Searching for Wisdom in America* (New York: Bantam Books, 1995), 169.

Chapter 7: Transforming Your Self

1. Di Stefano, *Holism*, 92.
2. Robert Audi ed., 'Sufism,' *The Cambridge Dictionary of Philosophy*, 888–889.
3. Soren Ventegodt and Gary Orr, 'The future of traditional African healers,' *Journal of Alternative Medicine Research*, Vol. 2, No. 4 (2010), 361.
4. Donald Winnicott, 'Ego Distortions in Terms of True and False Self,' in *The Maturational Process and the Facilitating Environment: Studies in the Theory of Emotional Development* (New York: International UP Inc., 1960), 140–152.
5. Stanislav Grof, *The Adventure of Self-Discovery: Dimensions of*

Consciousness and New Perspectives in Psychotherapy and Inner Exploration (Albany: State University of New York Press, 1988).

6. Matz, *Art*.
7. Brennan, *Hands*.
8. Groopman, *Doctors*.
9. Chabris and Simons, *Gorilla*.
10. Gonzales, *Survival*.
11. Krishnamurti, *Freedom*.
12. Wilber, *Everything*.
13. Juan Mascaro, trans., *The Upanishads* (New York: Penguin Books, 1965), 132.
14. Epstein, *Thoughts*, 95.
15. Stephen S. Hall, *Wisdom: From Philosophy to Neuroscience* (New York: Alfred A. Knopf, 2010), 22.
16. Schwartz, *Wisdom*, 75.
17. Schwartz, *Wisdom*, 75.
18. Murphy, *The Future of the Body*, 555.
19. Murphy, *Body*, 556, emphasis his.
20. Philip K. Dick, cited in Lawrence Sutin, ed., *The Shifting Realities of Philip K. Dick: Selected Literary and Philosophical Writings* (New York: Vintage, 1995), 187.
21. John Ratey and Eric Hagerman, *Spark: The Revolutionary New Science of Exercise and the Brain* (New York: Little, Brown, and Company, 2008).
22. Goswami, *Doctor*, 213.
23. Jon Kabat-Zinn, *Full Catastrophe Living* (New York: Delta, 1990).
24. Lee Lipsenthal, *Finding Balance in a Medical Life* (San Anselmo: Finding Balance, Inc., 2007).
25. Mark Epstein, *Thoughts without a Thinker: Psychotherapy from a Buddhist Perspective* (New York: Basic Books, 1995).
26. Griffith and Wilson, 'Idealism.'
27. Griffith and Wilson, 'Idealism throughout Internship.'

28. M.S. Krasner, R.M. Epstein, H. Beckman, et al. 'Association of an Educational Program in Mindful Communication with Burnout, Empathy, and Attitudes among Primary Care Physicians,' *Journal of the American Medical Association*, Vol. 302, No. 12 (2009), 1291.

29. Mohandas K. Gandhi, *An Autobiography: The Story of My Experiments with Truth* (Boston: Beacon Press, 1957), 93–95.

30. Gandhi, *Autobiography*, 25.

31. Gandhi, *Autobiography*, 12, 24–25, 91.

32. Pema Chodron, 'Loving Kindness Meditation,' *The Places That Scare You* (Boston: Shambhala, 2001), 41–47, and 130.

33. Martia Nelson, *Coming Home* (Mill Valley: Nataraj, 1997), 74.

34. Nelson, *Home*, 74, emphasis hers.

35. Jarow, *Creating*, 7.

36. Jarow, *Creating*, 6.

37. Julia Cameron, *The Artist's Way: A Spiritual Path to Higher Creativity* (New York: J.P. Tarcher/Putnam, 2002).

38. Friedrich August Kekule von Stradonitz, 'Famous Dreams.' Dream Interpretation-Dictionary website, accessed January 6, 2013, http://www.dreaminterpretation-dictionary.com/famous-dreams-friedrich-von-stradonitz.html.

39. Kekule von Stradonitz, 'Famous Dreams.'

40. 'Archimedes,' Wikipedia website, accessed January 12, 2013, http://en.wikipedia.org/wiki/Archimedes.

41. Judith Orloff, *Second Sight: An Intuitive Psychiatrist Tells Her Extraordinary Story and Shows You How to Tap Your Own Inner Wisdom* (New York: Three Rivers Press, 2010).

42. Norman Shealy, *Medical Intuition: A Science of the Soul* (Virginia Beach: A.R.E. Press, 2010).

43. Larry Dossey, *The Science of Premonitions: How Knowing the Future Can Help Us Avoid Danger, Maximize Opportunities, and Create a Better Life* (New York: Plume, 2009).

44. Carl Gustav Jung, *Memories, Dreams, Reflections* (New York:

Vintage, 1989), 4.

45. Reinhold Niebuhr, 'The Serenity Prayer,' Wikipedia, accessed January 30, 2012. http://en.wikipedia.org/wiki/Serenity_Prayer

46. Talking Heads, 'Once in a Lifetime,' from the album *Remain in Light*, Sire Records, 1980.

47. David Whyte, *The Three Marriages: Reimagining Work, Self and Relationship* (New York: Penguin, 2009), 313.

48. Whyte, *Marriages*, 313.

49. John Ralston Saul, *On Equilibrium* (Ringwood: Penguin Books, 2001), 317.

50. Saul, *Equilibrium*, 317.

51. Whyte, *Marriages*, 137.

52. Rebecca Solnit, *A Field Guide to Getting Lost* (New York: Penguin, 2005), 5.

53. Thoreau, cited in Solnit, *Lost*, 15.

Part IV: RE-HUMANIZING YOUR PRACTICE

1. Gautam Naik, 'Faltering Family M.D.s Get Technology Lifeline: Doctors Think Small to Revive Solo Role for Primary Care,' *The Wall Street Journal* online, February 23, 2007, accessed April 7, 2012, http://online.wsj.com/article/SB117201140861714109-search.html.

2. Benjamin Brewer, 'Satellite Office Could Lower Costs, Allow More Time for Patients: Country Doctor Determined to Try New Practice Model,' *The Wall Street Journal* online, January 10, 2006, accessed April 7, 2012, http://online.wsj.com/article/SB113683811203541840.html.

3. L. Gordon Moore, 'Going Solo: Making the Leap,' *Family Practice Management*. February 2002, American Academy of Family Physicians website, accessed April 7, 2012. http://www.aafp.org/fpm/2002/0200/p29.html.

Chapter 8: My Journey in Creating a Holistic Practice

1. Carl Jung, originally from *The Structure and Dynamics of the Psyche*, cited in Schwartz, *Matters*, 421.
2. Klamen (1995).
3. Kopacz (1999).
4. Klamen (1999).
5. Klamen (1996).
6. Shunryu Suzuki, *Zen Mind, Beginner's Mind* (New York: John Weatherhill Inc., 1986), 76–77.
7. Mark Thorpe and Miranda Thorpe, 'Immigrant Psychotherapists and New Zealand Clients,' *The Journal of the New Zealand Association of Psychotherapists (Inc.) Te Ropu Whakaora Hinengaro*, Vol. 14 (December 2008): 30–45.
8. Mila Goldner-Vukov, 'A Psychiatrist in Cultural Transition: Personal and Professional Dilemmas,' *Transcultural Psychiatry*, 41 (September, 2004): 386–405.
9. Patte Randal, M.W. Stewart, D. Lampshire, J. Symes, D. Proverbs, and H. Hamer, 'The Re-covery Model: An integrative developmental stress-vulnerability-strengths approach to mental health,' *Psychosis: Psychological, Social, and Integrative Approaches*, 1(2), (2009): 122–133.
10. Jovanotti, 'Fango,' from the album *Safari*, Decca International, 2008. Lyrics translated on LyricsTranslate.com, accessed March 27, 2012, http://lyricstranslate.com/en/fango-mud.html.

Chapter 9: Transforming Your Practice

1. Samuel Shem, 'Fiction as Resistance,' *Annals of Internal Medicine*, Vol. 137, No. 11 (Dec. 3, 2002), 934.
2. *Tabula Smaragdina (The Emerald Tablet)*, attributed to Hermes Trismegistos, cited in Carl Jung, *Mysterium Coniunctionis, The Collected Works of C. G. Jung, XIV* (Princeton: Princeton University Press: 1989), 115fn. Jung frequently referenced this book in his later, alchemical writings. He believed that

the more perceptive alchemists were concerned with purifying and transforming the inner (spiritual and psychological) substance of the practitioner, rather than changing physical lead into gold.

3. 'Uncle Ben,' Wikipedia website, accessed January 12, 2013, http://en.wikipedia.org/wiki/Uncle_Ben#.22With_great _power_comes_great_responsibility.22.

4. Gardiner Harris, 'More Doctors Giving Up Private Practices,' *The New York Times*, March 25, 2010.

5. Naik, 'Faltering.' Also see 'Family Practice Management: Solo Practice,' American Academy of Family Physicians website, accessed April 7, 2012, http://www.aafp.org/fpm/topicModules/viewTopicModule. htm?topicModuleId=53.

6. L. Gordon Moore, Ideal Medical Practice website, accessed April 7, 2012, http://www.idealmedicalpractice.com/info.htm.

7. L. Gordon Moore and John H. Wasson, 'The Ideal Medical Practice Model: Improving Efficiency, Quality and the Doctor-Patient Relationship,' *Family Practice Management*, 14(8) (September 2007), 20–24, Academy of American Family Physicians website, accessed April 7, 2012, http://www.aafp.org/fpm/2007/0900/p20.html#fpm20070 900p20-bt1.

8. Morgan and Simmons, *Health Cheque*, 197.

9. Morgan and Simmons, *Health Cheque*, 183.

10. Peck, *Road*, 28–29.

11. For a review of the use of electricity and electromagnetic fields in medicine, see Robert O. Becker and Gary Selden, *The Body Electric*.

12. M.H. Cohen, Ruggie, Micozzi, *The Practice of Integrative Medicine: A Legal and Operational Guide* (New York: Springer, 2007), 88.

13. CAMLAW blog website,

http://www.camlawblog.com.

14. *The I Ching: Or Book of Changes*, trans. from Chinese to German by Richard Wilhelm, trans. from German to English by Cary Baynes (Princeton: Princeton University Press, 1977), 191.

Chapter 10: Holistic Decision Making

1. Carl Bode, ed. *The Portable Thoreau* (New York: Penguin Books, 1984), 20–21.
2. Howard Thurman, Wikipedia, accessed April 22, 2012. Wikipedia gives the print reference for this quote as being in Gil Baille's *Violence Unveiled*, p. xv.
   http://en.wikipedia.org/wiki/Howard_Thurman#Quotations.
3. Philip K. Dick, 'Man, Android, and Machine' (1976), in *The Shifting Realities of Philip K. Dick: Selected Literary and Philosophical Writings* ed. Lawrence Sutin (New York: Vintage Books, 1995), 211–212.
4. Gandhi, *Autobiography*, 25.
5. Shem, 'Fiction,' 936.
6. Storr, *The Essential Jung*, 21.
7. Carl Jung, *C.G. Jung Speaking* (Princeton: Princeton University Press, 1987), 111.
8. Andrea Joy Cohen, *Blessing in Disguise*, xxv.
9. Havel, *Disturbing*, 180–181.
10. Esther Sternberg, *Healing Spaces: The Science of Place and Well-Being* (Cambridge: The Belknap Press of Harvard University Press, 2009).
11. Shem, 'Fiction,' 936.
12. Jung scarab beetle reference. Originally from *Collected Works*, Vol. 8, paragraphs 843–5, cited in Anthony Storr, *The Essential Jung* (Princeton: Princeton University Press, 1983), 339–340.
13. *The I Ching*, 191.
14. *Adaptation*, 2002, directed by Spike Jonze, written by Charlie

Kaufman, distributed by Columbia Pictures.

15. Jung, *Memories, Dreams, Reflections*, 196.

16. Randal, '*Re-covery*.'

Part V: RE-HUMANIZING THE CULTURE OF MEDICINE

Chapter 11: Leading the Transformation of Medicine

1. Larry Dossey, 'A Conversation about the Future of Medicine,' accessed December 9, 2012, http://www.dosseydossey.com/larry/QnA.html.

2. Carol Hanisch, 'The Personal is Political,' Carol Hanisch website, accessed February 26, 2013, http://www.carolhanisch.org/CHwritings/PersonalisPol.pdf.

3. The Institute of Medicine, in *Crossing the Quality Chasm*, lists 'Ten Rules to Guide the Redesign Health Care,' cited in Harding and Pincus, 'Improving.'

4. American Holistic Medical Association website, 'Principles.'

5. Gandhi, *Truth*, 134.

6. 'Mahatma Gandhi,' Wikipedia website, accessed March 10, 2013, http://en.wikipedia.org/wiki/Mahatma_gandhi.
'Jan Smuts,' wikipedia website, accessed March 10, 2103, http://en.wikipedia.org/wiki/Jan_smuts.

7. Wilber, in Schwartz, *Matters*, 353.

8. Peter Senge, C. Otto Scharmer, Joseph Jaworski and Betty Sue Flowers, *Presence: Human Purpose and the Field of the Future* (New York: Crown Business, 2004), 193.

9. Peter Block is the author of a number of books, including *The Abundant Community; Community: The Structure of Belonging; The Answer to How Is Yes: Acting on What Matters; Stewardship: Choosing Service Over Self-interest;* and *The Empowered Manager*, among others.

10. Frances Westley is the co-author of *Getting to Maybe: How the World Is Changed*.

11. Peter Drucker authored many books in his life, including: *Managing in the Next Society*; *The Ecological Vision*; *Managing for the Future*; *Managing the Nonprofit Organization*; *Innovation and Entrepreneurship*, to name just a few.

12. Margaret Wheatley is the author of *So Far from Home: Lost and Found in Our Brave New World*; *Leadership and the New Science: Discovering Order in a Chaotic World*; and *Finding Our Way: Leadership for an Uncertain Time*, to name a few.

13. Peter Senge is the author of *The Necessary Revolution: How Individuals and Organizations Are Working Together to Create a Sustainable World*; *Presence: An Exploration of Profound Change in People, Organizations, and Society*; and *The Dance of Change*, among others.

14. Adam Kahane is the author of *Solving Tough Problems: An Open Way of Talking, Listening, and Creating New Realities* and *Power and Love: A Theory and Practice of Social Change*.

15. Notes taken from 'The Resilient Community' lecture by Peter Block, June 18, 2012, at the Authentic Leadership In Action Summer Institute in Nova Scotia.

16. Peter Senge, C. Otto Scharmer, Joseph Jaworski and Betty Sue Flowers, *Presence: Human Purpose and the Field of the Future* (New York: Crown Business, 2004).

17. Schwartz, Gomes, and McCarthy, *Working*, 168–169.

18. Schwartz, Gomes, and McCarthy, *Working*, 162.

19. Arbuckle also calls for a 'transforming style' of leadership that he calls 'paramodern' leadership. This shares significant features with Palmer's, Youngson's and my own writing. Arbuckle, *Humanizing*, 165, 172.

20. Palmer, *Courage*, 202.

21. Palmer, *Courage*, 173.

22. Parker Palmer, 'All *the* Way Down,' W.M. Eades website, accessed March 10, 2013, http://www.wmeades.com/id220. htm.

23. For a good summary of Palmer's life and work, see 'Parker J.

Palmer: Community, Knowing and Spirituality in Education,'
The Encyclopedia of Informal Education, accessed March 10,
2013,
http://www.infed.org/thinkers/palmer.htm.

24. Palmer, *Courage*, 103.
25. Palmer, *Courage*, 199.
26. Palmer, *Courage*, 207.
27. Palmer, *Courage*, 209.
28. Palmer, *Courage*, 200.
29. Palmer, *Courage*, 201.
30. Palmer, *Courage*, 202.
31. Palmer, *Courage*, 204.
32. Palmer, *Courage*, 206.
33. Palmer, *Courage*, 205.
34. Youngson, *Care*, 216–220.
35. Youngson, *Care*, 184.
36. Youngson, *Care*, 131.
37. Youngson, *Care*, 133.
38. Berrett and Spiegelman, *Patients*,
    http://patientscomesecond.com/, accessed December 12,
    2012.
39. Robin Youngson, *Time to Care: How to Love Your Patients and Your Job* (Raglan: RebelHeart Publishers, 2012), 165.
40. Arbuckle, *Humanizing*, 182.
41. Gandhi, *Experiments*, 25.
42. Gandhi, *Experiments*, 318–319.
43. This was 19th-century German philosopher Hegel's view of the development of culture. Hegel's concept of dialectical progression influenced Marx in terms of economic analysis and Jung in terms of psychological analysis. The more complex, synthetic view includes explanatory models that can appear contradictory if not placed within a larger framework. See Audi, *Dictionary* entries for 'Hegel,' 365–370, and 'dialectic,' 232–233.

Chapter 12: Reconnection and Re-humanization in Medicine

1. Di Stefano, *Holism*, 172.
2. Philip K. Dick, 'The Android and the Human,' (1972), in *The Shifting Realities of Philip K. Dick: Selected Literary and Philosophical Writings*, ed. Lawrence Sutin (New York: Vintage Books: 1995), 183.
3. Stoller, *Observing*, 32, emphasis added.
4. Palmer, *To Know*, 26.
5. Palmer, *To Know*, 23.
6. Michael Murphy, *The Future of the Body: Explorations into the Further Evolution of Human Nature* (New York: Jeremy Tarcher/Putnam, 1992), 558–559.
7. Cohen, *Healing*, 16.

Bibliography

American Board of Integrative and Holistic Medicine website. Accessed April 1, 2012.
http://www.abihm.org/.

American Academy of Family Physicians website. 'Family Practice Management: Solo Practice.' Accessed April 7, 2012. http://www.aafp.org/fpm/topicModules/viewTopicModule. htm?topicModuleId=53.

American Academy of Family Physicians website. 'Patient Centered Medical Home (PCMH).' Accessed November 19, 2012.
http://www.aafp.org/online/en/home/membership/initiatives/ pcmh.html.

American Academy of Family Physicians website. 'Patient-Centered Medical Home Checklist.' Accessed November 19, 2012.
http://www.aafp.org/online/etc/medialab/aafp_org/documents/ membership/pcmh/checklist.Par.00001.File.tmp/PCMHCklist. pdf.

American Holistic Medical Association website. '10 Principles of Holistic Medicine.' Accessed April 1, 2012.
http://www.holisticmedicine.org/content.asp?pl=2&sl=22& contentid=22.

Angell, Marcia. 'The Epidemic of Mental Illness: Why?' *The New York Review of Books*, June 23, 2011.

Angell, Marcia. 'The Illusions of Psychiatry.' *The New York Review of Books*, July 14, 2011.

Antonioli, C. and M. Reveley. 'Randomised controlled trial of animal facilitated therapy with dolphins in the treatment of depression.' *British Medical Journal*, 26; 331(7527) (2005): 1231.

Arbuckle, Gerald. *Humanizing Healthcare Reform*. London: Jessica Kingsley Publishers, 2013.

Arizona Center for Integrative Medicine website. Accessed April 1, 2012. http://integrativemedicine.arizona.edu/about/index.html.

Audi, Robert, ed. *The Cambridge Dictionary of Philosophy*. New York: Cambridge University Press, 2009.

Australasian Integrative Medicine Association (AIMA) website. Accessed April 1, 2012. http://www.aima.net.au/about_aima.html.

Bach, Richard. *Illusions*. New York: Dell/Eleanor Friede, 1977.

Baikie, Karen and Kay Wilhelm. 'Emotional and Physical Health Benefits of Expressive Writing. *Advances in Psychiatric Treatment*, 11 (2005): 338–346.

Barnes, Patricia, Barbara Bloom and Richard Nahin. 'Complementary and Alternative Medicine Use among Adults and Children: United States, 2007.' *National Health Statistics Report*, No. 12, December 2008, from the National Center for Complementary and Alternative Medicine website, pdf available at, http://nccam.nih.gov/news/camstats/2007.

Barrett, William. *The Illusion of Technique: A Search for Meaning in a Technological Civilization*. New York: Anchor Press, 1978.

Beahrs, John O. *Limits of Scientific Psychiatry: The role of uncertainty in mental health*. New York: Brunner/Mazel, 1986.

Becker, Robert O. and Gary Selden. *The Body Electric: Electromagnetism and the Foundation of Life*. New York: Harper, 1985.

Belli, Angela and Jack Coulehan (eds.). *Blood and Bone*. New York: Persea Books, 1989.

Berrett, Britt and Paul Spiegelman. 'Patients Come Second' website. Accessed 3/1/13. http://patientscomesecond.com/

Berrett, Britt and Paul Spiegelman. *Patients Come Second: Leading Change by Changing the Way You Lead*. Austin: Greenleaf Book Group Press, 2013.

Bivens, Roberta. *Alternative Medicine? A History*. Oxford: Oxford

University Press, 2007.

Bode, Carl. Editor, *The Portable Thoreau*. New York: Penguin Books, 1984.

Brennan, Barbara, *Hands of Light*. New York: Bantam, 1988.

Brennan, Troyen, David Rothman, Linda Blank, David Blumenthal, Susan Chimonas, Jordan Cohen, Janlori Goldman, Jerome Kassirer, Harry Kimball, James Naughton and Neil Smelser. 'Health Industry Practices That Create Conflicts of Interest: A policy proposal for academic medical centers.' *Journal of the American Medical Association*, Vol. 295, No. 4 (January 25, 2006): 429–433.

Brewer, Benjamin. 'Satellite Office Could Lower Costs, Allow More Time for Patients: Country Doctor Determined to Try New Practice Model.' *The Wall Street Journal* online, January 10, 2006. Accessed April 7, 2012.

http://online.wsj.com/article/SB113683811203541840.html.

Brown, Dee. *Bury My Heart at Wounded Knee*. New York: Holt, 2001.

British Medical Association website, 'Issues facing the NHS,' (26, September 2008). Accessed March 25, 2012.

http://www.bma.org/uk/healthcare_policy/nhsissuesfaqs.jsp.

Burbeck, R., S. Coomber, S. Robinson and C. Todd. 'Occupational Stress in Consultants in Accident and Emergency Medicine: A National Survey of Levels of Stress at Work.' *Emergency Medicine*, Vol. 19 (2002): 234–238.

Cameron, Julia. *The Artist's Way: A Spiritual Path to Higher Creativity*. New York: J.P. Tarcher/Putnam, 2002.

Cameron, William. *Informal Sociology: A Casual Introduction to Sociological Thinking*. In Quote Investigator website. Accessed February 21, 2012.

http://quoteinvestigator.com.

Chabris, Christopher and Daniel Simons. *The Invisible Gorilla*. New York: Broadway Paperbacks, 2009.

Chodron, Pema. *The Places That Scare You*. Boston: Shambhala, 2001.

Chopra, Deepak. Foreword to *The Quantum Doctor*, by Amit Goswami. Charlottesville: Hampton Roads, 2004.

Choudhry, Niteesh, Henry Stelfox and Allan Detsky. 'Relationships between Authors of Clinical Practice Guidelines and the Pharmaceutical Industry.' *Journal of the American Medical Association*. Vol. 287, No. 5 (February 6, 2002): 612–617.

Cohen, Andrea Joy. *A Blessing in Disguise*. New York: Berkley Books, 2008.

Cohen, J.M. and J-F. Phipps. *The Common Experience*. Los Angeles: J.P. Tarcher, 1979.

Cohen, Marc, Vicki Kotsirilos, Tim Bajraszewski and Craig Hassed. 'Long consultations and quality of care: Australasian Integrative Medicine Association position statement.' August 31, 2009.

Cohen, Michael H. *Healing at the Borderland of Medicine and Religion*. Chapel Hill: University of North Carolina Press, 2006.

Cohen, Michael H. *Legal Issues in Alternative Medicine: A Guide for Clinicians, Hospitals, and Patients*. Victoria: Trafford, 2006.

Cohen, Michael H., Mary Ruggie and Marc S. Micozzi. *The Practice of Integrative Medicine: A Legal and Operational Guide*. New York: Springer Publishing, 2007.

Dana, Jason, and George Lowenstein. 'A Social Science Perspective on Gifts to Physicians from Industry.' *Journal of the American Medical Association*, Vol. 290, No. 2 (July 9, 2003): 252–255.

Di Stefano, Vincent. *Holism and Complementary Medicine: Origins and Principles*. Crows Nest: Allen & Unwin, 2006.

Di Stefano, Vincent. *The Meaning of Natural Medicine. An Interpretative Study*. Accessed April 3, 2012. http://thehealingproject.net.au/Thesis/Chapter10.html.

Dick, Philip K. 'The Android and the Human,' (1972). In *The Shifting Realities of Philip K. Dick: Selected Literary and*

Philosophical Writings, edited by Lawrence Sutin. New York: Vintage Books, 1995.

Dick, Philip K. 'Man, Android, and Machine,' (1976). In *The Shifting Realities of Philip K. Dick: Selected Literary and Philosophical Writings*, edited by Lawrence Sutin. New York: Vintage Books, 1995.

Dowell, Anthony, Travis Westcott, Deborah McLeod and Stephen Hamilton. 'A Survey of Job Satisfaction, Sources of Stress and Psychological Symptoms among New Zealand Health Professionals.' *New Zealand Medical Journal*, Vol. 114 (2001): 540–543.

Dossey, Larry. 'A Conversation about the Future of Medicine.' Accessed December 9, 2012.
http://www.dosseydossey.com/larry/QnA.html.

Dossey, Larry. *Reinventing Medicine: Beyond Mind-Body to a New Era of Healing*. San Francisco: HarperSanFrancisco, 1999.

Dossey, Larry. *The Science of Premonitions: How Knowing the Future Can Help Us Avoid Danger, Maximize Opportunities, and Create a Better Life*. New York: Plume, 2009.

Durie, Mason. *Mauri Ora: The Dynamics of Maori Health*. South Melbourne: Oxford University Press, 2001.

Durie, Mason. *Whaiora: Maori Health Development*, second edition. South Melbourne: Oxford University Press, 1998.

Edwards, Betty. *Drawing on the Artist Within*. New York: Fireside, 1986.

Eisenberg, David, R.B. Davis, S.L. Ettner, S. Appel, S. Wilkey, M. Van Rompay and R.C. Kessler. 'Trends in Alternative Medicine Use in the United States, 1990–1997.' *Journal of the American Medical Association*, 280 (1998): 1569–1575.

Elkins, David N. *Humanistic Psychology: A Clinical Manifesto*. Colorado Springs: University of the Rockies Press, 2009.

Encyclopedia of Informal Education, The. 'Parker J. Palmer: Community, Knowing and Spirituality in Education.' Accessed March 10, 2013.

http://www.infed.org/thinkers/palmer.htm.

Engel, George L. 'The need for a new medical model: A challenge for biomedicine.' *Science* 196 (1977): 129–136.

Epstein, Mark. *Thoughts without a Thinker: Psychotherapy from a Buddhist Perspective*. New York: Basic Books, 1995.

Eslick, Guy, Peter Howe, Caroline Smith, Ros Priest and Alan Bensoussan. 'Benefits of Fish Oil Supplementation in Hyperlipidemia: A Systematic Review and Meta-analysis.' *International Journal of Cardiology*, Vol. 136, No. 1 (July 2009): 4–16.

Fernandez, Richard. *Physicians in Transition: Doctors Who Successfully Reinvented Themselves*. Denver: Wise Media Group, 2010.

Forster, E.M. *Howard's End*. London: Hodder & Stoughton, 2011. Kindle Edition.

Foucault, Michel. *The Birth of the Clinic*. New York: Vintage Books, 1994.

Foucault, Michel. *The Foucault Reader*, ed. Paul Rabinow. New York: Pantheon, 1984.

Gandhi, Mohandas K. *An Autobiography: The Story of My Experiments with Truth*. Boston: Beacon Press, 1957.

Gandhi, Mohandas K. In 'Arun Gandhi Shares the Mahatma's Message,' by Michael Potts, in *India – West*. San Leandro: IndiaWest Publications, 2002. Cited on the Wikiquote website. Accessed April 22, 2012.
http://en.wikiquote.org/wiki/Mahatma_Gandhi.

Gerber, Richard. *Vibrational Medicine*. Rochester: Bear & Company, 2001.

Ghaemi, S. Nassir. *The Rise and Fall of the Biopsychosocial Model: Reconciling Art and Science in Psychiatry*. Baltimore: Johns Hopkins University Press, 2010.

Goldner-Vukov, Mila. 'A Psychiatrist in Cultural Transition: Personal and Professional Dilemmas.' *Transcultural Psychiatry*, 41 (September, 2004): 386–405.

Gonzales, Laurence, *Deep Survival: Who Lives, Who Dies, and Why*.

New York: W. W. Norton, 2005.

Goswami, Amit. *The Quantum Doctor*. Charlottesville: Hampton Roads, 2004.

Gray, Terry. Website accessed April 3, 2012. http://staff.washington.edu/gray/misc/which-half.html.

Griffith, C.H. and J.F. Wilson. 'The Loss of Idealism throughout Internship.' *Evaluation and the Health Professions*, 26 (2003): 415–426.

Griffith, C.H. and J.F. Wilson. 'The Loss of Student Idealism in the 3rd Year Clinical Clerkships.' *Evaluation and the Health Professions*, 24 (2001): 61–71.

Grof, Stanislav. *The Adventure of Self-Discovery: Dimensions of Consciousness and New Perspectives in Psychotherapy and Inner Exploration*. Albany: State University of New York Press, 1988.

Groopman, Jerome. *How Doctors Think*. Boston: Mariner Books, 2007.

Gu, Qiuping, Charles Dillon and Vicki Burt. 'Prescription Drug Use Continues to Increase: U.S. Prescription Drug Data for 2007–2008,' *NCHS Data Brief*, No. 42, September 2010. U.S. Department of Health & Human Services. Accessed March 25, 2012. http://www.cdc.gov/nchs/data/databriefs/db42.pdf.

Halbesleben, Jonathon R.B. and Cheryl Rathert. 'Linking Physician Burnout and Patient Outcomes: Exploring the Dyadic Relationship between Physicians and Patients.' *Health Care Management Review*, Vol. 33, Issue 1 (January/March 2008): 29–39. doi: 10.1097/01.HMR.0000304493.87898.72.

Hall, Stephen S. *Wisdom: From Philosophy to Neuroscience*. New York: Alfred A. Knopf, 2010.

Hanisch, Carol. 'The Personal is Political.' Carol Hanisch website. Accessed February 26th, 2013. http://www.carolhanisch.org/CHwritings/PersonalisPol.pdf.

Harding, Kelli and Harold Pincus. 'Improving Quality of Psychiatric Care: Aligning Research, Policy, and Practice.'

Focus, Vol. 9, No. 2 (Spring 2011).

Harris, Gardiner. 'More Doctors Giving Up Private Practices.' *The New York Times*. March 25, 2010.

Havel, Vaclav. *Disturbing the Peace*. Translated by Paul Wilson. New York: Vintage, 1990.

Henning, Marcus, Susan Hawken and Andrew Hill. 'The Quality of Life of New Zealand Doctors and Medical Students: What Can Be Done to Avoid Burnout?' *The New Zealand Medical Journal*, Vol. 122, No. 1307 (2009): 102–110.

Hickey, Steve and Hilary Roberts. 'Evidence-Based Medicine: Neither Good Evidence nor Good Medicine.' *Journal of Integrative Medicine, Official Journal of the Australasian Integrative Medicine Association*. Vol. 16, No. 3 (2011): 22–25.

Holt, Shaun and Iona MacDonald. *Natural Remedies That Really Work: A New Zealand Guide*. Nelson: Craig Potton Publishing, 2010.

Hyde, Lewis, *The Gift: Creativity and the Artist in the Modern World*. New York: Vintage, 1979.

The I Ching: Or Book of Changes. Translated from Chinese to German by Richard Wilhelm. Translated from German to English by Cary Baynes. Princeton: Princeton University Press, 1977.

Ideal Medical Practice website. Accessed April 7, 2012. http://www.idealmedicalpractice.com/info.htm.

Illich, Ivan, *Limits to Medicine, Medical Nemesis: The Expropriation of Health*. New York: Marion Boyers, 1976.

Jarow, Rick. *Creating the Work You Love*. Rochester: Destiny Books, 1995.

Jovanotti. 'Fango,' from the album *Safari*. Decca International, 2008. Lyrics translated on LyricsTranslate.com. Accessed March 27, 2012. http://lyricstranslate.com/en/fango-mud.html.

Judith, Anodea. *Eastern Body, Western Mind*. Berkeley: Celestial Arts, 1996.

Jung, Carl Gustav. *C.G. Jung Speaking*. Princeton: Princeton University Press, 1987.

Jung, Carl Gustav. 'In memory of Sigmund Freud' (1932), *The Collected Works of C. G. Jung, vol. 15: The Spirit in Man, Art, and Literature*. Princeton: Princeton University Press, 1971.

Jung, Carl Gustav. *Memories, Dreams, Reflections*. New York: Vintage, 1989.

Jung, Carl Gustav. *Modern Man in Search of Soul*. Orlando: Harcourt Harvest, 1955.

Jung, Carl Gustav. *Mysterium Coniunctionis, The Collected Works of C. G. Jung, XIV*. Princeton: Princeton University Press: 1989.

Jung, Carl Gustav. *The Psychology of Kundalini Yoga*. Princeton: Princeton University Press, 1999.

Jung, Carl, *The Structure and Dynamics of the Psyche*, cited in Schwartz, Tony. *What Really Matters: Searching for Wisdom in America*. New York: Bantam Books, 1995.

Kabat-Zinn, Jon. *Full Catastrophe Living*. New York: Delta, 1990.

Kavar, Louis. *The Integrated Self: A Holistic Approach to Spirituality and Mental Health Practice*. Washington: O-Books, 2012.

Kaiser Family Foundation website. 'National Survey of Physicians, Part III: Doctors' Opinions about their Profession.' Accessed April 3, 2012, pdf available at: http://www.kff.org/kaiserpolls/20020426c-index.cfm.

Kekule von Stradonitz, Friedrich August. 'Famous Dreams.' Dream Interpretation-Dictionary website. Accessed January 6, 2013. http://www.dreaminterpretation-dictionary.com/famous-dreams-friedrich-von-stradonitz.html.

Kennedy, Michael. *A Brief History of Disease, Science, and Medicine*. Mission Viejo: Asklepiad Press, 2004.

King, Michael. *The Penguin History of New Zealand*. Camberwell: Penguin, 2003.

Klamen, Debra, Linda Grossman and David Kopacz. 'Attitudes about Abortion among Second-Year Medical Students.'

Medical Teacher, Vol. 18, No. 4 (1996): 345–346.

Klamen, Debra, Linda Grossman and David Kopacz. 'Medical Student Homophobia.' *Journal of Homosexuality*, Vol. 37, No. 1 (1999): 53–63.

Klamen, Debra, Linda Grossman and David Kopacz. 'Posttraumatic Stress Disorder Symptoms in Resident Physicians Related to Their Internship.' *Academic Psychiatry*, Vol. 19, No. 3 (Fall 1995): 142–149.

Kluger, M., K. Townend, and T. Laidlaw. 'Job Satisfaction, Stress and Burnout in Australian Specialist Anaesthetists.' *Anaesthesia*, Vol. 58 (2003): 339–345.

Kopacz, David. *Finding Your Self*. Unpublished, limited number of copies printed by Stipes Publishing, 2008, 2009 for a class at Parkland College, Champaign, Illinois.

Kopacz, David, Debra Klamen and Linda Grossman. 'Medical Students and AIDS: Knowledge, Attitudes and Implications for Education.' *Health, Education and Research*, Vol. 14, No. 1 (1999): 1–6.

Kozak, Leila, Lorin Boynton, Jacob Bentley, and Emma Bezy, 'Introducing spirituality, religion and culture curricula in the psychiatry residency programme.' *Medical Humanities*, 36 (2010): 48–51.

Krasner, Michael, Ronald Epstein, Howard Beckman, Anthony Suchman, Benjamin Chapman, Christopher Mooney and Timothy Quill. 'Association of an Educational Program in Mindful Communication with Burnout, Empathy, and Attitudes among Primary Care Physicians.' *Journal of the American Medical Association*, Vol. 302, No. 12 (2009): 1284–1293.

Krishnamurti, J. *Total Freedom*. San Francisco: HarperSan Francisco, 1996.

Lawrence, D.H. *D.H. Lawrence: The Complete Poems*, 1977. p. 620, cited in David Elkins, *Humanistic Psychology: A Clinical Manifesto*. Colorado Springs: University of the Rockies Press, 2009.

von Laue, Max. Wikiquote website, accessed August 27, 2013, http://en.wikiquote.org/wiki/Talk:Quantum_mechanics.

Lee, F. Joseph, Moira Stewart and Judith Brown. 'Stress, Burnout, and Strategies for Reducing Them: What's the Situation among Canadian Family Physicians?' *Canadian Family Physician*, Vol. 54 (2008): 234–235.e1–5.

Levinson, Wendy, Debra Roter, John Mullooly, Valerie Dull and Richard Frankel. 'Physician-Patient Communication: The Relationship with Malpractice Claims among Primary Care Physicians and Surgeons.' *Journal of the American Medical Association*, Vol. 277, No. 7 (Feb. 19, 1997): 553–559.

Lipsenthal, Lee. *Finding Balance in a Medical Life*. San Anselmo: Finding Balance, Inc., 2007.

Mainguy, Barbara, Michael Valenti Pickren and Lewis Mehl-Madrona. 'Relationships Between Level of Spiritual Transformation and Medical Outcome.' *Advances in Mind-Body Medicine*, 27(1) (2013): 4–11.

Mascaro, Juan, trans. *The Upanishads*. New York: Penguin Books, 1965.

Matsumoto, David, ed. *The Cambridge Dictionary of Psychology*, New York: Cambridge University Press, 2009.

Matz, Susan. *The Art of Energy Healing, Volume 1: The Foundation*. Nevada City: Blue Dolphin, 2005.

Miller, Phillip, Louis Goodman, Tim Norbeck. *In Their Own Words: 12,000 Physicians Reveal Their Thoughts on Medical Practice in America*. Garden City: Morgan James, 2010.

Mischoulon, David. 'Ask the Expert: Depression and Dysthymia.' *Focus*, Vol. 10 (2012): 461–462.

Moore, L. Gordon. 'Going Solo: Making the Leap.' *Family Practice Management*. February 2002. American Academy of Family Physicians website. Accessed April 7, 2012. http://www.aafp.org/fpm/2002/0200/p29.html.

Moore, L. Gordon, and John H. Wasson. 'The Ideal Medical Practice Model: Improving Efficiency, Quality and the Doctor-

Patient Relationship.' *Family Practice Management*, 14(8), (September 2007): 20–24. Academy of American Family Physicians website. Accessed April 7, 2012. http://www.aafp.org/fpm/2007/0900/p20.html#fpm20070900p 20-bt1.

Morgan, Gareth, and Geoff Simmons, with John McCrystal. *Health Cheque: The truth we should all know about New Zealand's public health system.* Auckland: Public Interest Publishing, 2009.

Moynihan, Ray and Alan Cassels. *Selling Sickness: How drug companies are turning us all into patients.* New York: Nation Books, 2005.

Mudge-Riley, Michele. Foreword to Richard Fernandez, *Physicians in Transition: Doctors Who Successfully Reinvented Themselves.* Denver: Wise Media Group, 2010.

Murphy, Michael. *The Future of the Body: Explorations into the Further Evolution of Human Nature.* New York: Jeremy Tarcher/ Putnam, 1992.

Naik, Gautam. 'Faltering Family M.D.s Get Technology Lifeline: Doctors Think Small to Revive Solo Role for Primary Care.' *The Wall Street Journal* online, February 23, 2007. Accessed April 7, 2012. http://online.wsj.com/article/SB117201140861714109-search. html.

National Center for Complementary and Alternative Medicine (NCCAM). Accessed April 1, 2012. http://nccam.nih.gov/.

NGM Blog Central, *National Geographic*, 'The Cost of Care,' Posted Dec 18, 2009, cited in The Society Pages. http://thesocietypages.org/graphicsociology/2011/04/26/cost-of-health-care-by-country-national-geographic/.

Nelson, Martia. *Coming Home.* Mill Valley: Nataraj, 1997.

New Zealand History Online, The. '100 Maori words every New Zealander should know.' Accessed January 2, 2013.

http://www.nzhistory.net.nz/culture/maori-language-week/ 100-maori-words.

Niebuhr, Reinhold. 'The Serenity Prayer.' Wikipedia. Accessed January 30, 2012.

http://en.wikipedia.org/wiki/Serenity_Prayer.

Niemi M.B., M. Harting, W. Kou , A. Del Rey, H.O. Besedovsky, M. Schedlowski and G. Pacheco-Lopez. 'Taste-immunosuppression Engram: Reinforcement and Extinction.' *Journal of Neuroimmunology*. 188 (1–2) (2007): 74–79.

Nietzsche, Friedrich. *Thus Spake Zarathustra*, Part I, Chapter XXII, Section 2. In *The Portable Nietzsche*, edited and translated by Walter Kaufmann. New York: Penguin Books, 1982.

'No Free Lunch' website. Accessed January 5, 2013.

http://www.nofreelunch.org.

Orloff, Judith. *Second Sight: An Intuitive Psychiatrist Tells Her Extraordinary Story and Shows You How to Tap Your Own Inner Wisdom*. New York: Three Rivers Press, 2010.

Ornish, Dean. *Love and Survival: 8 Pathways to Intimacy and Health*. New York: HarperCollins, 1998.

Palmer, Parker. 'All *the* Way Down.' W.M. Eades website. Accessed March 10, 2013.

http://www.wmeades.com/id220.htm

Palmer, Parker. *The Courage to Teach: Exploring the Inner Landscape of a Teacher's Life*. San Francisco: Jossey-Bass, 2007.

Palmer, Parker. *To Know As We Are Known: Education as a Spiritual Journey*. New York: HarperOne, 1983.

Partnership on the Health of the NHS Workforce. *Improving the Health of the NHS Workforce*. London: The Nuffield Trust, 1998.

Pearson, Nancy and Margaret Chesney. 'The CAM Education Program of the National Center for Complementary and Alternative Medicine: An Overview.' *Academic Medicine*, Vol. 82, No. 10 (October 2007): 921–926.

Peck, M. Scott. *The Road Less Travelled*. London: Arrow, 1978.

Pert, Candace. *Molecules of Emotion: The Science Behind Mind-Body*

Medicine. New York: Simon and Schuster, 1999.

Peterkin, Allan D. *Staying Human During Residency Training*. Buffalo: University of Toronto Press, 2008.

Police, The. 'Rehumanize Yourself,' from the album, *Ghost in the Machine*. A&M Records, 1981.

Randal, Patte, M.W. Stewart, D. Lampshire, J. Symes, D. Proverbs, and H. Hamer. '*The Re-covery Model* – An integrative developmental stress-vulnerability-strengths approach to mental health.' *Psychosis: Psychological, Social, and Integrative Approaches*, 1(2), (2009): 122–133.

Ratey, John and Eric Hagerman. *Spark: The Revolutionary New Science of Exercise and the Brain*. New York: Little, Brown and Company, 2008.

Roy, Ranjan. *Social Support, Health, and Illness: A Complicated Relationship*. Buffalo: University of Toronto Press, 2011.

Salgo, Peter. 'The Doctor Will See You for Exactly Seven Minutes.' *The New York Times*, March 22, 2006.

Salovey, Peter, Jerusha Detweiler, Wayne Steward and Alexander Rothman. 'Emotional States and Physical Health.' *American Psychologist*, Vol. 55, No. 1 (January 2000): 110–121.

Saul, John Ralston. *On Equilibrium*. Ringwood: Penguin Books, 2001.

Schwartz, Mark, Steven Durning, Mark Linzer and Karen Hauer. 'Changes in Medical Students' Views of Internal Medicine Careers From 1990 to 2007.' *Archives of Internal Medicine* 171(8), (2011): 744–749.

Schwartz, Tony. *What Really Matters: Searching for Wisdom in America*. New York: Bantam Books, 1995.

Schwartz, Tony, Jean Gomes and Catherine McCarthy. *The Way We're Working Isn't Working*. New York: Free Press, 2010.

Seligman, Martin E. *Flourish: A Visionary New Understanding of Happiness and Well-being.*' New York: Free Press, 2011.

Senge, Peter, C. Otto Scharmer, Joseph Jaworski and Betty Sue Flowers. *Presence: Human Purpose and the Field of the Future.*

New York: Crown Business, 2004.

Shapiro, Johanna. *The Inner World of Medical Students: Listening to Their Voices in Poetry*. New York: Radcliffe Publishing, 2009.

Shealy, Norman. *Medical Intuition: A Science of the Soul*. Virginia Beach: A.R.E. Press, 2010.

Shehabi Y., G. Dobb and I. Jenkins. 'Burnout Syndrome among Australian Intensivists: A Survey.' *Critical Care and Resuscitation*, Vol. 10 (2008): 312–315.

Sheldrake, Rupert. *The Science Delusion: Freeing the Spirit of Enquiry*. London: Coronet, 2012.

Shem, Samuel. 'Fiction as Resistance.' Annals of Internal Medicine, Vol. 137, No. 11 (Dec 3, 2002): 934–937.

Shem, Samuel. *The House of God*. New York: Dell, 1978.

Solnit, Rebecca. *A Field Guide to Getting Lost*. New York: Penguin, 2005.

Solnit, Rebecca. *Hope in the Dark: Untold Histories, Wild Possibilities*. New York: Nation Books, 2006.

Solnit, Rebecca. *A Paradise Built in Hell: The Extraordinary Communities That Arise in Disaster*. New York: Penguin, 2009.

Starr, Paul. *The Social Transformation of American Medicine: The rise of a sovereign profession and the making of a vast industry*. New York: Basic Books, 1982.

Sternberg, Esther M. *Healing Spaces: The Science of Place and Well-Being*. Cambridge: The Belknap Press of Harvard University Press, 2009.

Stoller, Robert. *Observing the Erotic Imagination*. New Haven: Yale University Press, 1992.

Storr, Anthony. *The Essential Jung*. Princeton: Princeton University Press, 1983.

Sulmasy, D.P. 'A biopsychosocial-spiritual model for the care of patients at the end of life,' *Gerontologist*, 42 Spec No. 3 (Oct 2002): 24–33.

Surgenor, Lois, Ruth Spearing, Jacqueline Horn, Annette Beautrais, Roger Mulder and Peggy Chan. 'Burnout in hospital-based medical consultants in the New Zealand Public Health System.' *New Zealand Medical Journal*, Vol. 122, No. 1300 (2009): 11–18.

Sutin, Lawrence (editor). *The Shifting Realities of Philip K. Dick: Selected Literary and Philosophical Writings*. New York: Vintage, 1995.

Suzuki, Shunryu. *Zen Mind, Beginner's Mind*. New York: John Weatherhill Inc., 1986.

Swensen, Stephen J., Gregg S. Meyer, Eugene C. Nelson, Gordon C. Hunt, Jr., David B. Pryor, Jed I. Weissberg, Gary S. Kaplan, Jennifer Daley, Gary R. Yates, Mark R. Chassin, Brent C. James and Donald M. Berwick. 'Cottage Industry to Postindustrial Care – The Revolution in Health Care Delivery.' *New England Journal of Medicine* 2010; 362:e12, February 4, 2010, http://www.nejm.org/doi/full/10.1056/NEJMp0911199.

Tacey, David. *Gods and Diseases: Making Sense of our Physical and Mental Wellbeing*. Sydney: HarperCollins, 2011.

Talking Heads. 'Once in a Lifetime.' From the album *Remain in Light*, Sire Records, 1980.

Thommasen, H., M. Lavanchy, I. Connelly, J. Berkowitz and S. Grzybowski. 'Mental Health, Job Satisfaction, and Intention to Relocate: Opinions of Physicians in Rural British Columbia.' *Canadian Family Physician*, Vol. 47 (2001): 737–744.

Thomson Healthcare. *PDR for Herbal Medicines*, fourth edition. Montvale: Thomson Reuters, 2007.

Thoreau, Henry David. Cited in Solnit, Rebecca. *A Field Guide to Getting Lost*. New York: Penguin, 2005.

Thorpe, Mark and Miranda Thorpe. 'Immigrant Psychotherapists and New Zealand Clients.' *The Journal of the New Zealand Association of Psychotherapists (Inc.) Te Ropu Whakaora Hinengaro*, Vol. 14, December 2008.

Thurman, Howard. Wikipedia. Accessed April 22, 2012. http://en.wikipedia.org/wiki/Howard_Thurman#Quotations.

Tzu, Chuang. *Basic Writings*. Translated by Burton Watson. New

York: Columbia University Press, 1964.

Tzu, Lao. *Tao Te Ching*. Translated by D.C. Lau. New York: Penguin Classics, 1963.

US Department of Health and Human Services, 'Health, United States, 2007,' 24. Available at, http://www.cdc.gov/nchs/data/hus/hus07.pdf.

Ventegodt, Soren and Gary Orr. 'The future of traditional African healers,' *Journal of Alternative Medicine Research*, Vol. 2, No. 4, (2010): 359–362.

Watters, Ethan. *Crazy Like Us: The Globalization of the American Psyche*. New York: Free Press, 2010.

Wazana, Ashley. 'Physician and the Pharmaceutical Industry: Is a Gift Ever Just a Gift?' *Journal of the American Medical Association*, Vol. 283, No. 3 (January 19, 2000): 373–380.

Whyte, David, *The Three Marriages: Reimagining Work, Self and Relationship*. New York: Penguin, 2009.

Wikipedia website. 'Archimedes.' Accessed January 12, 2013. http://en.wikipedia.org/wiki/Archimedes.

Wikipedia website. 'Mahatma Gandhi.' Accessed March 10, 2013. http://en.wikipedia.org/wiki/Mahatma_gandhi.

Wikipedia website. 'Jan Smuts.' Accessed March 10, 2103. http://en.wikipedia.org/wiki/Jan_smuts.

Wikipedia website. 'Uncle Ben.' Accessed January 12, 2013. http://en.wikipedia.org/wiki/Uncle_Ben#.22With_great_power _ comes_great_responsibility.22.

Wilber, Ken. *A Brief History of Everything*, second edition. Shambhala, Boston, 2011. Kindle Edition.

Wilber, Ken. Ken Wilber Online, Shambhala Publications website. Accessed April 21, 2012, http://wilber.shambhala.com/html/books/kosmos/excerpt6/ part1.cfm/

Wilson, Kris, Claire Dowson, and Dee Mangin. 'Prevalence of complementary and alternative medicine use in Christchurch, New Zealand: children attending general practice versus

paediatric outpatients.' *Journal of the New Zealand Medical Association*, Vol. 120, No. 1251, March 23, 2007. Accessed online, April 3, 2012.
http://journal.nzma.org.nz/journal/120-1251/2464/

Winnicott, Donald. 'Ego Distortions in Terms of True and False Self.' In *The Maturational Process and the Facilitating Environment: Studies in the Theory of Emotional Development.* New York: International UP Inc., 1960.

Youngson, Robin. *Time to Care: How to Love Your Patients and Your Job.* Raglan: RebelHeart Publishers, 2012.

Index

hospital, 40, 156, 261, 265; contextual dimension, 131, 140-142, 198-200, 279-280; corporate, 7; emotional dimension, 137; individual and, 80, 194, 298; healing interconnection, 9, 86, 106; internal and external, 135; interventions, 220; learning, 311; new medical models, 91; psychoneuroimmunology, 110; sociological and ecological, 79; systems, 98; traditional model, 2, 79-80

Epstein, Mark, 180

Errors, cognitive, 47-49, 335

Evidence-based medicine, 14, 17-20, 28, 32; as a tool, 166; biomedical model, 103-104; critique of, 47-48, 106, 151; eclipsing other human dimensions, 150; health care reform, 38; technicians, 149

Facing the Pain Exercise, 185-186

Faith, hope and healing, 110; in technique, 20, leadership, 301; scientific, 51; spiritual dimension, 196, 278; *taha wairua*, 81

'Fango,' 225, 232-233

Fetish, 34-35

Field Guide to Getting Lost, A,

203

Finding Balance in a Medical Life, 41, 174, 269

Finding Your Self Across Time Exercise, 204-205

Forster, E. M., xx

Foucault, Michel, 39, 70-72, 78

Foundational model of medicine, 2, 10-13, 24, 38-39, 86, 122-123, 162, 182, 217, 269, 327

Full Catastrophe Living, 173

Gandhi, Mohandas K., 183, 269-270; holistic leadership, 294-297, 299, 311

Gifts, gift economies, 107-108; pharmaceutical companies, 31-33

God, 59- 60, 115-116, 194-195

Gonzales, Lawrence, 157

Goswami, Amit, 53-57, 127, 134, 172, 321

Groopman, Jerome, 17-18, 20, 44, 47-51, 151

Havel, Vaclav, 111-112, 121, 278, 279

Healing, and love, 106-108, 137, 156; bone and wound, 49, 253; connection, xxii, 144, 148, 317; consciousness, 53-57; continuous healing relationship, xiv, 41-42, 292;

AYNI
BOOKS

"Ayni" is a Quechua word meaning "reciprocity" – sharing, giving and receiving – whatever you give out comes back to you. To be in Ayni is to be in balance, harmony and right relationship with oneself and nature, of which we are all an intrinsic part. Complementary and Alternative approaches to health and well-being essentially follow a holistic model, within which one is given support and encouragement to move towards a state of balance, true health and wholeness, ultimately leading to the awareness of one's unique place in the Universal jigsaw of life – Ayni, in fact.